CHALLENGES IN REFORMING
THE HEALTH SECTOR
IN AFRICA

REFORMING HEALTH SYSTEMS
UNDER ECONOMIC SIEGE

THE ZIMBABWEAN EXPERIENCE

SECOND EDITION

PAULINUS LINGANI NCUBE SIKOSANA

Order this book online at www.trafford.com
or email orders@trafford.com

Most Trafford titles are also available at major online book retailers.

© Copyright 2009 Paulinus L. N. Sikosana.

Note for Librarians: A cataloguing record for this book is available from Library and Archives Canada at www.collectionscanada.ca/amicus/index-e.html

Printed in Victoria, BC, Canada.

ISBN: 978-1-4269-1519-2 (sc)
ISBN: 978-1-4269-1520-8 (dj)

Library of Congress Control Number: 2009933018

Our mission is to efficiently provide the world's finest, most comprehensive book publishing service, enabling every author to experience success. To find out how to publish your book, your way, and have it available worldwide, visit us online at www.trafford.com

Trafford rev. 8/26/2009

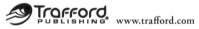

www.trafford.com

North America & international
toll-free: 1 888 232 4444 (USA & Canada)
phone: 250 383 6864 ✦ fax: 812 355 4082

CONTENTS

8 THE SECTOR WIDE APPROACH (SWAp)

9 REGULATION, COMMERCIALIZATION AND SUBCONTRACTING

10 COMMISSION OF REVIEW INTO THE HEALTH SECTOR IN ZIMBABWE

11 HEALTH REFORMS AND EQUITY

PREFACE

Health sector reforms have in some instances been relegated to the realm of the mysterious, making it difficult for most people to grasp the intentions behind their implementation. One of the aims of this book is to make the subject of health reforms much more understandable even to those people who do not work in the field of health.

The subject of health reforms in developing countries has, to an extent, mainly been approached from a rather theoretical perspective, mostly by consultants and researchers who may be far removed from the day to day implementation of such reforms. The main objective of this book is to provide a view from within. It tackles the subject of health sector reforms by blending the theory behind health reform with practical examples and experiences from a country which has implemented health reforms for almost a decade. The book tells the story behind the demise of Zimbabwe's health delivery system, once considered to be a good example of best practices in the delivery of primary health care services in the Sub-Saharan region.

What evolves is a typical textbook experience of a health delivery system caught up in economic and political turmoil and struggling to apply the theory of reforms in the context of a real world. The author tackles the subject from a narrative and analytical point of view through the description of common and popular health sector reform elements, their practical implications on the health system, advantages expected from their implementation, pitfalls and potential outcomes, based on the Zimbabwean experience, and indeed that of any other developing country.

For those in the know, the book reiterates the fact that health reforms in a developing country setting have a different approach and emphasis from those in developed countries, though both aim to improve efficiency in the allocation and utilization of resources within the health sector. It is important that individual countries adopt and adapt those reform elements that suit the uniqueness of their own circumstances.

Whilst the book is a rare dossier on the dramatic rise and meteoric fall of a health delivery system in a developing country, it also serves as a reference text on the diverse nature of health reforms and their implementation.

The impact of reforms can only be assured if countries actually implement what they propose as proposals are only intentions.

ACKNOWLEDGEMENTS

Many thanks go to MOHCW staff, past and present, members of the Local Government Capacity Building Coordinating Committee and all those who were actively involved in the development and implementation of the health sector reform process in Zimbabwe. My appreciation goes to Dr. Timothy Stamps, the former Minister of Health and Child Welfare, for his unwavering support to the change agenda within the health sector in Zimbabwe; and to Dr. R. Chatora, the former Secretary for Health for his role in the design of the health sector reform agenda.

Special thanks go to my wife Najma, the rest of the family; Phathisani, Majid, Melissa and Mahmoud who have all been supportive and a source of great inspiration.

Thank you all, Ngiyabonga! Tatenda, Ahsante!

This book is dedicated to my late brother, Father Titus Sikosana, who as a Catholic priest fought for justice and peace, and my late father, who lived a life of selfless dedication to improving the education of others.

INTRODUCTION

Context of Africa's health challenges

Slow economic growth and development

Poverty remains rampant in Africa, much more than in any other part of the world. Even though in many ways health still occupies center stage in the development agenda in Africa, there continues to be a crisis in the financing of health services in general and for the poor in particular. The reason advanced for this situation is the lack of resources. This is despite the variety of sources available for health financing. Health financing in Africa remains inadequate for several reasons, the major one being the continent's continued economic underdevelopment. The levels and rates of growth in per capita incomes in sub-Saharan Africa (SSA) have continued to lag behind those of the rest of the world. This has resulted in 10% of the world's population struggling to survive on 1% of the world's income. In this region more than 640 million people are poor, 90% of whom live in rural areas and earn less than 50 cents a day. With 10% of the world's population and only 1% of the world's income the SSA region accounts for 80% of AIDS deaths in the world. Measures of poverty have remained virtually the same at 44% in 2002 compared to 44.6% in the 1990s, (United Nations Economic Commission, Economic Report for Africa, 2007).

In the 1980s market prices for export commodities slumped, international interest rates short up and many African countries found themselves in economic crises and unable to repay their foreign debts. In desperation to get new capital to repay these loans African countries found refuge in the World Bank (WB) and the International Monetary Fund (IMF). These institutions were very willing to assist but only on their terms. African countries were required to implement economic policies called Economic Structural Adjustment Programs (ESAPs). This meant that they had to adjust their economies to suit the interests of the big powers in the global economy. Public sector job losses and wage cuts associated with these World Bank and IMF programs are well documented and have increased hardships in many of these countries.

In most of these countries the ESAPs have led to cuts in government spending on services to the poor, reduction in trade barriers and maintenance of their economies as sources of cheap labor and raw materials for multinationals. As a result conditions of poverty and underdevelopment have worsened and foreign debt increased. In the 2000-2001 period the World Bank provided loans totaling US$3.4 billion to countries in SSA, US$250 million less than what the African countries spent on debt repayments. Anecdotal evidence shows that World Bank policies have in some cases led to the closure of several hospitals and clinics, and also left some of them understaffed and lacking essential supplies. Under World Bank policies 42 poorest countries in Africa reduced their health expenditures by more than 50%.

Economic growth, especially in SSA, has generally been sluggish and where there has been some discernible growth the benefits have not been equitably distributed. Even after 20 years of Economic Structural Adjustment (ESAP) the average incomes in Africa are still at the level they were in the late 1960s. In the last decade poor people have increased both in proportional and absolute terms. Studies show that adjustment has contributed significantly to increased poverty levels in those countries whose economies are dependent on the exports of primary agricultural and mineral goods and where urban poverty is relatively high. Currency devaluation as part of ESAP has led to increased costs of imported foods and in some cases to an increase in the prevalence of wasting and stunting amongst children as households are forced to decrease food expenditures. A few countries have however demonstrated some successes in the use of social safety net strategies.

The economic report for Africa for 2000 painted a picture of slowed growth rates for the year and ranked African countries based on the performance of macroeconomic, poverty reduction and institution building policies. Top performers included those countries with lower foreign debt, lower budget deficits and lower interest rates and thus considered to have more advanced market liberalization, reliable infrastructure and effective pro-poor policies. The report also reveals that Africa's real GDP growth rate fell to 3.2% in 2002 from 4.3% in 2001. This meant that only 5 of the 53 countries in Africa achieved the 7% growth rate necessary to meet the Millennium Development Goals. According to the 2007 Africa economic report the overall GDP growth for Africa was 5.7% in 2005 and 5.8% in 2007. Relative to their development goals only 4 countries recorded an average GDP growth rate of 7% in the period 1998 – 2006 and were thus positioned to achieve their MDGs by 2015. Of particular significance during this period is the poor economic performance of Zimbabwe as the only country that recorded negative economic growth of -4.4 and -7.1 rate in 2005 and 2006 respectively.

The recommended minimum level of government expenditure for a developing country on an essential health package is estimated to be US$34 per person per year. Total per capita expenditures on health in 2000, from all sources, ranged from US$5 to US$28 amongst some 10 countries in Africa. 29 countries in Africa spent less than US$ 10 per person per year on health whilst only 9 spent US$37 or more. In 2007, the per capita public health expenditures on health amounted to about US$10 in low income countries (LICs) compared to US$ 2 000 in developing countries, (Schieber, G (2007)).

Whilst most African countries rely on external sources to finance their health sector there is convincing evidence that foreign aid in large quantities may weaken a country's economy by crowding out private investment. For example, information from National Health Accounts (NHA) shows that some countries have a very high proportion of external resources as a percentage of public expenditures on health. In 2000 this proportion was 86.7% in Malawi, 96% for Uganda, 24.1% for Ghana, 24.8% for Zambia and 6.8% in Lesotho. In 2007 external sources accounted for an average of only 6% of total health spending in LICs though in over 20 African countries this figure was more than 30%, with extreme cases reaching upwards of 60%. In 2007 the external component in Mozambique's public health financing was close to 70%.

In 2000 four countries in Africa spent less than 5% of their annual budget on health, 23 spent between 5% and 10% and 15 between 11% and 15%. Only 2 countries spent over 15% of their budgets on health. According to Schieber, G (2007) in 2007 public spending accounted for 25% of total health expenditures in low income developing countries compared to 60% in high income countries. This is against the background of African heads of state committing themselves in 2000 to allocate at least 15% of their annual budgets to the health sector.

In the past decade private expenditures on health in most developing countries rose from 42% to 52%. In the majority of countries in Sub Saharan Africa, the poor bear the brunt of the regressive nature of out of pocket payment which in 2007, on average, accounted for 70% of health spending in these countries compared to 15% in developed nations. These parameters are more an indication of the decline in government commitment to health financing than a positive move towards improved market orientation of the health sector. Social health insurance on the other hand accounted for only 1% of all health spending in LICs compared to 30% in the developed world.

Because of the slow progress towards the achievement of the MDGs in most developing countries, development assistance for health increased from US$ 2.5 billion in 1990 to almost US$ 14 billion (13% of global ODA) in 2005. According to the Global Monitoring Report (2006), ODA share going to HIV/AIDS more than doubled, at the expense of support to Primary Health Care which declined by almost 50%.

Reliance on Overseas Development Aid (ODA)

Improving the impact of development aid for health

Previously, multilateral aid was dominated by projects, conditional lending and technical assistance to developing countries. However with the recent dramatic increase in the volume of health aid and in the number and diversity of actors, there has been renewed effort to reduce poverty in order to improve the health of the poor. Increased aid volumes have also increased programming on specific diseases or interventions, especially focusing on immunizations (GAVI), core diseases (PEPFAR, GFATM, Rollback Malaria, Stop TB Partnership, UNAIDS, Malaria Booster Program) and health systems reforms, all of which have tended to distort the approach to aid disbursement.

These fragmented initiatives which are dominated by disease specific investments have weakened the public health systems of recipient countries. The Sector Wide Approach (SWAp) has been one of several attempts to integrate and coordinate development aid at country level and to demonstrate the need to improve the horizontal management of global health interventions as recipient countries continued to experience difficulties in managing all the new inputs. The Paris Declaration, complemented by a variety of aid management instruments, has become the main document that guides the process of improving the management of development aid in health.

The capacity of many developing countries to utilize resources made available through development aid has generally been beset by several problems which according to Schieber, G, (March 2007) include:

♦ Limited absorptive capacity to utilize the amount of aid that is made available to them

◆ Aid meant for one sector being used by the government to offset budget allocations to other sectors, e.g. defense.

◆ Poor policy environment for aid to achieve positive results

◆ Debt repayment having negative effects on the economic growth of countries

◆ Aid usually coming with high transaction costs for recipient countries

◆ Donor imposed conditionalities which rarely work.

◆ Highly aid dependent governments which, as a result, tend to be more accountable to donors than to their citizens

◆ Poor accountability on the impact of the aid provided

The Paris Declaration on Aid Effectiveness

The Paris Declaration was the result of a high level forum where ministers from developing and developed countries and heads of multilateral and bilateral development institutions resolved and committed themselves to reform ways in which international aid was delivered and managed. This meeting reaffirmed previous commitments to harmonize and align the delivery of aid. The declaration calls for a practical program of work which is based on five principles; ownership, alignment, harmonization, management for results and mutual accountability. According to the declaration donors are to be held publicly accountable to each other at the global level in complying with the commitments made at the meeting. At the country level donors and partners are expected to jointly assess progress in implementing agreed commitments on aid effectiveness by making the best use of local mechanisms. The follow up meeting, *Accra Agenda for Action on Aid Effectiveness*, noted progress in the implementation of the Paris Declaration and partners made commitments on further progress.

The International Health Partnership (IHP+)

This initiative is the brain child of the British Prime Minister, Mr. Gordon Brown, who launched it in September 2007. The initiative aims at driving forward work on the MDGs through a global partnership of leading donor nations and international agencies. Initially the IHP targeted first wave countries which included Burundi, Cambodia, Ethiopia, Kenya, Mali, Mozambique, Nepal, and Zambia. These countries developed country "compacts" - which are business models that build on lessons learned from the Sector Wide Approach (SWAp), aid harmonization (based on the Paris Declaration) and focusing on the achievement of health related

MDG goals. Each government and its development partners committed to develop and implement one comprehensive and costed national health plan based on long term flexible financing from both national and international sources and to achieve verifiable results monitored on the basis of mutual accountability and benchmarks. These countries are expected to increase investment in their own health systems, address any policy constraints and strengthen planning and accountability mechanisms. Civil society and other stakeholders are expected to be provided with enough space to participate in the design and review of the country IHP compacts.

Potential areas of consensus in development assistance

There seem to be several areas on which donors have a potential to reach consensus at both the global and country levels. In the area regarding approaches to strengthening health systems the following areas seem to emerge:

- ◆ Improving the performance of health systems through reform and capacity building
- ◆ Recognition of the role of multiple determinants of health
- ◆ Strengthening the role of partnerships amongst donors, partner countries and other development initiatives
- ◆ Guaranteeing sustainable health financing

With respect to health priorities there is room for consensus with respect to the following areas:

- ◆ Strengthening public health functions and focusing on the prevention of communicable diseases and disease surveillance
- ◆ Increasing access to health care by the poor through social protection and pro-poor health financing
- ◆ Focus on the rights based approach to Reproductive and Sexual health
- ◆ Health reforms and strengthening institutional capacity
- ◆ Increased support and collaboration with the private sector
- ◆ Increased role of NGOs in the implementation of development aid.

Increasing levels of poverty

Highly Indebted Poor Country Initiative (HIPC)

Apart from having a huge external debt burden African countries have also accumulated fiscal deficits which have increased their domestic debt. Attempts to finance this debt have crowded out credit to the private sector. Because some of these areas of expenditures cannot be easily cut back they have seriously diminished the country's fiscal space.

The foreign debt in particular has left some African countries with significant debt servicing obligations. The poor fiscal state of these countries has led the World Bank and the IMF to develop the HIPC initiative, which "forgives" a significant proportion of the country's multilateral and bilateral debt. The idea is for the countries to use funds freed by debt relief to implement social programs that contribute to poverty reduction. At the end of the process it is envisaged that the country will achieve sector sustainability and thus not require further rounds of debt relief. This initiative has however focused only on external debt relief.

Poverty Reduction Strategy Paper (PRSP)

The PRSPs are World Bank and IMF instruments aimed at increasing the focus of public expenditure priorities on the poorest households and these usually go hand in hand with Heavily Indebted Poor Country debt relief. Countries receiving debt relief must first satisfy "creditors" that a PRSP is in place and that it will facilitate the allocation of new funds to intended poor households. In 2003 Africa had 23 of the 44 PRSPs operational worldwide. Because Zimbabwe was perceived to be mismanaging its economy as well as being in arrears to the Poverty Reduction and Growth Facility (PRGF), the IMF suspended technical assistance to the country and removed it from the list of countries eligible for the PRGF.

Accountability on the dock

Medium Term Expenditure Framework (MTEF)

These are instruments intended to identify the full budgetary resource envelop available to the government, inclusive of external resources. The instrument provides a framework of quantifying the proportions of resources going to the various sectors in government. The framework also provides an opportunity for the reconciliation of capital and recurrent expenditure needs and to specify targets to be achieved. Within this framework public expenditures are linked to policy priorities through a top down resource envelop and a bottom up estimation of recurrent and medium term costs of implementing existing policy and match these to available resources in the context of the annual budget process. The MTEF budget process involves the determination of the macroeconomic and public sector resource envelop, aligning policies and objectives under existing resource constraints, linking policies, resources and means for each sector, reconciliation of resources and means and finally reconciling strategic policy and available means.

Public Expenditure Review (PER)

This is another instrument used mainly by the World Bank and partner governments to analyze public sector expenditures by focusing on efficiency and equity in the use of resources within the country. The aim of the PER is to resolve some of the following issues:

 ♦ Determine the justification of public interventions within a sector on the basis of efficiency and equity and determine appropriate alternative strategies to deliver the interventions.
 ♦ To explore the sources of funding and if there are any fiscal deficits to determine their sustainability and consistency with economic growth, inflation and other macroeconomic objectives
 ♦ To determine if public expenditures have been prioritized across sectors and if they are consistent with any resource constraints.
 ♦ To determine whether public sector institutional arrangements and political incentives allow for efficiencies in public spending and what reforms are necessary to allow this to happen.

Factors besieging the health sector in Zimbabwe

Links between economic growth and health

High economic growth can result in improved health outcomes. The lack of adequate financial investment in health is one of the major causes of underdeveloped health systems in developing countries. Sustained economic growth has the potential to enable countries to increase both public and private investment in the health sector. Improved health has an intrinsic economic value in that it produces well being which has a direct impact on labor productivity and ultimately, economic growth. Good health influences the productivity of workers by increasing their physical strength, endurance and mental capacity. Workers with good health have fewer episodes of absenteeism from ill health and those whose health improves are able to re-enter the labor market. Existing workers on the other hand remain in employment for longer periods without going into early retirement as a result of poor health.

Economic growth also has the potential to improve the health of a nation by removing people out of poverty and creating opportunities for a better life. Because a market economy can be "an engine of fast economic growth and expansion of living standards", Sen, A (1999), it is reasonable to infer that policies which restrict market opportunities can constrain the realization of some social benefits that would normally accrue from a market system through overall economic growth. The market system is however not a panacea to resolving all economic problems as there are situations where it is legitimate to argue for market regulation, especially where there are market failures.

Whilst low income can be a major contributor to illiteracy, ill health, hunger and malnutrition; better education, on the other hand, can help individuals to earn higher incomes. Improved health in children has a direct impact on school attendance and the performance of students. Poor health lowers the potential for educational attainment and subsequently leads to lower social status in adult life. Many diseases that affect society can be prevented by educating the general public, especially women and children. A better educated individual is more likely to assess the costs and benefits of actions which have health implications than a person with lesser education. Mothers who have attained higher levels of education are more likely to seek medical help for their children and teach them healthy habits. If individuals do not demand health care when they require it immediately, they actively jeopardize their own health and that of others, especially if they suffer from a communicable condition.

There is enough evidence that an increase in a country's average income reduces poverty and that an increase in per capita income is associated with an increase in a country's expenditures on health. A 10% increase in a country's income reduces poverty rates by between 20% and 30% and leads to a projected increase of about 11.4% in health expenditures. After all, wealthier countries have fewer diseases and studies in these countries have demonstrated that life expectancy is positively related to the level of per capita income.

According to Sen, A., (1999) poverty should not only be viewed in terms of low income but must be considered "as a deprivation of basic capabilities". Consequent to this concept, if poor people are deprived of basic opportunities this tends to reflect in premature death, severe malnutrition in children, an increase in the burden of disease, illiteracy and other social ills.

Economic growth increases the country's tax revenue base and thus making it possible for the government to allocate and spend more resources on public services such as health and education. Therefore, by increasing the incomes of poor people economic growth enhances their ability to pay for goods and services that contribute to the improvement of their health and education levels. The state of a country's economy thus affects the demand or amount of health services individuals or households will purchase or consume, given the price of the health services, the prices of alternatives or related items, the income of individuals or households.

A poorly performing economy affects more the private medical sector whose development plans are premised on the demand for health services. The provision of health services by the government or public sector, on the other hand, is based on perceived need, which is the level of health services which good medical opinion deems necessary to meet particular health targets. Even if the government provided these services free of charge at the point of consumption, such services would undoubtedly not be free as clients or patients bear transport and other related opportunity costs. Utilization rates and demand for health services are affected by, amongst other factors, direct out of pocket expenses, household income and wealth, travel time, and transport costs to health facilities.

Economic growth and an increase in health expenditures, each on its own, are not sufficient enough to contribute to improved health and health status. There must be effectively functioning institutions and appropriate policy choices in place. For example, the GNP per head increases life expectancy through the intermediary of increasing the incomes of the poor and public expenditures on health. Appropriate policy choices may relate to increased investment in cost effective health interventions that target the poor and/or basic education policies that target the girl child. Cumulatively, the effect of economic growth depends on how a country distributes and utilizes the fruits of its economic growth. Furthermore, where there is no rule of law and there is poor governance it is almost impossible for the seeds of economic growth to germinate into improved social services.

Economic growth and the health sector in Zimbabwe

The government of Zimbabwe has never been able to mobilize sufficient local resources to provide or purchase enough health care services for its population. Even if enough financial resources were to be made available for the delivery of the required health services, the health sector would probably not have adequate capacity to effectively utilize all the available resources. The macro economic instability which began in the late 1990s increased the risks associated with investment in the country. Poor monetary policies and a skewed exchange rate regime contributed to the country's hyperinflationary environment. The government resorted to printing money in order to finance its ballooning budget deficit, a situation which compromised its capacity to manage its taxes and expenditures. The combination of mismanagement, over expenditures by government, corruption and open ended borrowing strained the economy to the limit resulting in balance sheets that no longer balanced. In the end it became impossible to borrow in order to pay old debts and lenders were no longer willing to come forward and assist.

Internal and external factors that characterize the economic crisis affecting the country's health sector:

Internal factors:

♦ Contraction of the GDP at an average rate of 5.8% per annum between 2000 and 2005. As a result, between 1998 and 2006 Zimbabwe's GDP contracted by 23%.

♦ Retrograde economic policies of government, e.g. Statutory Instrument 159A of 2007, Amendment of National Incomes and Pricing Commission Act and Education Act Regulations 2007.

♦ Fiscal and monetary mismanagement which resulted in a large budget deficit, and a hyperinflation estimated to be over 230 million% (September 2008).

♦ A huge external debt burden of over US$ 4.7 billion in 2006 with arrears amounting to US$ 2.7 billion.

♦ A 3.6% annual decline in exports between 2001 and 2006 resulting in a critical shortage of gross foreign reserves, which in 2007 averaged only 0.8 months cover.

♦ Increasing poverty levels with 75% of the population falling below the poverty line as defined in terms of total consumption.

♦ An unemployment rate of more than 70% which resulted in massive losses of income

♦ A mismanaged land reform program compounded by unpredictable weather patterns, leading to poor agricultural yields, food shortages and declining export earnings.

External factors:
♦ Loss of support from the international community which resulted in a decline in donor contributions to public health expenditures from 13% in 1997 to less than 1% in 2002.
♦ Suspension of technical assistance from the IFM and removal of Zimbabwe from the list of countries eligible to benefit from the Poverty Reduction and Growth Facility (PRGF).
♦ Suspension of European Development Fund (EDF) assistance to Zimbabwe in 2002 and the subsequent freezing of EURO 127 million to Zimbabwe and the 9th EDF program.
♦ Legislated restrictions (sanctions) under the Zimbabwe Democracy Economic Recovery Act (2001) against the government of Zimbabwe, which, *inter alia*, bar multilateral lending institutions with dealings with the United States from extending lines of credit to Zimbabwe.
♦ Ineligibility of the country to fully benefit from some global health and development initiatives.

In light of the above economic arguments and links between economic growth, health and the general well being of a nation, it is worth reiterating that Zimbabwe's economy shrunk by almost 40% between 2000 and 2008, and continued to do so beyond this period. Such a massive shrinkage in any economy has the potential to significantly constrain the ability of any government to deliver social services to its population. Downstream effects include the consequences of increasing poverty, an increasing burden of disease and in the long run, a decrease in life expectancy. The associated decline in health expenditures has resulted in all aspects of the health delivery system in Zimbabwe being severely weakened.

Serious shortages of food have resulted in increasing levels of malnutrition and child mortality rates. As the crisis continues to unfold, basic commodities have disappeared from retail outlets. The prices of those items that happen to be available are beyond the reach of many. The shortage of foreign currency to import raw materials compounded by a severely reduced purchasing power, and the collapse of small and medium scale businesses has led to an increased pool of people that do not have any means to support the livelihoods of their families.

Specific to the health sector, the crisis has resulted in severe shortages of essential drugs and medical supplies particularly affecting public health institutions. *"The country's health delivery system has deteriorated over the past decade. A lack of essential drugs, a brain drain from the health sector, corruption and misplaced priorities by government are some of the problems"* (anonymous, 2007). Patients suffering from chronic illnesses such as diabetes, hypertension, cancer and AIDS have difficulties in obtaining medication to maintain their health. Individuals with chronic kidney disease are particularly compromised by the frequent breakdown of dialysis machines and the shortage of renal dialysis solutions. The cancellation of emergency and non emergency surgery has become the order of the day at most public health institutions which increasingly rely on financial and material donations from well wishers. Patients are compelled to provide their own medical supplies such as gloves and syringes and in some cases relatives have to provide food for inpatients.

The cost of drugs in the private sector has increased to levels beyond the reach of the majority of the population, even those covered by private health insurance schemes. The cost of private medical care outstrips the capacity of health insurance schemes to reimburse private health providers for services rendered to their members. Private providers of care are now compelled to demand cash up front even from members of private health insurance schemes before they attend to them. Patients who previously could afford and relied on private health care are now forced by circumstances to seek medical care from public health facilities. This has put more pressure on the already strained and underfunded public health sector whose quality of care has continued to deteriorate mainly as a result of a lack of adequate funding, equipment, medicines, and increasingly as a result of a severe shortage of staff to run them.

The deterioration in the function of the health delivery system is part of a system wide failure in government machinery. Considering that the effective development and function of a health system depends on cross sector synergies. Thus, in order to have a clear picture, one must necessarily analyze the impact of the economic crisis on the other sectors that have a direct or indirect impact on the overall function of a health system.

Physical capital such as health facility buildings and plant equipment which are the responsibility of the ministry responsible for infrastructure development, have rapidly deteriorated as a result of poor maintenance and disrepair. The government simply does not have the money to invest in the repair and/or rehabilitation of aging infrastructure across all the sectors, including the road network. Poor infrastructure has impacted negatively on the quality of care by affecting structure and process factors. Poor roads have meant that patients have difficulties in accessing medical care facilities, especially in rural areas. A poor road infrastructure also means that patients cannot be easily referred to the next level of care in cases of complications, thus contributing to an increase in hospital deaths. The distribution of medical supplies to health facilities throughout the country has become a challenge. The erratic generation of electricity in the country, its distribution and frequent fuel shortages contribute to the poor function of critical care hospital departments, including the function of ambulance services.

Human capital development has also been significantly and adversely affected by the poor state of the economy. The shortage of resources has jeopardized the ability of government to invest in education infrastructure. The ability of parents and guardians to pay school fees for their children has also been diminished. Declining school enrolment and completion rates mean that the education system may no longer able to produce enough students with qualifications necessary to pursue careers in the health profession. There is ample evidence that poor education attainment by the girl child has a potential impact on family wellbeing and contributes to high maternal and infant mortality rates.

The hyperinflationary environment has severely diminished the value of the salaries and other means of live hood for professionals, forcing them to leave the country in search of better employment opportunities in other countries. *"I can't blame the health personnel for leaving this country,... These conditions are not bearable and the situation is deteriorating"* (anonymous, 2004). As a result the country has been experiencing a very serious human resources crisis which, considering the lead time it takes to train experienced health professionals, seems unlikely to be solved in the immediate future.

Summary of the impact of economic decline on the health delivery system:

  ♦ Shortages of pharmaceuticals and drug supplies
  ♦ Poor quality of care at public health institutions
  ♦ Old medical equipment in disrepair
  ♦ Deteriorating physical infrastructure and lack of repair
  ♦ Human resources crisis as a result of out-migration
  ♦ Power blackouts affecting the function of health facilities
  ♦ Fuel shortages affecting patient referral

- Compromised and inadequate health insurance coverage
- Compromised access to health services by the poor
- Inability of the sector to acquire up to date health technology
- Shortage of water purification chemicals as a public health problem

It is important to note that governance failures have a significant and adverse effect on a country's investment climate. In this context, Zimbabwe's governance record has not been a rosy one, tarnished by increasing levels of corruption in both the public and private sectors. High levels of corruption in the public sector have resulted in instances where the poor have not been able to easily benefit from government services such as birth and death registration, passports, vehicle licenses, free medical treatment at public health institutions without having to make side payments to public officials. Overall, it would appear that state systems have become seriously compromised and ineffective in ensuring transparency and accountability in both public and private institutions. The question which arises is whether the "rule of law" still prevails in Zimbabwe or not. The persistent inability of the judiciary system to protect private property has seriously affected investor confidence and dampened the prospects of economic growth and consequently, health development.

Anecdotal evidence points to the fact that there have been increasing quantities of public sector drugs that have being illegally siphoned into the private sector by unscrupulous health staff. "*Corruption is deeply rooted in the public service, contributing to the poor health services, drugs are being looted and tender regulations in purchasing drugs are not being followed, resulting in government losing millions of dollars*" (anonymous, 2004). In some instances public sector staff have colluded with "brief case" business persons who sell the same stolen public sector drugs back into the public health system. In some cases public sector clinicians use their privileged positions at public hospitals to recruit patients for their private surgeries whilst others use government facilities and resources to treat their private patients. Due to poor salaries some consultants and specialists over extend the privilege granted to them to do private practice by spending more time at their personal surgeries than they do at their places of work and thus fraudulently prejudicing the state by claiming full salaries for little or no work being done for the state. The absence of some consultants at work also means that junior professionals are not supervised or given bed side training. Such incidences should however not tarnish the good image of the majority of those health professionals who continue to dedicate their services towards the well being of the poor in Zimbabwe. Special mention goes to the Zimbabwe Medical Association (ZIMA) which regularly organizes and carries out free medical treatment campaigns targeted at populations living in the rural areas of the country.

Zimbabwe's response to the health sector crisis

The health sector response to economic shocks brought about by ESAP was first of all at the macro level through the development and institutionalization of health sector reforms. This was however a slow, deliberate, measured and evolving process. At the macroeconomic level, the government responded by designing and implementing several emergency economic turnaround programs. This process started with the ESAP in the early 1990s followed by ZIMPREST, Vision 2020, the Millennium Economic Recovery Plan, the National Recovery Program, and the 9 month National Economic Development Priority Program of 2008. Unfortunately, despite all these efforts and initiatives, the failure of government to attract balance of payment support and foreign investment, the economic crisis continued unabated, at times exacerbated by way ward monetary and economic policies.

In the midst of a visibly deteriorating health system it would appear that business continued as usual within the public health sector. A response that relied on the slow pace of reform was not a viable option. There was a need to accelerate and expand pro-poor safety net programs to ensure that the poor continued to have unimpeded access to primary health care and referral services. A revision of the national health strategy and the development of a national emergency health plan would have been a good option, with clearly defined short term objectives and strategies, at least to ensure the availability of essential supplies for the core health service package.

Finding itself in a severe economic crisis that threatened the integrity of its health delivery system, the Ministry of Health and Child Welfare (the government of Zimbabwe) should have embarked on a deliberate and aggressive response to mitigate its impact on the health of the population. Facing a similar crisis that arose from the economic embargo imposed by the USA, the Cuban response was swift, with the government declaring the health status of its people a national priority and demonstrating this fact by increasing the health budget in local currency, as a share of GDP. The national strategic and operational plans were redrawn in light of the changed circumstances. There was emphasis to achieve and maintain equity in access to scarce health resources in hand, and to ensure that everybody benefited from whatever little health resources and services were available. (UNDP, 1990). Regular meetings were convened (weekly) by the Minister to assess available foreign currency resources and decisions made to prioritize only life saving purchases and medications that were not covered by urgent international appeals.

Though working under very difficult conditions, Cuban health professionals demonstrated exceptional dedication, with some of the clinicians in institutions across the country phoning local colleagues, the ministry, and colleagues abroad to find lifesaving antibiotics for their patients, (Reed, G. and Frank, M, 1997). Apart from the fact that the population was very literate and trusted the system to deliver for them, universal access to a community oriented primary health care network by every family contributed significantly to the resilience of the Cuban health delivery system.

The poor state of Zimbabwe's health delivery system and its lack of attention to the potential for health disasters are evident in the manner the country responded to the cholera epidemic that occurred in 2008 and spilling over into 2009. The unprecedented number of cholera cases which in only six months had exceeded 65000 cases and 3500 deaths, clearly demonstrated the total lack of capacity for disease surveillance, epidemic preparedness and case management within the health sector as well as the poor state of the country's inter-sectoral disaster management systems. The unprecedented nature and extent of this cholera epidemic is the ultimate testimony of a health delivery system that is totally dysfunctional as a result of years of neglect and underfunding by the government.

Prospects for improved health in Africa

First and foremost there must be recognition that health is a pre-condition for economic development and poverty reduction. The health sector must also be recognized as an integral part of the design and implementation process of poverty reduction strategies.

Jeffrey D. Sachs (2003) is quoted to have said, *"critics of foreign assistance sometimes mistakenly argue that the basic problem of health care in the poorest countries is mismanagement of health systems. I want to reject that view categorically. There is no way to manage an efficient health system at US$7.50 per capita. And there is no way that the world's poorest societies, just barely surviving at current income levels, or perhaps not surviving, can manage much* more than that out of their own resources".

According to the UNDP the world has enough resources to be able to eliminate the worst forms of poverty from the planet. Africa needs a major health and economic development process through massive investments in its economy and the health development process. The MDG approach has renewed interest in health development through linking it to education, water, sanitation, poverty reduction and growth.

In the context of health reforms Africa needs to develop strategies that focus on putting in place sustainable health financing, health provision structures and viable public management systems. Macroeconomic policies must be designed and implemented in ways that enhance the development of efficient health sectors. Most African countries require strategies that will ensure an absolute increase in expenditures on health from local resource mobilization. Appropriate fiscal policies can be used to improve the allocation and utilization of resources. Local resources mobilization efforts can be complemented by increasing development assistance to the levels needed to achieve globally agreed goals, and having external debt relief by the international community, improved market access and a reduction in the constraints that prevent African countries from fully realizing the benefits of globalization. Because African countries rely more on external trade, expanding market access for their exports remains a priority in ensuring increased economic growth.

Development partners must commit to and deliver predictable and sustainable health development aid in order to avoid disruptions in national programs and uncertainty in planning for the future. Donors must submit to being held accountable for delivering on their promises. The current lack of global coherence in aid delivery policies and fragmentation in donor assistance requires commitment to aid harmonization and improved donor coordination under the leadership of the ministry of health in recipient countries.

African countries must take full responsibility for good governance, the development of sound policies, tackling corruption and investing in people. Weak governance constrains the performance of health systems and has a serious impact on public health. Public health systems in some of these countries are plagued by political interference in the management of public institutions, poor human resources management such as corrupt practices in recruitment, promotion and transfer of staff. Poor governance affects efforts to achieve equity through the misallocation of resources.

It is essential that much more effort is invested in the reduction of inefficiencies in the utilization of available resources through eliminating waste and plunder within health institutions. Ministries of health may require restructuring in order to improve management and planning capacity and to streamline bureaucracy. Organizational restructuring improves accountability, reduces overlap and duplication and may restore the authority of the ministry of health within the sector. There must be renewed focus to remove bottlenecks that militate against the achievement of the MDGs such as; resolving human resources for health constraints, removing barriers to access to health care, strengthening supply and logistic systems and the adoption of effective macroeconomic and health sector policies and strategies.

On the home front countries need to strengthen their health systems by:

- Increasing investment in health and utilizing existing investments efficiently
- Investing in basic infrastructure to deliver health services, drugs and supplies
- Guaranteeing access to quality essential drugs (quality control)
- Ensuring universal coverage of basic health services (delivery of essential basic health packages)
- Dealing with the human resources for health issues
- Improving their governance record

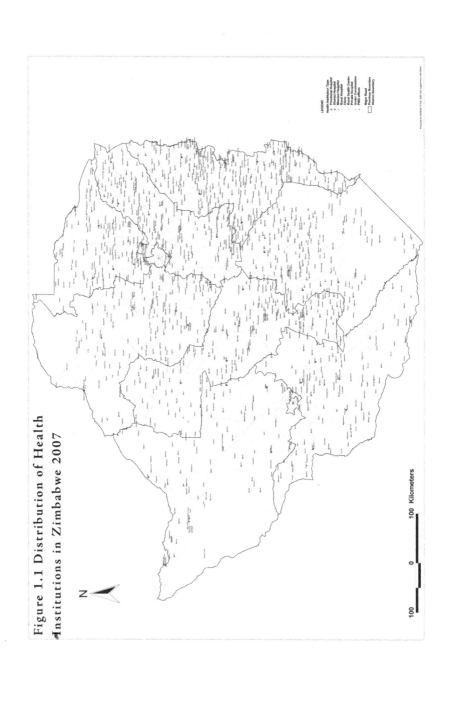

Figure 1.1 Distribution of Health Institutions in Zimbabwe 2007

1

OVERVIEW OF THE HEALTH SECTOR IN ZIMBABWE

Introduction

Zimbabwe attained its independence from Britain in 1980. It is a land locked country located north of the Tropic of Capricorn between the Limpopo River in the south and the Zambezi River in the north. The country borders Zambia in the north, Mozambique in the East, South Africa in the South and Botswana on the West. The total surface area of the country is 90 759 square kilometers and the population in 2008 was estimated to be 12.6 million people.

The majority of the population consists of two major Bantu-speaking people, the Shona who constitute about 70% and the Matebele about 16% of the total population. The country has a small minority of Europeans, Asians and persons of mixed race. Nearly three quarters of the people live in rural areas.

The country has had one of the most diversified economies of any African country with mining and agriculture as the most important sectors and a manufacturing sector that is well developed. The road network totals about 85 780 kilometers in length with 2 745 kilometers of railroad.

At independence Zimbabwe adopted Planning for Equity in Health as its policy framework. This policy statement was aimed at addressing the imbalances in which the rich and urban minorities enjoyed better health and other social amenities that included privileged access to the most sophisticated health care in the country. On the other hand the poor rural folks who constituted the majority of the citizens had minimum access to often poor health facilities.

The objective of government was to ensure that deprived populations received priority in the provision of health services. To achieve these objectives the government adopted Primary Health Care (PHC) as its main strategy of providing health services. The PHC approach is characterized by health care that is considered appropriate, accessible and affordable to both the state and the individual.

The government inherited what it termed a fragmented health care delivery system consisting of a variety of providers who include the Ministry of Health (MOH), local government, missions, industrial medical services, the private for profit sector and NGOs, all of whom were not well coordinated.

The role of the government has been to guide, support and be the lead agent within a multi-sectoral drive to provide health for all. Health was thus considered a developmental issue in which communities and other sectors are expected to participate in both its production and consumption. In addition to these core responsibilities the ministry of health has the duty to receive and transfer grant funds to municipalities, local councils, missions and other voluntary organizations.

The major health problems at the time were identified through a sectoral review that was conducted in 1980, soon after the country attained its independence. The problems identified indicated that Zimbabweans suffered and died from diseases of poverty, nutritional deficiencies, communicable diseases and conditions related to pregnancy, childbirth and the newborn period. Amongst the most important causes of childhood morbidity and mortality were diarrhea, pneumonia (whooping cough), measles, tetanus of the newborn, malaria and tuberculosis.

Available data on health indicators indicated that the coverage of Maternal and Child Health (MCH) services was generally inadequate. Estimates at the time indicated *'that up to 25% of the target groups in the rural areas were fully covered by immunizations against childhood diseases'.* (GOZ/MOH, 1984).

Before 1980 there had been a fee charged for all curative services provided at government institutions. In 1980 the new government abolished hospital and clinic fees for patients earning up to 150 Zimbabwean Dollars (US$390) per month. This policy decision resulted in a three-fold increase in outpatient consultations, mainly in the rural areas. Revenue collected from user fees at all other government institutions reverted to the treasury. However, revenue collected at the Parirenyatwa Group of Hospitals was retained by the hospital's Board of Governors for local use at the hospital.

The repeal of the Medical Services Act (1979) in 1981 ended the discrimination in access to health services which was officially based on racial lines. The hospital wards, which had hitherto been designated 'European Wards' became 'open wards' into which private practitioners could admit their private patients irrespective of race, color or creed. The wards previously designated as "African Wards" were re-designated 'closed' to private practitioners.

The immediate post independence developments and policies in Zimbabwe were motivated by the need to redress the inequities in access to social services. The implementation of these policies resulted in an increase of about 77% in real terms in government expenditures on health between 1980 and 1990. The number of staff within the public health sector also increased from about 12 000 to 23 000. The government's commitment to PHC saw the share of expenditures on preventive services almost doubling in the first five post independence years from 8% to 15%.

The Health Delivery platform - Infrastructure

Of the 316 Rural Health Centers (RHC) targeted to be constructed and 450 targeted to be upgraded, 246 had been constructed by 1998 and several more upgraded. The number of government hospitals increased during the same period from 43 to 60. These included 24 district hospitals which were either upgraded or constructed under the World Bank financed Family Health Projects (FHP) I and II, Table 1.1 (next page).

The Ministry of Health and Child Welfare's national health profile for 2006 provides information, though considered to be incomplete, on the number of health facilities operating in Zimbabwe. About 1331 of these are either RHCs, urban clinics or rural hospitals. About 200 of these facilities are government run hospitals consisting of district, general, provincial, infectious diseases hospitals and central hospitals. It is estimated that there are at least 25 722 hospital beds nationally in the public sector, Table 1.2. At some point this figure translated to a ratio of about one bed per 1000 population. In 1980 it was estimated that there were 836 health facilities in the public health sector in Zimbabwe.

Table 1.1: Distribution of health facilities by province

Facility	Manicaland	Mashonaland Central	Mash. East	Mash. West	Matabeleland North	Mat. South	Midlands	Masvingo	Harare City	Bulawayo City	Totals
Clinics, RHCs and Rural Hospitals	253	130	168	128	92	105	106	170	45	34	1331
District and Other Hospitals	36	13	22	22	17	18	28	23			179
Provincial Hospitals	1	1	1	1	0	1	1	1			7
Central, Infectious Diseases Hospitals	0	0	0	0	0	0	0	0	7	7	14
Total	290	144	191	151	109	124	235	194	52	41	1531

Compiled from MOHCW Health Profile for 2006

Table 1.2: Distribution of hospital/facility beds by province

Facility	Manicaland	Mashonaland Central	Mash. East	Mash. West	Matabeleland North	Mat. South	Midlands	Masvingo	Totals
Clinics RHCs	1327	550	453	645	466	510	900	730	5581
Rural Hospitals	645	84	195	351	260	332	213	447	2527
District & Other Hospitals	1406	625	821	1358	1545	1007	2345	2280	11387
Provincial Hospitals	290	120	178	407	0	186	432	271	1884
Central Hospitals	0	0	2448	0	1895	0	0	0	4343
Total	3668	1379	4095	2761	4166	2035	3890	3728	25722

Compiled from information in the MOHCW Health Profile 1999

Estimates indicate that religious missions operate at least 60 Rural Health Centers and 80 hospitals of various sizes. At least 13 of the mission hospitals are designated as district hospitals by the Ministry of Health and Child Welfare (MOHCW). In 1999 it was estimated that there were 35 private hospitals in Zimbabwe with a total complement of at least 1.152 beds.

By 1998, 50% of government health facilities outside the major urban areas were electrified, 55% had piped water and 60% had radio or telephone communications. The 2006 Zimbabwe health profile indicates that only 46% of rural health facilities were electrified, 53% had some telecommunications and that 48% had a reticulated water supply system. Matabeleland and the Midlands provinces had the least proportion of facilities that were electrified, 39.3% and 39.8% respectively. According to the 1999 health profile, the population per RHC was about 9 000 against a set target of 1 RHC per 10 000 population.

Organization of Health Services

The health delivery system is district based and consists of primary, secondary, tertiary and central hospital levels. These levels are expected to function as a referral chain consisting of facilities of increasing sophistication from the lower levels upwards. The primary level consists of a network of health centers and community based health workers. The secondary level consists of district hospitals which constitute the first referral hospital level. The tertiary level consists of provincial and general hospitals. Central hospitals are at the top of the hierarchy and offer specialist referral services. These institutions are also teaching hospitals for health professionals. This type of hospital is only found in urban areas.

At the lowest level of the health system, below the RHCs, is a network of community health workers consisting of Village Health Workers (VHW), Farm Health Workers (FHW) and Community Based Distributors (CBD). About 6 000 VHWs were deployed as early as 1981 under the then Ministry of Health (MOH). The Village Health Worker received basic training in preventive health, health promotion, first aid treatment and environmental health concepts. The VHWs were paid a modest allowance for their efforts and each supplied with a bicycle for increased mobility. According to the policy of government communities selected VHWs on the basis of agreed criteria.

This cadre of "volunteer" health workers was later transferred from the MOHCW to the Ministry of Community Development, Co-operatives and Women's Affairs. This move was viewed by many as being politically motivated and that it was meant for the government to utilize these cadres for political mobilization in rural areas. The move was also considered to be a major setback for the community health movement in Zimbabwe.

With regards the referral system, the reality on the ground is that the patient referral system is not functioning well. This is because the lower levels of the health system are under utilized as most patients bypass them. This phenomenon has been attributed to the poor quality of care at health center level resulting from staff and drug shortages which have over the years become a common feature within the public health sector.

In most cases RHCs do not have electricity or any communication with the district hospital. In other cases the lower levels of the health system are bypassed because the nearest health facility is a district or central hospital which is perceived to be offering a better quality of services.

Major Providers of Health Care in Zimbabwe

Hospital Services

There are several sub-sectors involved in the provision of hospital services in Zimbabwe. The Ministry of Health and Child Welfare is the largest single provider of health care in Zimbabwe. The ministry operates close to 400 RHCs and rural hospitals, 60 hospitals, including 35 district and general hospitals, 7 provincial hospitals, 6 central hospitals, and 8 infectious diseases hospitals, including one national referral mental health institution.

Municipalities and Rural District Councils operate another approximately 600 urban clinics and Rural Health Centers between them. Religious Missions operate 60 RHCs and 80 hospitals of which 13 are designated as district hospitals. Missions are organized under an umbrella organization, the Zimbabwe Association of Church Related Hospitals (ZACH), which looks after their collective interests.

The private for profit sector in Zimbabwe has over the years been expanding at a phenomenal rate. This has been a response to an increasing demand for alternative quality services. In 2001 private health facilities included 35 hospitals, 768 establishments for private medical practitioners (GPs), 216 pharmacies, 88 dental practitioners' practices, 49 Nursing homes, 67 psychological services, 100 medical laboratories, 41 radiology services, 47 optical services and 65 physiotherapy and occupational therapy offices, (Source: Health Professions Council, 2001). Statistics from the 2006 health profile indicate that there are 338 private pharmacies in Zimbabwe.

Preventive Services

The implementation of preventive health services falls under the Provincial Medical Director (PMD) of the MOHCW who also oversees the function of tertiary and district hospital services within the province. At the MOHCW headquarters there are program managers who develop program policy frameworks, provide high level technical support and a strategic direction to the operational level with respect to preventive health programs.

The District Medical Officer (DMO) is in charge of coordinating the implementation of district health services. The PMD and his/her Provincial Executive provide overall technical and administrative supervision and support to the DMO and his/her District Health Management Team (DHMT).

The PMD heads a Provincial Health Executive Team which consists of several provincial program heads, namely:
- The Provincial Nursing Officer (PNO)
- The Medical Officer of Health (Maternal and Child Health)
- The Medical Officer of Health (Epidemiology and Disease Control)
- The Provincial Nutritionist
- The Provincial Health Education Officer
- The Provincial Environmental Health Officer (PEHO)
- The Provincial Pharmacist
- The Provincial Health Services Administrator (PHSA)

Preventive health services consist of a number of programs which include maternal and child health services, reproductive health services, behavior change communication services (health education), communicable disease prevention and control and environmental health services. Support systems for the delivery of these programs include drugs procurement, distribution and management; diagnostic and laboratory services; planning and budgeting; transport management; human resources development and management; infrastructure development and maintenance;

and general administration. Preventive programs and services are coordinated at national and provincial levels and delivered at the various levels of the health system which include the community level, RHCs and the district level under the direction of the District Medical Officer (DMO) and his/her team.

At the district level the DMO leads a core group of District Health Executive (DHE) members who together are in charge of coordinating the delivery of all health services in the district, including the provision of technical supervision and support to mission institutions, Rural District Council health facilities, the operations of health NGOs and the private medical sector operating within the district. The DHE is composed of the following officers:

+ District Medical Officer (DMO)
+ The District Nursing Officer (DNO)
+ The District Health Services Administrator (DHSA)
+ The District Environmental Health Officer (DEHO)
+ The District Pharmacy Technician (Pharmacist)
+ The Executive Officer responsible for health in the Rural District Council is a co-opted member of the DHE.

The DHE and PHE are expected to hold management meetings at least fort nightly. The District Health Team (DHT) and the Provincial Health Team (PHT) are collective management structures responsible for the planning and budgeting processes and monitoring progress in the implementation of health programs within the district and province respectively. These teams are expected to meet on a quarterly basis.

The Provincial Health Team is composed of all members of the Provincial Health Executive, members of the DHEs, representatives from mission institutions and other health providers within the province. The District Health Team (DHT) is composed of the DHE, representatives from all RHCs, Rural District Council clinics, religious mission institutions and all other providers of health within the district.

Religious missions in the health sector

At independence the government made a decision to integrate mission health facilities into the public health sector as part of its efforts to increase access to health care in rural areas. As an incentive for the missions to operate within the overall health sector policy framework, the government increased the annual grant it allocated for financing the operations of these institutions. Under the government policy framework religious missions have an obligation to provide free services to those patients considered eligible for such free services in terms of existing user fee policies. To facilitate compliance with this policy mission institutions are allocated a government grant based on the following criteria:

+ 100% salaries grant for approved staff posts.
+ 80% grant for other recurrent expenditures.
+ 100% grant for drugs purchased from the National pharmaceutical Company (Natpharm).
+ 100% grant for approved infrastructure development.

The financing agreement between the two parties is informal with no signed or legally binding contract document. Over the years it increasingly became apparent that the government grant allocated to religious missions was not enough to maintain the services they provided. The amount of money they collected from user fees did not amount to any significant proportion of their recurrent costs. Grant allocations from government were three to five times less than what the government allocated to its own institutions of comparable size and work load. Donations which mission institutions received from their overseas benefactors continued to decline.

Mission institutions have often been accused by the MOHCW of refusing to divulge the full amount of the financial and material resources they receive from overseas benefactors. Allegedly, this made it difficult for the MOHCW to find a rational basis upon which to review the amount of grant money it allocated to them. As a result a situation emerged where mission institutions have over the years become poorly maintained; offering poor quality hotel services as well as experiencing a comparatively higher staff turnover rate than government institutions. However since the donor community stopped direct financial support to the government of Zimbabwe in 2001, some mission institutions became favorite recipient intuitions of donor finances. This situation has greatly improved the lot of some of these mission and NGO establishments.

Local Government Authorities

In 1998 the country had 13 Municipalities and 58 Rural District Councils all providing health services as part of their statutory obligations. Health services provided by these institutions consist mainly of primary health services delivered through clinics.

As part of its responsibilities the MOHCW submits health budget estimates on behalf of missions and local authorities to the Treasury. On receiving these funds from the treasury the MOHCW transfers these grants to the respective local authorities and mission institutions on a monthly and/or quarterly basis.

The grant to urban local authorities is provided on the basis of a Public Finance Agreement entered into in 1976 between urban councils and the MOHCW on behalf of central government. This agreement was intended to guarantee that urban local authorities would receive 100% funding from central government for recurrent costs and 50% of the costs of approved capital development projects. The urban councils were in turn required to adhere to government policies, especially as they apply to the exemption of the poor and indigent patients from paying user fees on seeking health care from their facilities.

Facts on the ground indicate that over the years central government has failed to honor its obligations under this agreement. As a result urban councils have resorted to charging user fees for all health services in order to meet shortfalls in their health budgets. Urban local authorities have also over the years reviewed their staffing levels and capital development projects without applying for the necessary approval from the Secretary for Health. This effectively means that the MOHCW has no financial obligations in terms of the 1976 agreement to support staff salaries or new capital projects which over the years have not received the required approval by the Secretary for Health.

The Private for profit health sector

Soon after independence the government put in place bold measures to try and curtail the development of the private for profit sector. In its policy document, "Planning for Equity in Health" the government explicitly states that *"private medicine is wasteful of resources. It not only inflates total medical costs, but it uses up the country's limited foreign exchange allocations for pharmaceuticals......private practice for fulltime employees will be phased out..."* (GOZ/MOH, 1984). The government also proclaimed that *"government had a duty to control the size of the private medical sector in the public interest"*. The document also states that no further expansion of private sector facilities would be permitted and that private practice by full time government and university doctors would be phased out.

However, despite these initial pronouncements by government, the private medical sector supported by Medical Aid Societies (private voluntary health insurance schemes) steadily increased its share within the delivery of health care in Zimbabwe. There has been a dramatic increase in the number of general practitioners' surgeries, maternity homes managed by nurse-midwives and to some degree the number of industrial clinics. A significant number of large private hospitals offering specialist services have also been established in some urban areas. As is the case in many developing countries in the region the private health care sector has been mostly confined to urban areas of the country.

In 1999 it was estimated that as many as 1 million persons in Zimbabwe were covered by medical aid schemes. This meant that approximately 90% of private health facility users were covered by medical aid and that 75% of insurance payments were made to private practitioners.

The poor conditions of service in the public sector and the poor economic environment literally forced the majority of health professionals to explore employment opportunities in the private sector as well as outside the country. Over the years the government relaxed its restrictive policies on public sector employees wishing to engage in private practice. Consultants have been allowed half a day a week to engage in their personal private practice. The problem however is that in exercising this privilege some doctors have tended to take much more time than they are entitled to. This has meant that patients in public health institutions suffer and remained unattended.

The poor economic outlook in the country has over the years adversely affected patronage of the private medical sector in Zimbabwe. Membership in most of the medical insurance schemes has also decreased as a result of economic hardships and inflationary pressures that have seen medical insurance premiums go beyond the reach of many Zimbabweans. This environment saw some private medical establishments close down as a result of poor business. Others were taken over by one of the largest medical insurance schemes in the country which transformed them into managed care facilities.

Health financing in Zimbabwe

The operations of the public health sector in Zimbabwe are financed mainly from tax revenue allocated by the Treasury to the MOHCW. The salary budget is held centrally and salaries are paid to civil servants directly from the Salary Service Bureau (SSB). At the time of writing the only government institution that received both its general recurrent and salary budgets as part of a grant from central government was Parirenyatwa Central Hospital which is now managed by a Hospital Management Board. However because the grant from treasury is usually inadequate to support the hospital's running expenses this has at times resulted in the hospital being unable to pay its staff salaries on time.

Mission hospitals have over the years been financed through government grants which they supplement with donations from overseas as well as with revenue from user fees that they charge. A major problem has been that grant funds channeled from treasury through the MOHCW to missions and Rural District Councils have often been disbursed late, resulting in delays in the payment of salaries for staff at these institutions. In some cases RDCs have used monies meant for staff salaries for other council business. Such irresponsible acts have often resulted in a lot of frustration amongst health workers employed by these organizations. This is one of the reasons why staffs in the MOHCW are not willing to be transferred to RDCs as part of the decentralization process of government service delivery.

In fiscal year 1980-81 total government expenditures on health represented 4 percent of the gross national product, equivalent at the time to United States Dollars (US$) 16 per capita. This figure excluded expenditures on self-care and direct payments to private institutions and general practitioners. Amongst the different health providers, the government accounted for 71% of the total national expenditures on health in the same financial year. Between fiscal years 1980-81 and 1987-88 MOHCW expenditures rose by 94%, translating into an increase of 48% in real per capita expenditures. As a proportion of the GDP this translated to an increase from 2.2% of the GDP in the early 1980s to 3.1% in 1990/91. In 1990-91 government expenditures on health peaked at US$22 per capita, the highest ever achieved in Zimbabwe since independence. At the time health expenditures by the government of Zimbabwe compared favorably with those of other countries in the region. By 1995 this figure had however declined to US$13. In the 1996/97 fiscal year this figure rose to US$16. However, the rapid increase in the development of infrastructure contributed to health resources being spread too thin and thus effectively increasing the gap between demand and available resources

The general trend on health expenditures has been one of a noticeable decline since 1990/91. Between 1990 and the year 2000 government expenditures on health as a proportion of total public spending declined from 6.4% to 4.3%. As a proportion of the GDP this was a reduction from 3.1% to 2.1%. These figures translate into an average reduction in expenditures on health of about 33%. This decline in expenditures took place against an increasing burden of disease and workload in the public health sector mainly attributed to the HIV/AIDS epidemic.

National Health Accounts (NHA) conducted by the MOHCW in 2001 indicated that total health expenditures in the 1999 financial year in Zimbabwe accounted for 7.8% of the GDP. Public health expenditures accounted for 3.7% of the GDP, private health spending 4.1% and donor spending, 0.9% of the GDP.

Private sector spending constituted 50.1% of the total national health expenditures, whilst public and donor spending contributed 36.9% and 13% respectively. These figures translate to a total national per capita expenditure of US$37.26. Of this national per capita expenditure figure US$13.73 was contributed by the public health sector which consists of the government and donors (US$4.84) with the private sector spending US$18.68 per capita. Household expenditures contributed 45.8% of total private health spending and 23% of total health financing, translating to per capita spending of US$8.55, (Zimbabwe NHA, 2001).

According to the Zimbabwe Country Analytic Report (USAID, 2007), government expenditures on health increased from 2.1% of GDP in 2002 to 4.3% in 2006. This increase was however more apparent than real due to recent declines in real GDP. According to the publication, Health and Social Statistics, the Human Development Report of 2007 (available on line at: www.hdr.undp.org, accessed on 31 May 2007) the total per capita expenditures on health for Zimbabwe in purchasing power parity (PPP) terms in United States dollars was $PPP 139 compared to, for example, Zambia 63, Mozambique 58 and Kenya 86.

User fees

In 1980 access to public health services was declared free at the point of delivery for the vast majority of poor and unemployed Zimbabweans. Patients in formal employment who earned less Z$150 per month (at the wage structure prevailing at the time) were eligible for free health services at public health facilities. Fees were to be levied only on those patients who bypassed the referral system. In 1991 under pressure from the World Bank the government of Zimbabwe further enforced cost recovery at all levels of the health system and attempted to put in place effective exemption mechanisms to protect the most vulnerable. A letter from local community leaders or an officer from the Social Development Fund (SDF) was enough proof for free access to health services. Despite these exemption strategies the immediate impact of the enforcement of user fees was a noticeable decline in the utilization of public health facilities, especially in the rural areas. In November 1992 the cut off level for exemption to pay user fees was raised from Z$150 (US$27) to Z$400 (US$78). In 1993 the GOZ abolished fees at RHCs and rural hospitals. Those hospitals with no establishment for a medical doctor were classified as rural hospitals and thus did not charge any user fees. This review of user fees was partly to alleviate the effects of the drought that occurred in 1991-92 as well as to eliminate the high administrative costs associated with the collection of the proceeds from user fees. The other reason was an attempt by government to guarantee equity in access to health services. Despite the government policy to abolish user fees at public health facilities in rural areas, most Rural District Councils and religious missions have continued to charge user fees. In January 1994 the MOHCW revised its fees upwards to be in line with the economic costs of providing health care and to align them with those charged by the private for profit sector.

The total revenue collected from fees as a proportion of MOHCW recurrent expenditures never at any time exceeded 3.5%. The major reason for the poor yield of revenue from user fees was partly the result of poor billing methods at government institutions both for direct payments and for payments from medical aid schemes. The other reason was that all the revenue accruing from user fees reverted to Treasury. This acted as an obvious disincentive for institutions to effectively collect all the revenue.

Development Assistance

In fiscal year 1990/91 total government expenditures amounted to 49% of GDP, mostly funding a fiscal deficit. By 1995/96 the country's budget deficit had reached 10.1% of GDP despite the implementation of the Economic Structural Adjustment Program (ESAP). As a result in 1995 the International Monetary Fund (IFM) declared the Government of Zimbabwe (GOZ) "off tract" resulting in bilateral and multi-lateral donors and lenders suspending development aid and external official financial support to the country.

Up until the mid 1997 donor inflows contributed up to 13% to public health expenditures. By 2002 this figure had declined to 1% of MOHCW expenditures, though about 34% of all available donor resources flowed through the MOHCW.

Health Insurance

The health insurance industry in Zimbabwe is dominated by Medical Aid Societies whose resources mainly flow to the private for profit sector (75%) and 14% to government hospitals (NHA, 2001). The health insurance industry contributed about 45% to national health care financing in 2001.

Human Resources for Health

Zimbabwe has more than 50 registration categories of professional health workers all trained to very high standards within the country. The majority of these health workers are nurses who account for more than 80% of the total registrations. Medical doctors account for about 6% of the registrations. Due to the very poor personnel information systems within government it has remained a very difficult task to get the correct number of health professionals actually practicing in Zimbabwe at any one time. What is certain however is that since independence the number of categories of health professionals and the absolute number of health workers employed in the public health sector increased significantly to match the expansion in the health delivery system.

In Zimbabwe not all health professionals whose names appear on the Health Professions Council (HPC) register are actually practicing within the country at any particular time. Some health professionals maintain their names on the register in order to avoid the cumbersome process of re-registering when they come back into the country at a later date.

In 1995 the MOHCW employed an estimated 7 036 nurses (32% of those registered), 47% of registered doctors and 12% of registered pharmacists. The majority of those registered were either working in the private sector or were out of the country. In 1999 the total establishment of the MOHCW was 24 651. Approximately 9 903 of the established posts were for professional staff. When the government implemented its Civil Service Reforms and the Economic Structural Adjustment Program (ESAP) the MOHCW was compelled to retrench 25% of its staff working in the clerical and administrative areas. MOH records for 2006 show that the total establishment for medical doctors of all grades in the MOHCW was 1 562 of which only 703 (45%) were filled. The total establishment for all grades of nurses was 12 013 (including trainee midwives) of which 4 523 posts (35%) were occupied. These figures crudely translate to 1 medical doctor per 17 200 population and 1 nurse per 2 525 population. There are of course significant disparities in these ratios between urban and rural areas.

The attrition rate in the public sector has continued to increase over the years, especially in the nursing profession where it was estimated to be 11% per annum and that for medical doctors being 8%. The major contributing factor has been the poor conditions of service resulting from a decline in the buying power of the country's currency. The World Bank (WB) estimated that the real value of salaries of civil servants in Zimbabwe declined by more than 30% between 1991 and 1995. Because the issue of human resources for health has reached crisis proportions in most of the developing world, a separate chapter is dedicated to this subject.

Zimbabwe's health profile

Since the 1980s more than 80% of the population has had physical access to health services in Zimbabwe. However, as a result of the country's resettlement and land reform program, more than a million newly resettled farmers and their families have no access to basic services, including health services. This is largely because the government has not provided new health infrastructure since the land reform program was implemented.

From the Zimbabwe Demographic Health Surveys (ZDHS) undertaken to date the Total Fertility Rate (TFR) for the country has declined from 5.5 children in 1988, 4.0 in 1999 and 3.8 by 2006 (DHS 2005-06). This is a phenomenal achievement by the country's family planning program which has generally been considered to be one of the best performing in the sub-region. According to the same DHS figures the Contraceptive Prevalence Rate (CPR) for Zimbabwe in the 2005-06 period was 58%, a figure which is well above the regional average.

The Infant Mortality Rate (IMR) declined from 140 per 1 000 live births in 1979 to 66 per 1000 live births in 1992. In 1999 this figure was 70 per 1 000 live births declining to 60 deaths per 1 000 live births by 2005 (DHS, 2005-06), Table 1.3. The life expectancy at birth increased from 57 years in 1979 to 62 years in 1988. By 1999 the demographic impact of HIV/AIDS had reduced the life expectancy for Zimbabweans to as low as 40 years. UN Population Division estimates for 2006 indicate that the average life expectancy of Zimbabweans is 42 years.

Table 1.3: Trends in Infant Mortality Rates (IMR) in Zimbabwe (1978-2005/06)

Year	1979	1981	1984	1986	1988	1992	1995	1999	2002	2005/06
IMR /1000 live births	140	79	69	64	61	66	80	70	67	60

Childhood mortality rates declined soon after independence from 37 per 1 000 live births to 23 per 1 000 live births in 1988. By 1999 (DHS) the child mortality rate had however deteriorated to 26 per 1 000 live births. The mortality rate in children under the age of five years in 1980 was 108 per 1 000 and by 1999 this had increased to 118 per 1 000. According to the DHS (2005-06) the overall under-five mortality rate declined to 82 per 1 000 in 2006. This should be considered significant progress considering the poor socio economic environment prevailing in the country. The DHS (2005-06) also showed that child mortality rates decreased in all categories, except for post neonatal mortality, which remained at 36 deaths per 1 000 live births.

The proportion of children who are nutritionally wasted in the age group below 3 years initially declined from 9% in 1982 to 1% in 1988 (DHS). By 1994, 5.5% of the children under the age of 3 years were wasted. In 1999 this figure had risen to 6% and remained the same in 2006. In 1988, 20.3% of children under the age of five years were stunted, 21.4% in 1994 (DHS) and 27% in 1999 (DHS). Figures from the UNFPA online source (2003) indicated that of the children under the age of five years, 13% were under weight, with more males being in this category compared to their female counterparts, 9.4% severely malnourished and 1.6% severely wasted. The proportion of stunted children declined from 36% in 1982 to 23% in 1994 and rose to 35% in 1999 (DHS). The DHS (2005-06) indicates that 29% of children under the age of five years were stunted, with 17% found to be below two standard deviations for weight for age, which was an increase from 13% in 1999 (DHS).

Vaccination coverage in children between 12-23 months increased from 25% in the pre-independence era to 80% in 1994 (DHS) and declined to 75 % in 1999 (DHS). In 1999 only 66% of these children had completed their vaccination schedule by the time they turned one year. There was a further decline to 53% in 2006 with only 75% of the children having received BCG, 63% having completed DPT vaccination and 66%

having been immunized against measles.

Adult mortality rates have been rapidly increasing since the advent of the HIV/AIDS epidemic in the late 1980s. The Crude Death Rate per 1000 population (CDR) for Zimbabwe initially showed a decline from 10.8 in 1982 to 6.1 in 1995 but rose again to 12.2 by the end of 1997. Current estimates indicate that the CDR has increased from 17.99 (2002) to 19 (2006) mainly due to HIV/AIDS, (UN Population Division), and possibly compounded by the deteriorating socio economic environment.

Estimates of Maternal Mortality Rate (MMR) in Zimbabwe have generally been characterized by inconsistencies depending on the sources of data quoted. At independence the MMR was estimated to be 90 deaths per 100 000 live births. In 1994 the DHS reported a MMR of 283 deaths per 100 000 live births, in 1999 (DHS) the MMR was 695 deaths per 100 000 live births and in 2006 the rate was 555 deaths per 100 000 live births. This figure is not significantly different from the one in the 1999 DHS. According to the 2001 World Development Indicators from the World Bank, the adjusted MMR for Zimbabwe in 1999 was 610 per 100 000 live births. An in depth analysis of the 1999 DHS data indicated that non-maternal female mortality rose more rapidly than overall mortality. This has been interpreted to mean that the rise in MMR is most likely a direct result of the HIV/AIDS epidemic.

The utilization of Antenatal Care (ANC) services has remained very high over the years. In 1990 the proportion of pregnant women who attended ANC at least once was 89% and by 1995 this figure had declined to 78%. The 1999 DHS reported that 93 per cent of pregnant women received ANC from trained health workers with a median of 4.7 visits per pregnancy. In 2006 95% of women received ANC from a trained health professional at least once. The proportion of pregnant women reported to be delivering at health facilities was 69% in 1994, 72% in 1999 (DHS) and declining to 68% in 2006 (DHS). According to the 2001 World Development Indicators skilled health workers attend to 84% of births in Zimbabwe. The disparities between rural and urban areas continue with 64% of pregnant women delivering at health facilities in rural areas compared to 89% in urban areas. In 2006, 81% of mothers received at least one tetanus toxoid injection during pregnancy with only 43% receiving iron supplements. Women in rural areas were more likely to receive iron supplements than their urban counterparts.

Table 1.4 Trends in selected health indicators for Zimbabwe (1980-2006)

Indicator	1980	1988	1994	1999	2005-06 (ZDHS)
Total Fertility Rate		5.5	4.3	4.0	3.8
Infant Mortality Rate/1 000 live births	140 (1979)	53 (DHS)	53 (DHS)	65 (DHS)	60
Child Mortality Rate per 1 000	37	23	36 (1997)	26	
Under five mortality	108	75 (DHS)	77 (DHS)	102	82
Life expectancy (yrs)	57 (1978)	62 (1988)	61 (1990-92)	40 (W/B 2001)	*40
Maternal Mortality Rate/100 000 births.	90	570 (1990 UNICEF)	283 (DHS)	695 (DHS)	555 (DHS) *880
Deliveries in Health facilities (%)	-	-	69	72	68
Crude Death Rate	10.8 (Census)		6.1 (1997)	12.2 (ICDS/1997)	12.8
Antenatal Care Coverage		89% (1990)	78% (1997)	93% (DHS)	94%
Immunization coverage	25% (1979)		80%	75% (DHS)	52.3 (DHS)
Measles	-	-	86.3 (DHS)	79.1 (DHS)	65.6(DHS)
BCG	-	-	95.7 (DHS)	88(DHS)	75.7 (DHS)
Contraceptive prevalence rate	38% (1984)	43% (DHS)	48% (DHS)	54% (DHS)	58%(DHS)

Sources: ZDHS 1988, 1994 and 1999; 1992 census, Inter-census Data 1997, ZDHS 2005-06,
*UNDP- HDR 2007-08)

HIV/AIDS in Zimbabwe

Zimbabwe is one of the 189 signatories to the United Nations General Assembly Session's (UNGASS) Declaration of Commitment to fight HIV/AIDS. The Zimbabwe National AIDS Coordination Program (NACP) was established in 1987 to coordinate HIV/AIDS prevention and control activities. The NACP developed a Short Term Emergency Plan (STEP) which was succeeded by the first Medium Term Plan (MTP1) implemented from 1988 to the end of 1993. The second Medium Term Plan (MTP2) was implemented between 1994 and 1998 and emphasized an inter-sectoral approach to the prevention and control of HIV/AIDS. In 1996 the government began its preparations for strategies beyond the MTP2 by putting in place a multi-sectoral consultative process.

The consultative process proposed the establishment of an inter-sectoral body, the National AIDS Council (NAC), to be located in the Office of the President. The Office of the President however declined to house the NAC citing inadequate human resources capacity and time constraints. The NAC was eventually established by an Act of Parliament in 1999 as a supra ministerial body managed by a board which is responsible to the Minister of Health and Child Welfare.

Most of the development partners, UNAIDS and civil society groups have over the years accused the government of Zimbabwe and blaming it for not doing enough to prevent and control the spread of HIV/AIDS in the country. The major weakness identified was that for a very long time HIV/AIDS activities had been left solely to an underfunded and under staffed MOHCW to coordinate. However, in 1995 Zimbabwe became one of the first few countries to apply for and be granted a World Bank loan (US$ 60 million) to implement HIV/AIDS/STI prevention and control activities. The framework of implementation of this agreement was the Sexually Transmitted Infections (STI) Project.

Despite the efforts by government, donors and NGOs HIV/AIDS has become a very serious cause of morbidity and mortality in Zimbabwe. Estimates and projections undertaken by the MOHCW in 1998 indicated that by the end of 1997, 12 years after the first case of AIDS was identified in Zimbabwe, there were about 320 000 cases of full blown AIDS.

However, only 70 000 of these had been reported by the MOHCW through its routine health information system. Several reasons contributed to this state of affairs, including incomplete reporting, poor access to health facilities, poor diagnostic capacity, denial of the existence of HIV by the then minister of health and the unwillingness of some health professionals to be open about HIV/AIDS diagnoses.

Zimbabwe established an HIV sentinel surveillance system in 1990 to track the progress of the epidemic. Sentinel surveys were conducted in 1991, 1993, 1994, 1995, 1997 and 2000. The surveillance data were based on HIV prevalence rates in pregnant women attending antenatal care clinics and in some cases patients reporting for STI treatment and/or Tuberculosis (TB). Zimbabwe was one of the first few countries to introduce HIV screening in its Blood Transfusion Services as early as 1985. Data from the Blood Transfusion Services has also been used to track the prevalence and incidence of HIV infection in this select population group over the years.

HIV prevalence rates in women attending ANC have ranged over the years from 7.6% to 20.3 % in 1993 and 18.7% to 32% in 1994/95. In 1994 the estimated national HIV prevalence in adults was 20%. In 1999 this figure had increased to over 25%. The ANC sentinel surveillance conducted in 2000 showed very high HIV prevalence rates of up to 35% compared to 29% in 1997. Typically the HIV prevalence was highest in the 30-34 year age group (43.5% in 2000) and lowest among women of ages between 40-44 years. Prevalence figures among women have generally been taken to suggest that recent infections are high and that young women are more vulnerable to HIV infection than their male counterparts. According to figures from the UNFPA (2003), HIV prevalence amongst adolescents (15-24 years) ranged between 26.40% and 39.61% for females and 9.90% and 14.85% for males.

The DHS (1999) reported that 1% of men and 4% of women either did not know about AIDS or were not aware of it. 17% of women and 7% of men were not able to cite a single way to avoid HIV/AIDS. Between 1994 and 1999 the proportion of people with knowledge about the condom as a means to avoid HIV infection increased from 57% to 66 % in women and from 66% to 76 % in men.

Information available in the mid 2000s indicated that overall, the prevalence of HIV in Zimbabwe was on the decline. According to the DHS (2005-06) adult HIV prevalence was 18%, based on a representative sample. 21% of women were found to be HIV positive compared to 15% for males. HIV prevalence increased with age and peaked at age 24-34 in women and 35-39 in men. However according to Ministry of Health estimates for 2007 the HIV prevalence rate in adults between 15-49 years of age had declined to 15.6%.

According to the Government of Zimbabwe's UNGASS Report on HIV/AIDS covering the period January 2006 to December 2007, the Ministry of Health and Child Welfare reported a steady decline in HIV prevalence among pregnant women (15-49 years) attending antenatal clinics from 25.7% in 2002, 21.3% in 2004 and 17.7% in 2006. Similar trends were observed among "pregnant women (15-24 years) where the prevalence declined from 20.8% in 2002, 17.4% in 2004 to 13.1% in 2006".

Evidence of a decline in HIV prevalence in the general population was supported by the 2007 EPP and Spectrum software, which estimated HIV prevalence in Zimbabwe to have been 26.5% in 2001, declining to 23.2% in 2003, to 19.4% in 2005 and to 15.6% in 2007. Data from several studies gathered by an epidemiological review commissioned by the MOHCW and published in 2005 firmly supported the decline in HIV prevalence. This decline was further supported by data from the ZDHS (2005/06).

Previous cumulative estimates of the number of persons living with HIV indicated that these would increase from 1.56 million in 1997, 1.8 million in 2000 and 2.3 million by year 2005. However later estimates indicated that there were 1 320 793 adults and children living with HIV/AIDS in 2007 in Zimbabwe. This pool of individuals with the potential to suffer from opportunistic infections exerted additional pressure on an already over stretched health delivery system. The case load of AIDS cases saw many children losing their parents and continued to create a huge pool of orphans and child headed families.

1998 projections indicated that the infant mortality rate would, as a result of the HIV/AIDS epidemic, increase to 64 per 1000 live births by the year 2005. The DHS (1999) reported an infant mortality rate which had already reached 65/1000 live births and an under-five mortality rate of 102 per 1000 live births. This figure was already much higher than the projected under five mortality rate of 80 per 1000 predicted for the year 2005, Table 1.5. According to figures from the DHS (2005-06) the overall child mortality rates in Zimbabwe declined during the five year period preceding the DHS, with an IMR of 60 deaths per 1 000 live births and under five mortality of 82 per 1 000 births.

Table 1.5 Projected impact of HIV/AIDS on health indicators in Zimbabwe (1998)

Year	Life Expectancy		Crude Death Rate		Infant Mortality Rate		Child Mortality	
	With AIDS	Without AIDS	With AIDS	Without AIDS	With AIDS	Without AIDS	With AIDS	Without AIDS
1988	39.8	64.9	20.1	6.2	61.8	35.9	123.4	50.5
2010	38.8	69.5	22.5	4.9	53.7	24.0	115.4	31.8

Based on information from: US Census Bureau and MOHCW 1998

The impact of the increase in mortality is being felt most severely in the age group of adults in the prime of their working life and amongst children under the age of five years. This is already having serious consequences on the economy and the social development of the country. The crude death rate had been expected to increase to 23 per 1000 by 2005. Many of the adult deaths were attributed to opportunistic infections, especially tuberculosis whose prevalence rate rose by 550 percent since the first case of HIV infection was reported in 1985. By 1999 the incidence of tuberculosis had reached 543 per 100 000 with up to 70% of TB cases reported to be HIV positive. This situation created a potential for multi-drug resistant tuberculosis which is very difficult and expensive to treat.

Whilst the general global opinion was that political involvement in HIV/AIDS prevention was at the periphery of the political agenda in Zimbabwe, the country eventually declared HIV/AIDS a national disaster in 2001. This move facilitated the country to secure antiretroviral drugs (ARVs) through parallel importation of generic forms of ARVs. An HIV/AIDS Trust Fund was established in 1999 whose main purpose was to finance the national multi-sectoral response to HIV/AIDS. The fund is raised from a compulsory and ear marked health levy collected as a payroll tax. When in 1999 Zimbabwe introduced the AIDS levy the country was probably the first and only country that raised funds for HIV/AIDS prevention and control through direct taxation of its citizens. In its first year of operation the levy collected close to US$ 20 million in revenue. An analysis of information from the Zimbabwe UNGASS Country Report (2006-2007) indicates that the country spent between US$7, 5 and US$11, 0 per capita on HIV/AIDS programs during the same period, from various sources, including the AIDS Trust Fund. Zimbabwe was amongst the first countries to have donated to the "Global AIDS and Health Fund" on the 25th of June 2001, when it contributed US$1,000,000.

Apart from the health delivery system having to cope with the treatment of opportunistic infections and STIs, the advent of Antiretroviral Therapy brought with it hope to many individuals living with HIV. ART has also resulted in a significant increase in the number of individuals voluntarily seeking to be tested for HIV. As these drugs continued to be relatively cheap and affordable the public health sector increasingly had to shoulder the responsibility and obligation to be the major provider of ART. By 2001 the MOHCW was already piloting a program to prevent mother to child transmission (PMTCT) of HIV using Nevirapine at selected health facilities. By the first quarter of 2004 the MOHCW had introduced ARV therapy in the public sector at two central hospitals and some urban clinics as part of the WHO 3 by 5 initiative. Apart from other sources, the government has used a significant portion of funds from the AIDS Trust Fund to support the purchase of ART and by mid 2004 a pharmaceutical company in Zimbabwe had started manufacturing antiretroviral drugs in country. The shortage of foreign currency in the country made it very difficult for resources from the HIV Trust Fund, which is collected in local currency, to be used directly in the purchase of ARTs.

The Government of Zimbabwe however managed to implement strategies and programs that contributed significantly to its efforts to scale up the response to HIV/AIDS in line with the country's National HIV/AIDS Strategic Plan (ZNASP, 2006-2010) which was launched in July 2006. The strategic plan takes the view that the HIV/AIDS problem is an emergency that requires the involvement of all stakeholders in the mobilization of the necessary resources.

One of the major goals of HIV/AIDS programs is to achieve universal access to treatment and care. In 2004 Zimbabwe had an estimated 510 356 adults (age 15-49 years) who required antiretroviral therapy (ART). Whilst in 2007 a total of about 102,566 individuals needed to be commenced on first line therapy, only 86,000 were able to receive the ART through the public sector rollout program which started in 2004. Between 2005 and 2007 the number of persons receiving ART increased from 25 000 adults to a combined total of almost 100 000 adults and children, including patients accessing treatment from the private sector[1].

---

1 Ministry of Health Estimates that 10 000 patients access treatment in the private sector.

Table 1.6: A comparison of regional health and health related indicators (2005)

Indicators 2000	Zimbabwe	Malawi	Kenya	Zambia	R.S.A.	Uganda	Mozambique	Tanzania	Botswana	Namibia
GDP per capita (2005).	2038	667	1240	1023	11110	1454	1242	744	12387	7586
Population/Millions	13.1	13.2	35.6	11.5	47.9	28.9	20.5	38.5	1.8	2.3
Per capita expenditures on health (PPP US$)	139	58	86	63	748	135	42	29	505	407
Public Health Exp. (as % of GDP 2004)	3.5	9.6	1.8	3.4	3.5	2.5	2.7	1.7	4	4.7
Private Health Exp. (as % of GDP 2004)	4.0	3.3	2.3	2.9	5.1	5.1	1.3	2.3	2.4	2.1
IMR/1000 live Births (2000-05)	81	79	79	102	55	79	100	76	87	46
Life Expectancy at Birth.	40.0	45.0	51.0	39.2	50.8	47.8	44	49.7	46.6	51.5
<5 year mortality rate/ 1000 live births	132	125	120	182	68	136	145	122	120	62
% <5 years under weight for age	34	53	36	53	31	45	47	44	29	30
Adjusted Maternal Mortality Rate/100 000 live births *Reported MMR	880 *1100	1100 *980	560 *410	830 *730	400 *150	550 *510	520 *410	950 *580	210 *270	210 *270
% births by skilled health attendants	73	56	42	43	92	39	48	43	94	76
Contraceptive prevalence rate (%)	58	33	39	34	60	60	17	26	48	44
0-12 months BCG immunization (%)	98	97	85	94	97	92	87	91	99	95
0-12 months Measles immunization (%)	85	82	69	84	82	86	77	91	90	73
Physician/100 000 people (2000-04)	16	2	14	12	77	8	3	2	40	30
Adult literacy (%)	89.4	64.1	73.6	68.0	82.4	66.8	38.7	69.4	81.2	85

Sources: UNDP: Human Development Report 2007-2008: www.undp.org/

According to the report, 1,422 health institutions offered Prevention of Mother to Child Transmission (PMTCT) services by the end of 2006. During this period "comprehensive PMTCT services" which consist of "on site HIV testing and counselling and ARV prophylaxis" were being offered in 547 of these facilities with the rest offering a limited package which excluded testing. For this category of facilities testing was done at those facilities that had the capacity to do so on their behalf. By 2007 98% of health facilities in Zimbabwe were offering PMTCT services. More than 98% of women delivering at health facilities received PMTCT services in 2007. The percentage of HIV positive women receiving ART therapy to reduce MTCT of HIV increased from 40% in 2005, 60% in 2006 and 67% by end 2007.[2]

The major challenges confronting the country in this area include those of guaranteeing sustained availability of funding for ART and an adequate human resources base. Such guarantees can only be realized through an environment of sustained economic growth and political stability in the country.

WHO performance assessment of the health sector performance in Zimbabwe (2000)

The World Health Report 2000 ranked the overall performance of Zimbabwe's health system at 155 out of a total of 191 member states of the World Health Organization (WHO), Table 1.7. The WHO performance system assessed the extent to which health systems convert health system resources into outcomes. The outcomes were measured in terms of health status, health system responsiveness and fairness of financial contribution. This performance was measured by what the country actually achieved as a percentage of what it could achieve with the level of resources or inputs available to it. The general opinion amongst critics of the methodology was that the league tables were spurious, misleading, based on crude data and in some cases entirely on opinions. Some of these critics were of the view that the exercise should not have been done at all (Institute for Health Sector Development, 2000).

The poor macroeconomic environment in Zimbabwe contributed significantly to the decline in the quality of care in the public health system. The public expressed their dissatisfaction with the health system through the print media and other forms of expression. They complained about the

---

2 PMTCT Program Annual Report 2007.

poor state and disrepair of rural, district, provincial and central hospitals throughout the country.

Table 1.7: Zimbabwe's health sector WHO performance ranking (2000)

Performance indicator	Indices of Performance	Rank
Overall level of Health DALE (Years)	32.9	184
Distribution of health in the Population [Index of Equality of child survival]	.785	98
Overall level of responsiveness [Index of level of responsiveness]	4.94	122
Distribution of responsiveness In population [Index of distribution of responsiveness]	.792	166-167
Fairness of financial contribution [index of fairness of financial contribution]	.850	175
Overall health system attainment [index of overall health system attainment]	62.3	147
Health expenditure per capita in international dollars	130	110
Performance on level of health	.80	191
Overall health system performance.	.427	155

Based on information in the World Health Report 2000

With the deterioration in health service delivery, the voices of dissatisfaction with the poor attitudes of nurses and doctors towards patients continued to haunt the authorities. There have also been allegations of health workers who lack empathy, who are rude and demonstrate irresponsible behavior which at times borders on outright negligence. Pregnant women seem to bear the brunt of ill treatment.

Conclusion and the way forward

By the year 2000, the state of the health sector and the indicators of health status in Zimbabwe were in contrast to what the once acclaimed health delivery system had achieved in the years following the attainment of the country's independence. At that time the health system boasted of a rapidly expanding health infrastructure, increasing access to quality health care by the majority of people in both rural and urban areas, an increasing number of locally trained health professionals who were adequate to the tasks in both numbers and quality and a very effective community health movement that propelled the country's Primary Health Care strategy to dizzy heights. As a result Zimbabwe's health delivery system was at the time considered to be amongst the best organized and performers in the sub region.

However with the advent of the HIV/AIDS pandemic in combination with opportunistic infections, including tuberculosis, the fragile social, economic and political situation in the country things began to fall apart in all sectors of government. As a result of dwindling internal and external financial resources the country's per capita expenditures on health declined. Whilst some of the indicators of health status have held their ground, there has been a rapid deterioration in all aspects of the quality of health care delivered through public health facilities. Physical access to health care has also been affected by the relocation of populations as a result of the land reform program.

The way forward depends on the achievement of a rapid economic turnaround, the achievement of political stability, stable human resources for health base and the development and implementation of a coherent program of work for the recovery of the health sector to its former glory and beyond.

2

AN OVERVIEW OF HEALTH SECTOR REFORMS IN DEVELOPING COUNTRIES

Introduction

Reform of the health sector has become a universal theme that attracts broad support in both developing and developed countries. Reforms have become a fashion internationally as almost all health systems are under constant pressure to contain costs, raise additional resources, increase efficiency, raise standards and improve equity. It is now very hard for any developing country to oppose implementing some kind of health reforms not only because reform implies positive and purposeful change but also because of new approaches to reforming the health sector.

The question to ask is whether the reforms undertaken to date have had a positive impact on health sector performance or not. This is not an easy question to answer because very few, if any, comprehensive evaluations of Health Sector Reforms (HSR) have been undertaken in Africa. Furthermore it may not be possible to disentangle the effects of one set of policies from those of others, especially where no baseline information is available and given that most countries have used a cocktail of approaches to their reforms. The question as to how and by whom public services should be provided and managed continues to be debated in many countries. Sector adjustment has been advocated to create an enabling environment and an institutional structure that is accountable and focuses on changes to the role of the state and its key institutions. State institutions must be rendered more responsive and less offensive to the public and consumer interests.

One way of viewing health sector reforms is to imagine them as part of overall social transformation and an attempt to respond to challenges posed by several factors which include historical, structural deficiencies in the health sector and changes in political systems.

Governments want to ensure that an appropriate share of public funds is allocated to health and that the benefits of publicly funded health care are equitably distributed. They also want to ensure that resources are used as effectively as possible, both in terms of health gain for the funds invested and minimum cost for the package of services provided. Unfortunately scarce resources often seem to benefit the better off rather than the poorest because of inherently inefficient patterns of resource allocations and poor targeting.

Because public sector services do not often respond to what people want, people will not accept substandard services without questioning them just because they are easily accessible. Poor quality health care has resulted in services that are grossly under-utilized as people are faced with long waiting times, inconvenient clinic hours and inadequate supplies and drugs. Whilst services in the private sector are perceived to be of a better quality patients may however be exposed to the risks of financial exploitation, with little or no safeguards against potentially dangerous health interventions.

Experience shows that *'all successful health care policies are piecemeal and that there is no perfect health care system. The choice should not be between an imperfect integrated system and a perfect market system or between an imperfect market system and a perfect integrated system. Both systems are imperfect.'* (Saltman, R, 1995).

The message is that before a decision is made to embark on reforms it is important to understand the goals of the health system in place and how the current system has performed in achieving these goals and the reciprocal relationships between what existed previously versus what is proposed to come later. Past policies may affect current policies negatively or positively with respect to the implementation of reforms.

Health Reform experiences in East, Central and Southern Africa

Reform tools in developing countries are universal and include some or all of the following combinations:

Civil Service Reforms

In many countries the ineffectiveness of the civil service constrains most development as well as public administration efforts. There is often inadequate capacity to formulate and implement policy, poor revenue collection and poor morale and motivation leading to reduced production across the board. The civil service in Africa has been viewed as being used to reward people for political patronage and guaranteed employment. Botswana, Mauritius, Namibia and South Africa have been classified as having advanced civil service reforms and Kenya, Tanzania and Zambia as committed reformers. Zimbabwe has been classified as being amongst those that are hesitant reformers, (African Development Bank, 2005).

These reforms attempt to improve the performance of the civil service so as to reduce the constraints within which the health sector functions. These reforms aim at reviewing the structure, functions, management practices and processes with the view to improving efficiencies in decision-making and resource utilization. In more cases than not this process has resulted in the retrenchment of civil servants as a cost cutting measure and the introduction of performance management systems within the public sector. The general view is that civil servants have brought the state into disrepute by perpetuating patrimonial bureaucracies which emphasize control and exercise of excessive power. The belief is that the more powerful public officials become the less effective and productive they are, and that they tend to achieve the opposite of what is expected of them. Most of these reforms have revolved around accountability, distortions in resource mobilization and management, the rule of law, incentive systems and the regulatory environment affecting private sector development. These reforms have advocated for downsizing, provision of incentives and improving management and accountability.

New Public Management

This is considered to be a new model of state management based on a shift from "government by control to government by contract". The model is characterized by organizational restructuring such as managerial autonomy of public enterprises and privatization within the sector, purchaser-provider split and decentralization. Government assumes the role of stewardship, oversight and regulation.

Purchaser-Provider Split

This is the creation of separate agencies to purchase and provide services – the former contracting with the latter on the basis of expected outputs and not on the basis of hierarchical relations. The purchaser-provider split is wholly within the public sector. Contracting on the other hand involves not only public-public contracts but also the use of private companies to deliver government services.

Management autonomy

This is as in semi-autonomous hospitals and gives managers the freedom to manage resources and develop implementation strategies without interference. Managers can adapt services to local conditions. However the downside of this arrangement is the potential for fragmentation in implementation and corruption.

Performance linked payment

The performance of civil servants is linked to pay and bonus, though it is very difficult to apply to public health services than to curative services. Public health services with clear outputs such as immunizations, family planning are easier to apply though it is possible that they can be tainted by falsification in reporting.

Reorganization of health systems

Initiatives in this area have centered on policies that aim at increasing the responsibilities and capacity of the lower levels of government such as districts and provinces. Decentralization is based on the notion of government close to the people. Some countries have gone a step further and granted autonomy to facilities such as large tertiary and teaching hospitals.

Experience from some countries in Africa suggests that decentralization faces problems of a lack of appropriate technical expertise to assume the new responsibilities. Powerful interest groups such as civil servants who may not be willing to be employed by local governments often undermine any attempts to decentralize decision making to the districts or local authorities. Ministries of health would like to keep the financial power but decentralize only the delivery of services. Local governments on the other hand have been accused of affording low priority to health issues.

Ndengwa, SN (2002) measured the extent of decentralization in some African countries based on 3 indices; political, administration and fiscal decentralization. The assessment found that South Africa, Uganda and Namibia had high scores on political decentralization with Zimbabwe attaining a very low level of political decentralization. In terms of administrative decentralization, South Africa and Uganda scored highly whilst Zimbabwe, Kenya and Tanzania had moderate scores. The administrative score indicates where the responsibility, for example, for hiring and firing civil servants resides. Fiscal decentralization was measured based on the proportion of public expenditure controlled by localities and arrangements for fiscal transfer from central government to localities. In the SADC region, only South Africa had a very high degree of fiscal decentralization followed by Zimbabwe. Overall South Africa and Uganda had high levels of decentralization, Zimbabwe, Namibia and Tanzania falling in the moderate category and Zambia, Malawi, Mozambique and Angola in the low level.

In Zambia it was demonstrated that policies on decentralization are popular because they provide district managers with greater capacity to manage their own budgets. In Uganda decentralization resulted in improved management, increased construction of Rural Health Centers and a 200% increase in hospital allocations at the expense of preventive services. According to Akin, Hutchinson and Strumpt, (2001), local government spent less on public goods after decentralization than before it, resulting in the under provision of public health services.

In Zambia and Uganda there was an improvement in the salaries and incentives of hospital based staff. However, Uganda experienced a decline in the utilization of Primary Health Care services. There are mixed results from experiences with hospital autonomy. In Kenya, Uganda and Zambia where major teaching hospitals were granted autonomy there was evidence, in some cases, of improved management and technical efficiency. Generally improvements were more in the areas of general management, finance and accounts, monetary control and general maintenance. In Tanzania the experience with hospital autonomy was different and not very encouraging. In all the cases of hospital autonomy equity in access was compromised.

In the majority of the cases local governance structures often lack the ability to collect and manage revenue from local taxes and user fees. This has often led to inter-regional equity suffering as a result of different capacities in various districts to generate their own revenue to run health care services.

Most decentralization activities in the Eastern, Central and Southern African (ECSA) region have been more at the intermediate level of management and largely excluding community involvement initiatives. There has been little focus on re-establishing local structures to support Primary Health Care and public health services.

The major lesson from these experiences is that whilst decentralization itself does not solve problems, local managers are in a better position to respond quickly to local needs. It is also necessary for local management to develop the capacity to respond appropriately to such local demands.

Application of competitive forces

Experience with the application of competitive forces to improve efficiency and consumer responsiveness shows that such management processes are not a panacea to the problems of the public sector. The extent to which policies to regulate the private sector can be introduced in some countries is influenced by the limited development of the private sector itself. The following areas have been explored by some countries in this reform area: subcontracting non-core services of the ministries of health to the private sector, contracting clinical services or diagnostic services to the private sector and the privatization of some ministry departments.

Some of the countries that introduced subcontracting soon realized that they did not have the capacity to assess the market, to design contracts, to regulate the complexities of the private sector and to monitor the opportunistic behavior of contractors. In most cases where non-clinical services have been subcontracted results show that the effectiveness of service delivery has improved. The down side to this is that the costs of delivering the contracted services have increased contrary to expected savings. This is the result of the tradeoff between savings on staff time and the anticipated improvement in the quality of contracted services.

The private medical sector in most African countries is characterized by inconsistencies in the quality of care. Some facilities are not registered, others employ un-registered or unqualified staff and in some cases there are no minimum standards to conform to. The regulatory framework in most of these countries is also very weak and ineffective. As a result of these shortcomings patients are often exposed to risks of clinical malpractice.

An overview of the reform elements that countries in the ECSA region have embarked on (2000) is summarized in Table 2.1.

Experience from other parts of the world shows that:

♦ It is often easier to expand access and develop system infrastructure than to control costs.

♦ Increases in expenditures on health do not necessarily translate into related increases in health outcomes.

♦ Administrative costs are higher in the private and social insurance based systems (compare the Beveridge and Bismarck forms of health delivery systems in Europe).

♦ Whilst publicly financed systems perform better in terms of assuring universal access, there is no systematic quality or efficiency evidence about public versus private provision.

♦ Efficient is not always sufficient. (Saltman, R. 1999).

Health financing options

The broadening of health financing options in developed countries has focused on the introduction of managed competition through contracting within the public sector or between the public and private sectors and by introducing complementary roles of private providers. Very few developing countries have attempted to follow the full path of managed competition. There are several categories of sources of financing health services which include:

♦ Public financing sources
  ♦ General taxation
  ♦ Income from sale of natural resources
  ♦ User fees
  ♦ Grant assistance
  ♦ Borrowing
  ♦ Efficiency gains in use of existing funds
♦ Private financing sources
  ♦ Private insurance
  ♦ Out of pocket expenses
  ♦ Grant assistance
  ♦ Borrowing
  ♦ Charitable contributions

User fees

The most popular financing reform implemented in the ECSA region is that of user fees or charges. Almost every country in the ECSA region has had a go at reforms which involve the introduction of user fees in one form or the other, Table 2.1. This is probably the only reform policy that has been extensively studied and evaluated.

For most countries in Africa, the policy objective in introducing user fees has been to raise revenue to pay for existing health services and improve the quality of care. Some countries, including Zimbabwe, claimed to have introduced user fees in order to improve the efficiency of the referral system. From a health sector point of view user fees have translated into a significant proportion of recurrent expenditures in very few countries. Instead such fees have tended to dissuade the poor more than the rich from using health services. For example, there were reductions in the utilization of health services soon after the introduction of user fees in Kenya, Lesotho, Mozambique, Swaziland, Zambia and Zimbabwe. Comparisons in the utilization of similar services in the private sector showed that the utilization remained steady during the same period despite higher fees. The introduction of user fees in Africa has compromised equity because of the difficulties in targeting and applying exemption policies. The costs of implementing a strict means-testing program in Lesotho and Zimbabwe were in some cases greater than the revenue collected from the fees.

Health insurance

Social Health Insurance (SHI) is a public compulsory health insurance scheme which covers a designated population whose contributions to the scheme are linked to a payroll system. Health care benefits are provided through own, public or private providers of health services. The scheme is established through some legal framework and is usually managed by a quasi-governmental organization which is autonomous from government. Only contributors to the scheme have a right to access specific health care benefits. The principle behind the scheme is that of social solidarity with high levels of cross subsidization across the system between the rich and the poor, low risk and high risk people and individuals and families. The scheme is required to maintain its own financial solvency.

Very few countries in the region have progressed beyond stating their intentions to introduce a social health insurance scheme. In 2001 Mozambique, Zambia, Tanzania, South Africa and Zimbabwe had developed proposals to introduce compulsory insurance schemes. Malawi expressed its intentions to consider the introduction of social health insurance in its 4th National Health Plan (1999-2004). Amongst the countries in this region of Africa, Kenya is on record as having introduced a compulsory insurance scheme as far back as 1966.

Voluntary health insurance is any health insurance that is paid for by voluntary contributions. Most private health insurance schemes are voluntary and benefits can be accessed from both private and public facilities.

In the majority of countries that have had a well established and substantial private medical sector (South Africa, Zimbabwe and Namibia) there are viable private health insurance schemes. In countries where the private medical sector has recently been establishing itself, Tanzania, Zambia, Mozambique and Uganda, employer based insurance schemes have recently been established.

Very few African countries have introduced legislation to regulate private insurance in order to deal with risk avoidance. Such regulation is necessary to ensure that because of increasing demands on medical services from patients with HIV/AIDS, these patients are not discriminated against by third party payers. Where insurance schemes are in operation most of them receive indirect subsidies from government through tax-deductible and tax-free benefits for employees, employers and providers of care. Such subsidies compromise equity in the allocation of public resources.

When health insurance schemes are in operation and user fees are an established phenomenon in the public sector, government facilities stand to benefit significantly from this source of revenue. The willingness to pay for insurance is however likely to be compromised in those countries where publicly provided health services continue to be provided 'free' at the point of delivery.

The major limiting factor in the introduction of health insurance in most African countries is the absence of an adequate population of people in formal employment that is necessary to support the number of active insurers in the market. Available evidence suggests that the expansion of health insurance beyond the formal sector of the economy may not be immediately feasible in most countries in Sub-Saharan Africa. This is in the main a result of increasing poverty in these countries.

Experiences with community based health insurance (CBHI) schemes can be found in the Democratic Republic of Congo, Zambia, Kenya, Tanzania and countries in Francophone West Africa. Such schemes are yet to be fully evaluated in the ECSA region. These are not for profit prepayment plans for health care which are controlled by the community and have voluntary membership. The membership is based on community membership and members generally share a set of common values. Experience shows that such schemes are usually not sustainable mainly because of their small size and that they do not always reach the very poor.

Core health service packages

The prioritization of health interventions has involved, amongst other options, the adoption of essential packages of health services. The package is considered to be a form of explicit health care rationing. The introduction of such a package effectively means that those services which are excluded from the publicly insured or financed package become inaccessible to the poor. In most cases it is not possible to avoid the rationing of health services delivery because of the mismatch between health resources, health needs and demands for health care. By implementing a health package it is possible to focus limited resources to a narrow range of effective interventions as opposed to providing all services.

The objectives of introducing essential health care packages are usually:

+ To improve technical and allocative efficiency in the delivery of health care
+ To ensure universal coverage with health services
+ To provide cost-effective interventions that can control the main causes of the burden of disease within a country.

Table 2.1: Elements of health sector reforms implemented in the ECSA Region

Reform Component	Characteristics of component	Countries implementing the Reform Component in ECSA
Improving performance of the civil service	Reduction in staff numbers. Improved salary packages and performance incentives. Better financial and management systems.	Tanzania, Botswana, Zambia, Zimbabwe, Mozambique, Uganda, Malawi, Swaziland, Namibia and Lesotho.
Decentralization.	Decentralizing responsibilities for management and revenue generation to lower levels of government (e.g. district) and to health facilities (e.g. hospitals)	**Zambia, **South Africa, Botswana, **Zimbabwe, **Uganda, **Tanzania, **Kenya, Namibia, **Malawi, **Mozambique.
Broadening choices for health financing	Introduction of user-fees. (most popular)	Lesotho, Kenya, Tanzania, Namibia, Swaziland, Uganda, Zambia, Zimbabwe, Mozambique, Botswana.
	Health Insurance.	*Kenya, Swaziland, Botswana, Uganda, Lesotho, *Zimbabwe, *Zambia, *Mozambique, *RSA, Namibia, *Tanzania.
	Community Financing Schemes.	Tanzania, Zambia and Kenya (pilot projects)
Introduction of managed competition.	Subcontracting and franchising the private sector and service agreements.	Namibia, Lesotho, Zambia, Zimbabwe, RSA, Mozambique, Tanzania, Malawi and Uganda.
Working with the private sector	Improving terms and regulations to private sector expansion and improved performance	RSA, Zimbabwe, Zambia, Tanzania, Namibia, Lesotho, Malawi, Mozambique
Sector Wide Approach	Improved donor co-ordination and aid management and effectiveness	Uganda, Mozambique, Malawi, Zambia, Tanzânia, Lesotho, Kenya.

* *Compulsory Social Health insurance (proposals).*
** *Experience with hospital autonomy*

The Sector Wide Approach (SWAp)

The objective of developing the SWAp was to improve the management and effectiveness of development aid to low income countries. The adoption of the Millennium Development approach brought with it significant increases in development aid targeted at the health sector in developing countries. As a result of this massive aid flow several problems have arisen, which include, a lack of global policy coherence; unpredictable aid at country level which is characterized by differences between donor pledges and actual disbursements at country level and an increase in vertical funds that are targeted at specific diseases or interventions. The large number of donors contributing to this increase has also brought problems of coordination at country level.

The SWAp approach is a policy and donor coordination framework or mechanism which is country driven and based on a shared vision developed through a comprehensive sector development strategy, agreed priorities, harmonization of financing, management and monitoring and evaluation systems.

Context of health reforms in Zimbabwe

Health reforms in Zimbabwe have been implemented in the context of the country's Economic Structural Adjustment Program (ESAP) which was developed and introduced in 1991. The components of the ESAP where based on the need to develop and implement strategies to reduce the country's budget deficit and also included:

+ Rationalization of the civil service (retrenchments)
+ Trade liberalization (price decontrols and removal of subsidies)
+ Devaluation of the local currency
+ Enforcement or introduction of cost recovery (in the health and education sectors)

At the end of the implementation period of the ESAP most of the expected results had not been achieved and the budget deficit exceeded the targeted 5% of GDP.

In 1987 the GOZ established a Public Service Review Commission to look into the functions of the civil service with the view to restructuring it. This process consisted of an in depth review of structures, functions and management processes in use in the public service. The commission found that the public service was:

+ Bloated and cumbersome
+ Managed by inexperienced officers
+ Characterized by an overlap and duplication of functions resulting in inefficiencies
+ Secretive and with very poor communication with the public
+ Inundated with complicated rules and procedures

In response to the observations and recommendations of the Public Service Review Commission government embarked on civil service reforms which were aimed at addressing the following issues:

+ Recruitment, motivation, personnel procedures and staff development
+ Functions and related administrative structures of the civil service as they affected its efficiency and effectiveness
+ Establishment of personnel information systems
+ Decentralization of operational and administrative functions hitherto carried out by the PSC to line ministries.
+ Decentralization of functions of line ministries from their headquarters to provincial and district offices
+ Introduction of performance management within the civil service

As part of this reform process all government ministries were required to develop mission statements and corporate plans. In 1989 the MOHCW developed its corporate plan, mission statement and a Patient's Charter. All these documents were aimed at creating an environment of accountability within government departments and facilitate the introduction of performance management. The PSC introduced a performance management-training program for the top three management levels within the various ministries of government, including the MOHCW. About 300 officers with managerial responsibilities within the MOHCW received this training. As a direct follow up to this exercise the government attempted to introduce a Performance Appraisal System within the public service. At the time of going to print, the performance appraisal system in government was still not yet fully established.

Regulations and procedures that governed personnel functions within government were reviewed and amended in line with the proposed performance management system. Following a job evaluation undertaken for the civil service the number of grades within the service was reduced from 120 to 18. As part of the civil service reform 23 000 positions were abolished from the public sector, including administrative staff in the MOHCW. Under these reforms the health sector was allowed to retain all professional staff in post though there was a freeze on the recruitment of new professional and clerical staff, even where there were vacancies.

The corporate plan of the MOHCW identified the need to improve financial management, general management and capacity for planning at all levels within the MOHCW. The MOHCW in conjunction with the University of Zimbabwe established a field based training program in public health, the Masters in Public Health (MPH) program. The modules on Planning and Management were used in the training of MOHCW staff in general management and planning skills.

The corporate plan identified several areas that needed attention, namely:

♦ Improving the efficiency and management of health expenditures
♦ Strengthening the link between planning and budgeting
♦ Introducing expenditure monitoring
♦ Decentralizing budget management to the lower levels of the health system
♦ Ensuring that managers have the necessary skills in financial management
♦ Delegating decision-making authority to lower levels
♦ Increasing the capacity to develop plans that focus on priority areas
♦ Several indicators of performance were introduced in order to monitor the performance of the sector through a benchmark system:
  ♦ Indicators of health needs.
  ♦ Indicators of resource availability and equity.
  ♦ Indicators of efficiency.
  ♦ Indicators of effectiveness and quality.

During this period government departments were required to develop and implement reforms which would complement the overall government reform agenda:

♦ Undertaking staff training in performance management
♦ Decentralizing and devolving responsibilities to the operational level
♦ Contracting some of their functions to the private sector
♦ Commercializing some of their departments

♦ Introducing expenditure monitoring and control systems to enhance financial accountability and performance
♦ Involving civil society more directly in the planning and execution of government programs
♦ Implementing communication strategies to disseminate information on the reforms that they were implementing

The initial ESAP phase (1991-1995) was succeeded by a second phase which the government and its local stakeholders called the Zimbabwe Program for Economic and Social Transformation (ZIMPREST). This phase covered the period between 1996 and 2000. ZIMPREST was aimed at consolidating whatever gains had been made in liberalizing the economy and the establishment of macro-economic stability. At the core of ZIMPREST was the restructuring and reorientation of government to achieve economic empowerment, social development to reduce poverty and the development of the private sector. Civil Service Reforms continued to be at the center of ZIMPREST. Whilst the GOZ had anticipated implementing ZIMPREST with financial resources from development partners, the World Bank and the International Monetary Fund (IMF), the anticipated funds never materialized. At the end of the plan period ZIMPREST did not achieve the desired results and the performance of the economy continued to decline resulting in the deterioration of the quality of social services.

In implementing ZIMPREST the Government of Zimbabwe (GOZ) replaced the 5-year National Development Planning strategy with an approach based on the formulation of a long-term national vision (Vision 2020). Sector plans were to be developed and updated on the basis of Medium Term Expenditure Frameworks, three year rolling plans and annual budget cycles.

The MOHCW developed its long-term strategy and vision for the health sector, the National Health Strategy (NHS) which it called "*Working for Quality and Equity in Health*". This National Health Strategy covering the period from 1997 to 2007 replaced and succeeded the MOHCW policy framework, "*Planning for Equity in Health*" which had been developed in the early 1980s to cover the plan period up to the end of the year 2000.

The policy framework, "*Planning for Equity in Health*" had been designed on the basis of the slogan, "Health for All by the Year 2000". Its implementation was based on the Primary Health Care approach. The

National Health Strategy (1997-2007) on the other hand based its approach on reforming the health sector and identifies key performance areas and challenges, namely:

+ Health determinants outside the traditional boundaries of the health sector
+ Declining health expenditures
+ Lack of community involvement and participation in the decision-making process related to health
+ The need to improve health sector management and the reorganization of the sector
+ Increased focus on quality and consumer satisfaction
+ Improvement in the conditions of service for health workers
+ The high prevalence of HIV/AIDS and the increasing burden of disease from other preventable conditions
+ Emerging and re-emerging infections
+ Improved coordination within the health sector

From a technical point of view the strategy identifies ten priority disease conditions to be tackled during the plan period:

+ HIV/AIDS, TB and STIs
+ Acute Respiratory Infections
+ Reproductive Health conditions
+ Cardiovascular conditions
+ Diarrheal diseases, including the prevention and control of cholera
+ Nutritional conditions, including the control of micronutrient deficiencies
+ Injuries
+ Mental disorders

At the time of going to print the health sector had started the consultation process towards the development of a national health strategy to succeed the 1999-2007 national health strategy.

Stages in the development of health reforms

The essential ingredients of health reforms include:
- Political will
- Leadership and capacity to implement the reforms
- Promotion of citizens' rights and participation
- Transformation of the health delivery structure
- Performance, accountability and improved health outcomes
- The redefinition of funding systems and resource allocation
- The changing role of the state

Sanford and Javier Martinez (1995) have outlined what they refer to as the stages in the development of health sector reforms. They describe stages 0 to 6 in this process. Stage zero consists of a situation where there are no plans or intentions by the government to embark on sector reforms. Stage 1 consists of the country undertaking a situation analysis or health sector appraisal with the specific objective of undertaking health reforms. The results of such a diagnostic exercise are to inform the process of health reform. Development partners with the full participation of the Ministry of Health finance such a study. Stage 2 involves the development of a clear plan that guides the implementation of the reforms and elaborates on key issues and intervention areas. At this stage of the process the document is official but has not yet been endorsed at the highest political level. Funds to implement the plan are not yet available.

According to the authors in stage 3 the plan document has received the necessary backing and consensus from politicians and civil society and financial support from development partners is assured. In stages 4 and 5 of the process financial resources for the reform agenda are available and the process of implementation has been agreed to. Responsibilities for the implementation of the various aspects of the reforms have now been assigned and some activities may already be on course. Stage 6 is the final stage which consists of the actual implementation of the program of reform with a committee of senior government officials in place to coordinate the whole process of reform.

No single principle for the goals of health sector reforms will be appropriate for all countries. Reforms must be characterized by locally determined compromises and trade-offs. Individual processes must be synchronized and organized appropriately not only for the reforms to take place but to avoid a chaotic sequence of unrelated events. The crucial characteristics of the reform process are the timing, consideration between short-term versus long-term strategies and the scale - pilot models versus full-scale countrywide implementation.

Economic, political circumstances and leadership are the most powerful forces in providing the impetus for a reform movement, the adoption of an agenda and the implementation of change. An armed struggle and the advent of democracy may lead to a need to develop new national health policies for the first time as a component of wider programs of economic and social reconstruction in all sectors. This was the case in Mozambique, South Africa and Zimbabwe. It is likely that a similar situation will arise in Angola. In other cases, changes in government have provided an opportunity for the introduction of radical reforms as was the case in Zambia.

Conclusion and the way forward

Whilst it is generally agreed that the principles underlying health reforms are well founded, there are however specific health sector reform strategies such as new approaches to health care financing, privatization and other familiar themes which do not benefit from the same unanimity of support. Unwanted or differing outcomes from health reforms result from differences in focus, the pace, sequence and entry points to such reform changes. Radical reforms have the potential to further penalize the poor and threaten political stability. One of the major conceptual problems with the design of health reforms is that in most cases the slogans of change are defined not by stating positive gains in the future but rather what should be thrown overboard.

Each country must develop its own individual set of values, vision and instruments to drive the reform process in order to achieve adequate access to quality care for its people, especially the most vulnerable groups. At the same time it is crucial that countries share intelligence on health care reforms, provide information and together analyze major issues on reforms. The idea of partners in health and a network for health reform is extremely appealing.

A mere transfer of responsibility to private financing sources exacerbates inequities and in itself will do nothing to improve performance in the public sector. Whilst African countries lack the capacity to regulate the complex private sector, this is compounded by the lack of essential elements of functioning governments, in some cases poor maintenance of the rule of law, the inability to levy and collect tax and the inability to administer the basic functions of government.

In most African countries the willingness to engage in serious structural reforms is often linked to conditions established by donors or lending agencies that link future aid disbursement to sector reforms being taken on board.

It is important that as the reform agenda progresses future events are based on conclusive evidence about earlier reforms. There must be a benchmark system developed to monitor and evaluate the process and outcome of such reforms. The extent to which extraneous factors influence the reforms must also be evaluated so as to accurately determine the extent of bias in interpreting the impact of reforms.

The shortage of resources and poorly functioning health systems will continue to be a major driving force for reform in Zimbabwe, and indeed in Africa. It is also unlikely that because of this lack of resources there will be a retreat from the principles of universality and comprehensiveness within the health sector in African countries.

It has been said that, *"More countries are dealing with health care reforms as if each was on Mars. Few have tried to learn from others… Instead of each country trying out its own experiments, they should be studying each other for ideas and pitfalls."* (Saltman, R, 1995).

Even though the impact of health sector reforms in most developing countries has not been fully evaluated, evidence points to mixed results.

The importance of political leadership to the success of reform initiatives and the understanding of issues cannot be over emphasized. It is necessary and an advantage to have politically supported and publicly debated reform strategies. Policy makers must appreciate that no single principle for the goals of reform will be appropriate for all countries. The success of reforms depends on the constraints facing the government, policy instruments available and the macroeconomic environment within which they can operate.

Review questions

1. Discuss some of the reasons why African countries embark on health reforms.
2. Market oriented reforms have the potential to restrict access to public health services by the poor. Discuss the logic of this statement.
3. Discuss the advantages and disadvantages of the following approaches to health reforms:
   + Big bang reforms
   + Incremental reforms
   + Pilot versus countrywide implementation of health reforms
4. Discuss the context, objectives and recommendations of Civil Service Reforms in a country of your own choice.
5. What do you understand by the term Economic Structural Adjustment Program (ESAP)?

3

ORGANIZATIONAL RESTRUCTURING

Introduction

One of the objectives of health reforms is to strengthen policy and planning functions, the setting of standards for health care provision and the development of appropriate systems for monitoring and evaluating performance. Many countries have restructured their ministries of health by making them smaller, leaner and less hierarchical. Others have separated the functions of service provision from those of purchasing services by introducing service contracting, autonomous hospitals, joint ventures and setting up management boards. In some cases central ministries have opted to reorient their functions by emphasizing management, financing and planning of human resources development as opposed to direct service provision. Decentralization is probably the most common structural reform strategy that has been implemented by ministries of health in Africa.

The health policy framework of the government of Zimbabwe, *Planning for Equity in Health,* was based on the economic policy framework of the early 1980s, *Growth with Equity.* Primary Health Care (PHC), which calls for communities to accept responsibility for their own health and aims to address broad issues of distributive justice, was chosen as the appropriate strategy to deliver health services in Zimbabwe. In the context of PHC the role of government was seen as that of creating an enabling environment for the provision of a comprehensive package of promotive, preventive, curative and rehabilitation services.

The Ministry of Health and Child Welfare (MOHCW) has since the early 1990s embarked on a health reform program in the context of Civil Service Reforms and the implementation of the Economic Structural

Adjustment Program (ESAP). To create the necessary conditions for the pursuit of its reform agenda the MOHCW formulated its National Health Strategy (NHS) 1997-2007; '*Working for Quality and Equity in Health*'. This strategy succeeded the post independence policy framework, "*Planning for Equity in Health*". The content, context and pace of the ministry's health reform agenda was also influenced by the Recommendations of the Presidential Review Commission on Health which were adopted by government in 1999.

The process of restructuring the ministry of health in Zimbabwe started with the policies developed by the government soon after independence in 1980. There was a need for the MOH to respond to the needs of the most vulnerable groups in society, especially those living in rural areas. The measures adopted resulted in a health system which was organized at four levels, each level delivering an appropriate mix of promotive, preventive and curative services. The higher levels of the system provide support, supervision and referral services to the levels below them. Each level of the health system developed horizontal links with corresponding structures in the political system so as to ensure political, community and inter-sectoral collaboration with other health related agencies.

Over the years the organization has evolved on the basis that the MOH must have the ability to fulfill its responsibilities to execute strategic and operational functions. However, with a shift towards devolution an appropriate structure needed to be designed to enable each level to play its own distinctive role within a devolved health system. The challenge for the MOH was that of developing a structure which would facilitate rather than impede coordination cross activities as well as across the different levels of the organization. With the proposed introduction of performance management within the public sector it was also necessary for the MOH to evolve beyond its bureaucratic structure, function and orientation. Any emerging structure needed to accommodate as well as reign in on the domineering culture of the medical profession established within the health system.

Any reorganization of the ministry of health had to be supported by evidence derived from a functional review process. A functional review is necessary to establish the state of existing organizational functions and relate these to the existing organizational structure. Such an analysis should identify any shortcomings in the current structure that justify proposals for organizational change. Furthermore, the analysis should also identify where the responsibilities for the core functions of the ministry lie within the organization, and indicate areas of overlap, duplication or omission where they exist. At the end of it all the functional review must place the organization in a context of both the present and the future environment. The organization must have a well-defined leadership level, middle level management, an operational level and an environment where intellectual management and activities can function effectively. Organizational tasks must match the core functions of the MOH and personnel specifications must also be based on the skills that match the requirements of the organization.

Figure 3.1 Functional linkages within the MOHCW (2000)

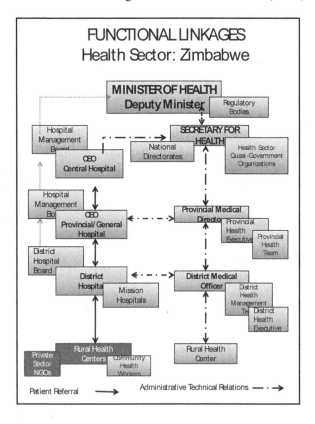

In conducting an organizational analysis it is crucial, amongst other things, to review some of the following issues, DFID (2003):

+ Current structure of the organization.
+ Consistency of the structure with organizational purpose and its operating environment.
+ Definition of the roles and responsibilities of individuals and their job descriptions.
+ The allocation of key functions/processes within the organization.
+ Lines of management accountability and systems for vertical communication within the organization.
+ Overlap or duplication between departments/units within the organization as well as the systems for horizontal communication.
+ Frequency of organizational restructuring, the rationale and process used for organizational review.
+ Reaction of people in the organization to any new structure.
+ The number of management levels in the organization.
+ The average span of control at each level.
+ Centralized or decentralized processes, decision making structures and their appropriateness to the organization's purpose.

Re-organization of the Ministry of Health in Zimbabwe

Functions of the Ministry of Health

In terms of the restricted government document; "Handbook on the Functions of the Minister of Health and Child Welfare" of March 1993, the following are the functions of the Ministry of Health and Child Welfare:

1. *Service Functions:*
   + Preventive Services
   + Curative Services
   + Health and Management Information Systems
   + Laboratory services
   + The supply of safe blood
2. *Training Functions*
3. *Regulatory Functions*
4. *Obligations to International health*

In terms of the Public Health Act (Chapter 15:09) and the Health Service Act, the functions of the Ministry of Health and Child Welfare can be summarized as follows:

Headquarters
+ To provide leadership for the sector
+ To coordinate the development and enforcement of health policy, national *s*tandards, norms and guidelines
+ To undertake strategic planning for the sector
+ To monitor disease trends, quality of care and health status of the nation
+ To consolidate budget estimates, undertake budget analysis, mobilize and allocate resources for the sector and institute expenditure controls.
+ To plan for human resources requirements, management and development
+ To regulate the operations of both private and public health sectors.
+ To commission research and ensure effective interagency coordination
+ To liaise with international health organizations and development partners.

Operational level
+ To implement government health policies and programs
+ To undertake operational planning and budgeting
+ To deliver the agreed package of health services
+ To provide support and supervision
+ To manage health resources effectively and efficiently
+ To monitor and evaluate service and program delivery
+ To undertake biomedical and operational research

The organizational structure of the MOH must reflect its values and facilitate the attainment of its vision and mission. It must reflect the strategic role of the central level and the decentralized operational functions of the district level. The central MOH has the responsibility to ensure that all levels of the organization have a clear definition, division and coordination of responsibilities and functions:
+ General administration
+ Financial management, including internal audit duties

- Health policy, norms, standards development and quality assurance
- Preventive programs
- Curative services
- Support systems
- Resource mobilization and allocation
  - Health financing
- Health planning and coordination
  - Programs and services
  - Human resources
  - Essential supplies
  - Infrastructure
  - Equipment
- Organizational performance
  - Health Information Systems and Surveillance
  - Monitoring & Evaluation
- Research and analysis
- International relations

In fulfilling these functions and responsibilities the central MOH must adopt a strategic and leadership role and leave health facilities, provincial and district offices to play an implementation role. The structure must demonstrate an effective division of labor within the organization through the establishment of appropriate divisions, departments and/or units. The most obvious variants for a ministry of health include divisions responsible for:

- **General Administration**
- **Financing and financial management** – ensuring that adequate financial resources are available by predicting anticipated operational costs, determining requirements for capital expenses, predicting how much and when cash is required over given periods.
- **Technical Programs** – e.g. Preventive and Curative Services in terms of development of policies, content, norms and standards at the strategic level and service delivery at the operational level. Technical programs are based on the core functions and priorities of the MOH.
- **Support systems**
  - *Laboratory services* – clinical and public health
  - *Planning & Budgeting* – strategic and operational planning and

budgeting. The MOH should have the capacity to define its objectives, what to do to meet the objectives, to determine how long it will take and how much it will cost. At the central level this many include *policy reforms, donor coordination, legislation* and *systems development*.

+ *Pharmaceuticals and supplies logistics* – policy, quantification, procurement and distribution.

+ *Human resources* – the most valuable resource in any organization is its human resources. There must be capacity to develop appropriate policies, to plan and project human resources needs, and the ability to nurture staff performance, to train staff, to develop systems for assessing and rewarding staff in order to retain and motivate them.

+ *Infrastructure and technology assessment* – to reflect responsibilities and capacity for policy development, planning, development, procurement and maintenance in this area.

+ *Monitoring and Evaluation* – determining how the organization will know if it is meeting its objectives, operating a health management information system, and supervision and support systems.

+ *Research* – gathering evidence for policy formulation and decision making

The organizational structure of the MOH in Zimbabwe has undergone several transformations since the country's independence. Suffice it to say that all the phases of restructuring, except the one soon after independence, were not backed by any functional review of the MOH. At independence the structure of the MOH was district based and supported by a Regional Health Authority structure. This structure was however reorganized soon after independence in line with the policy to adopt and implement the Primary Health Care strategy.

The Provincial Medical Director (PMD) replaced the Provincial Medical Officer of Health (PMOH) as head of provincial health services. The PMD was underpinned by two Medical Officers of Health, one responsible for Epidemiology and Disease Control and the other for Maternal and Child Health Services.

In 1985, the MOH organized a meeting on strengthening district health systems in Zimbabwe which took place at Juliasdale in Nyanga. The meeting adopted a district health organizational structure and agreed on the roles and responsibilities of the district health management teams (DHMTs). The management structures for the district health system were established and roles clearly defined. The roles and responsibilities of the core members of the District Health Executive, the District Hospital

Executive and the District Health Management Teams (DHMT) were outlined. The District Hospital Secretary post was the responsibility of the district hospital pharmacist, who was later replaced by a Health Services Administrator.

In the early 1990s there was reorganization at the MOH headquarters which established the post of Principal Medical Director: Health Care Services which was responsible for the coordination of medical/clinical services and disease prevention programs. The Principal Medical Director was a medical doctor who reported directly to the office of the Secretary for Health. PMDs and Medical Superintendents of Central Hospitals reported to the Principal Medical Director.

The Deputy Secretary: Finance, Administration and Planning and the Deputy Secretary: Health Support Services also reported directly to the Secretary for Health. The Deputy Secretary (Health Support Services) was responsible for coordinating technical support services which included diagnostic laboratories, environmental health services, radiological services and health related research institutions. This phase of the restructuring process did not involve restructuring at the operational level of the health system. The main objective was to strengthen program leadership in the technical areas of clinical and preventive services, infrastructure and investment planning by elevating the posts higher in hierarchy of the MOHCW.

Another significant phase in the reorganization of the MOH occurred in 1993 when the Ministry of Health was assigned additional responsibilities for coordinating child welfare functions. These responsibilities required the MOH to coordinate the multi sectoral National Program of Action for Children (NPA). This was in line with the 1990 World Summit for Children during which it was agreed that countries would put in place mechanisms and develop National Plans of Action to achieve the goals and objectives of the World Declaration on the Survival, Protection and Development of Children. With these additional responsibilities the MOH became the Ministry of Health and Child Welfare (MOHCW) and established a unit responsible for coordinating child welfare functions. This unit also provided secretariat services to the multi sectoral forum on the National Program of Action for Children.

At the time there was a realization in government that people appointed to the positions of Finance and Administration did not always have the necessary qualifications, capacity and skills to effectively manage government finances. It was also felt that the combination of general administration, financial management and planning functions overstretched the capacity of the post.

A decision was made to "professionalize" financial management responsibilities in all government ministries. As a result the posts of Deputy Secretary: Finance and that of Deputy Secretary: Administration, Policy and Planning were established in the MOHCW. The MOHCW incorporated the function of coordinating its reform agenda, policy development and analysis into the office of the Deputy Secretary: Administration, Policy and Planning. The post of Deputy Secretary: Health Support Services was abolished and its responsibilities taken over by the office of the Principal Medical Director: Health Care Services. Because of the additional responsibilities the span of authority for the Principal Medical Director became over extended. A decision was made to the effect that the PMDs and Medical Superintendents of Central Hospitals would report directly to the office of the Secretary for Health and Child Welfare.

Yet another reorganization of the MOHCW was undertaken in 2000 in line with the recommendations of the Review Commission on Health. The reorganization included:

♦ Revival of the Community Health Movement through the establishment of a central level post to coordinate community participation

♦ Establishment of a quality assurance framework within the sector; a Quality Assurance unit was established

♦ Strengthening collaboration between the public and private sectors by proposing the establishment of a National Health Coordinating Council within the MOHCW.

♦ Establishment of Hospital Management Boards as part of changes to the management structures of Central and Provincial Hospitals and their transformation into semi-autonomous central and provincial hospitals

♦ De-linkage of the health sector from the Public Service Commission (PSC) and the establishment of a Health Services Board.

In line with government's decentralization policy, the MOHCW was to reorganize itself such that the central level relinquished the direct provision of health services and to focus more on strategic and leadership functions such as; policy development and analysis, health regulation, strategic planning, human resources planning and development, resource mobilization, management and allocation, high level coordination and technical support to the operational level. It was necessary for the MO-HCW to organize itself based on its core functions as opposed to being structured on professional lines of authority. During this reorganization the two Deputy Secretary posts and that of the Principal Medical Director post were abolished. The main objective was to "de-medicalize" senior posts in the MOHCW so as to facilitate entry of other professionals into top management and leadership posts in the sector.

The Review Commission on Health made a recommendation to abolish the post of Director of Nursing Services on the basis that nursing was a profession and not a core function of the MOHCW. After lengthy discussions with the Public Service Commission it was resolved that the post of Chief Nursing Officer would continue as part of the structure of the MOHCW in spite of the recommendations of the Review Commission on Health. According to the MOHCW the post of Chief Nursing Officer was essential to the development of nurse leadership, participation in health policy formulation, the delivery of high quality nursing care, the development of policies on nursing personnel and the redefinition and adaptation of nursing practice in the country. The proposed abolition of this post had escalated the tense relations that already existed between the MOHCW and the national association of nurses. It was also a fact that all the other countries in the region, and elsewhere, had posts of Chief Nursing Officers.

Reports from the Public Accounts Committee continued to indicate that government finances in many ministries were in shambles. As a result, yet another decision was made to upgrade the post of Deputy Secretary: Finance to that of Director of Finance. This was meant to attract professionals qualified in accountancy and financial management to these posts. The elevated posts of Director: Technical Support and Director: Policy and Planning were also established. This was to move away from common service posts of "Deputy Secretary" and to create health sector specific posts. The Director for Policy and Planning was charged with the responsibility to coordinate the planning process and to ensure that the operational level adhered to the planning cycle. This directorate was also responsible for coordinating the reform agenda, health legislation, donors, human resources planning and development, hospital planning and projects development.

After the dissolution of the National AIDS Coordination Program (NACP) the MOHCW integrated the HIV/AIDS/STI programs and established an HIV/AIDS/TB/STI unit. The MOHCW was responsible for implementing the biomedical (health) response to HIV/AIDS as part of the national multi-sectoral response. The post of HIV/AIDS/STI officer was established as a supernumerary post financed by the World Health Organization.

The implementation of the recommendations of the Review Commission on Health facilitated the transition of central and provincial hospitals into semi-autonomous institutions to be managed by Hospital Management Boards. The transformation started in earnest in 2006 with the establishment of Hospital Management Boards of central hospitals which were accountable to the Minister of Health and Child Welfare as opposed to reporting to bureaucrats at the MOHCW headquarters.

The commercialization of the Government Medical Stores (GMS) into a "not-for-profit" private company (Natpharm) meant that the MOHCW was no longer responsible for the procurement and distribution of drugs, surgical and medical supplies. These were now the responsibilities of the new company, Natpharm, a statutory body headed by a Chief Executive Officer (CEO) who is responsible to a Management Board. The MOHCW however continued to be responsible for the development and oversight of pharmaceutical policies and the quantification of public sector requirements for pharmaceuticals, surgical and medical supplies.

The head of Internal Audit in the MOHCW no longer reported to the Director of Finance but directly to the Secretary for Health. This move was to remove the conflict of interest that arose from an audit department being housed in a department of finance.

It was also proposed that clinical diagnostic services at central hospitals either continue to be part of the hospital departments or individual hospitals opt to purchase diagnostic laboratory services from the private sector. In the event that this happened, the MOHCW would continue to oversee the operations of the two National Reference Laboratories, namely; the National Microbiology Reference Laboratory located at Harare Central hospital and the National Tuberculosis Reference Laboratory located at Mpilo Central hospital in Bulawayo. It was proposed that the Blair Research Institute, (now the National Institute of Health Research) and the Government Analyst Laboratory would be considered for semi-autonomous status at an appropriate time in the future.

In 2005 the MOHCW embarked on yet another restructuring exercise which was approved for implementation in July 2007. This exercise consolidated and built on the reorganization process undertaken in 2000 which was based on the recommendations of the Review Commission on

Health. The approved structure took into consideration the new system of grading posts within the public sector. The exercise was a combination of the establishment of new posts and the re-establishment of posts that had been abolished in previous restructuring processes:

♦ Re-establishment of the post of Director of Finance and Administration, replacing the post of Director of Finance.

♦ Re-establishment of the posts of Director of Curative Services, previously Medical or Clinical Services.

♦ Directorate of Preventive Services (re-introduced).

♦ Director of Laboratory Services (re-established).

♦ Director of Traditional Medicine, new and reflecting a major policy shift on Traditional Medicine.

♦ Deputy Director of Nutrition Services (re-established)

♦ Director of Nursing Services, reverting to its previous name.

As expected in any process of change, all the restructuring exercises that have taken place in the health sector over the years have been embroiled in criticism, mainly on the grounds that they were neither transparent nor participative enough. There were concerns that the reformed structures did not adequately address all the priority functions of the public health sector. The main point of argument was that not all health professional categories were represented at unit or departmental level. To some this meant that there needed to be departments or units established on the basis of professional categories as well as managerial posts based on professional groupings. This is understandable for a technical organization like a MOHCW where professionals are concerned about the prospects of their career paths. This is more so in an organization that is dominated by the medical profession. As an example, the reorganization process in 2000 abolished the posts of Director of Pharmacy and the Director of Nutrition services. Despite the fact that these functions continued to be provided for within the organization there were concerns that the MOHCW had abandoned its responsibilities in these areas. The fact of the matter is that organizational restructuring is a dynamic process which is meant to ensure that the organization functions effectively and achieves its goals and objectives during all the stages of its evolution over time.

The generally slow progress in the implementation of the restructuring process has been attributed to the negative attitudes of some managers, especially those managing vertical programs. Staffs who work in project financed programs usually feel threatened by the potential of losing their privileged positions and benefits which arise from project financing. With restructuring such positions are usually abolished and/or absorbed into the public service establishment, without the special and privileged conditions.

The Provincial Medical Directors (PMD)

The Provincial Medical Director's office is responsible for coordinating the delivery of health services at the provincial level and provides technical supervision and support to the district health teams. The provincial hospital, proposed for semi-autonomy under the reforms, provides the first level of specialist referral support to the district level. The PMD is the accounting officer at this level.

The office of the PMD is responsible for:
+ Technical and logistic support to the district health teams
+ Ensuring the development of provincial plans and adherence to the planning cycle, national guidelines and policies
+ Monitoring the performance of the health delivery system and programs
+ Facilitating the development of budget estimates, equitable resource allocation, expenditure controls and revenue collection
+ Monitoring the distribution and availability of pharmaceuticals, health manpower and other resources

District Health Services

The District Medical Officer is in charge of the District Health Team (DHT) and the District Health Executive (DHE) which coordinate the operations of the health delivery system at this level. In terms of the reforms, the MOHCW is yet to implement its decision to move from a position where the head of district health services has always been a medical officer (the DMO) to that of accommodating other health professionals in this position. Professional jealousies amongst members of the District Health Management Team have delayed implementation of this reform. For example, the District Environmental Health Officer (DEHO) was prepared to go along with the idea of a District Health Director as long as it was the DEHO in charge but not any other health professional. The same applied to the District Nursing Officer (DNO) who was only agreeable if it was the DNO and not the DEHO or other health professionals occupying the post. However, all the professionals in the team seemed to rally around the medical doctor being the team leader, albeit, for the time being.

The major role of the district hospital is to provide referral medical support to Rural Health Centers (RHCs), clinics, mission institutions and the private for profit sector within the district. The DHMT provides technical support in program development and implementation to the lower levels of the health system within the district.

This district level is thus responsible for:

+ Coordinating and supervising the delivery of local health services and programs by the private, public and NGO sectors
+ Promoting and facilitating community participation in local health service planning, implementation and monitoring
+ Preparation of annual health plans, the preparation, management and control of local budgets
+ Collection, consolidation, analysis and local use of health information
+ Human resources management and development
+ Coordinating the training and supervision of community health workers

The health planning process

The overall planning process

The government financial year covers the period beginning on the 1st of January to the 31st of December. The planning framework for the health sector is guided by the health policy framework and the national health strategic plan which is implemented through successive annual rolling plans. The planning process in the MOHCW is both a top down and bottom up process:

+ The central level coordinates a consultative process to develop a national health strategic plan, usually covering a 5-10 year period. The strategic plan is implemented within the MTEF through successive annual rolling plans.
+ The prioritization of sector activities is based on the core health service package.
+ The central level develops and disseminates national planning, budgeting and program guidelines and a sector planning schedule which is based on the overall government planning cycle. This planning cycle synchronizes the bottom up planning process from district to provincial level with national level deadlines so as to give the national health level enough time to consolidate the

national plan and budget estimates in time for consideration as part of the national budget.

♦ Based on the planning guidelines, health centers, clinics and hospitals develop plans and budgets which are consolidated with those from the district office for onwards transmission to the provincial level where all district plans are consolidated into a provincial plan.

♦ Provincial plans are consolidated at the national level into a national sectoral annual plan and budget estimate. Ideally, activities and budgets for all health sector stakeholders (public and not-for-profit sector) are captured during this planning process.

♦ An annual consultative planning forum, the MODO, takes place between the Ministry of Health, donors, mission institutions, bilateral and multilateral organizations and other service providers to discuss progress in the implementation of the annual plan, priorities for the next plan period, and levels of financing from different sources. Donors are expected to provide information on indicative estimates of financial support to the sector in the coming plan period.

♦ All levels of the health system undertake monitoring through compiling and submitting progress reports on a quarterly and annual basis.

Every effort is made to plan within available resources from the government, NGOs, the private sector and development partners, where possible. This is meant to ensure that the planning exercise is based on realistic resource assumptions and that it is not a mere shopping list. District Health Management Teams (DHMTs) coordinate the planning process at the district level and submit their plans to the Provincial Medical Director who reviews, approves and consolidates them for consideration by the Provincial Development Committee. The PMD then submits the consolidated provincial plan to the MOHCW headquarters.

The monitoring process and budget controls are achieved through the compilation of monthly, quarterly and annual reports. Quarterly meetings of Ward Health Committees, the District Health Teams (DHTs), the Provincial Health Team (PHT) and national level biannual meetings between the MOHCW and development partners are convened to discuss the planning process and progress in the implementation of programs and services. The national biannual meetings also discuss health sector priorities and potential financial support for the next plan period.

Role of the health center level

All health centers within the district, including mission and NGO institutions, are provided with national guidelines to guide their planning process. Based on the district allocation, the DHMT provides budget estimates or ceilings within which each health center proposes its activities. At this level the process entails costing activities that are relevant to the health center core health package based on local program inputs such as; essential drugs and supplies, cold chain equipment and supplies, stationary, patient rations, purchase of minor equipment, minor maintenance of infrastructure, utility bills, supplies for village health workers and home based care programs, travel expenses and allowances, etc. Information gathered during this process from each health center is consolidated together with that from the district office and the district hospital into a district health plan.

Communities are involved at this level through their participation in Ward or Village Health Committee meetings which are attended by Rural Health Center and Clinic staff, village health workers, other community development workers, village elders, traditional healers, traditional midwives and local councilors. The monitoring and evaluation process takes place through supervision of community activities and regular meetings of local health committees. Health center staffs discuss health information collected by community health workers which is compiled as part of health centre information.

Role of the district level

District Health Management teams (DHMTs) conduct their first planning meetings between May and June and the second meetings between July and August in preparation for the next plan period. In the event of full devolution it is expected that the responsibility for coordinating district planning will rest with an appropriate committee of the Rural District Council (RDC). It is expected that the DHMT will continue to coordinate the planning process for the health department within RDC structures. The DHMTs interpret and disseminate the planning guidelines to the rest of the providers of health services within the district and coordinate the planning process through meetings of the District Health Team which consists of all health stakeholders within the district.

The DHMT consolidates the plans and budgets of the district office, all hospitals, health centers and clinics into a district plan. The provincial level ensures that the district plan is prepared in accordance with the decisions of the national planning forum and that it is within the budget ceiling. The district health plan must be presented to the district health committee or appropriate body within the RDC for final consideration and "approval" by the District Development Committee (DDC). After the plan has been finalized and approved by the DDC, the DHMT provides feedback the rest of the district team. The plan and budget are then submitted to the PMD with each member of the District Health Team retaining a copy of the plan. Monitoring is based on agreed indicators and targets, quarterly progress reports, supervision visits and the conduct of quarterly DHT meetings. Regular reports are submitted to the PMD who convenes quarterly Provincial Health Team meetings where the provincial progress report is discussed, finalized and then submitted to the head quarters of the MOHCW. An issue that remains unresolved is the role of the PMD with respect to that of the RDCs in the finalization and approval of the district health plans. Is the district health plan approved by the PMD and then submitted to the RDC? Is the plan approved by the RDC and then forwarded to the PMD for final submission to the MOHCW for consolidation into the health sector plan? It would appear however that a definitive decision can only be arrived at when the full extent and implications of the decentralization process are fully known.

Role of the provincial level

According to the planning timetable, the development of provincial plans must take place during the period of July to September. Common sense dictates that this process can only be completed after the districts have submitted their plans and budgets. It is generally expected that provincial plans are completed three months before the beginning of the next financial year (the 1st of January of each plan period). As earlier indicated, the PMD disseminates national planning and budgeting guidelines, agreed national priorities for the next plan period and budget ceilings (if available from treasury on time) to the districts. The provincial team provides technical oversight to the District Health Executive in their planning process.

The province convenes the Provincial Health Team (PHT) meeting where progress in the previous plan period is discussed; district plans are presented, discussed and consolidated into a provincial plan and budget. Program managers at the provincial level, provincial and general hospitals develop their plans which are an integral part of the overall provincial plan. Individual district plans are examined in terms of content, justification and compliance with the guidelines and budget estimates. The finalized (consolidated) provincial plan is presented by the PMD to the Provincial

Health and Social Services subcommittee of the Provincial Development Committee (PDC). Should the plan be approved, the PMD submits it to the MOHCW headquarters. At the end of each quarter the PMD convenes a PHT meeting where progress in the implementation of the various district plans and the overall provincial plan are discussed and a progress report submitted to the MOHCW headquarters.

Role of the MOHCW headquarters

The MOHCW has the responsibility to coordinate the development of a national health policy framework and a national health strategic plan; to develop and disseminate national planning and budgeting guidelines and to communicate budget ceilings for the plan period. The provinces are expected to submit their plans to the ministry headquarters between October and November for consideration by the ministry's top-level management team. The MOHCW holds biannual meetings in which all the eight provincial health teams, central hospitals and development partners are represented to discuss the national plan.The meeting in November/December discusses progress in the current plan period and agrees on priorities for the next annual plan period. Donors are expected to indicate the level of financing likely to be made available in the coming year. The meeting in July mainly focuses on mid term progress in program implementation and expenditure patterns. Program managers at the national level are responsible for developing strategic documents and plans, program policies, national program guidelines and act as technical resource persons to the provinces. The ministry's top-level management team (TMT) undertakes regular monitoring visits to selected districts during the course of the year to get first hand information on the implementation of programs and hospital services.

The planning department is responsible for coordinating the planning cycle and to ensure that the process is in synchrony with the rest of the government departments. The department also ensures that central level departments produce quality plans and in a timely manner and consolidates these into a central level plan and budget. In reality the process is not always as smooth as would be expected, especially at the community level where local participatory structures are not effective.

Planning for hospital services

Hospitals follow the same planning cycle as the provinces, districts and health centers. Prior to attaining semi-autonomous status central hospitals used to develop plans which they submitted directly to the MOHCW headquarters for approval and consolidation under the curative or medical services portfolio. With semi-autonomy these hospitals are expected to develop business plans which they submit to their Management Boards for approval. These hospital plans have to be within the budget made available to them and consolidated as part of the national health sector plan and budget. Hospital plans are divided into several "cost centers":

+ Maternal health, child health and family planning services
+ General medical services including pediatrics
+ Obstetrics and Gynecology
+ Pathology services, including the mortuary
+ General surgical and orthopedic
+ Theatre services
+ Oral health services
+ Pharmaceuticals and medical supplies
+ Radiology, Radiotherapy services
+ Hospital equipment and maintenance
+ Diagnostic laboratory services
+ Physiotherapy and rehabilitation services
+ Hospital based mental health services
+ Hospital catering
+ Accident and Emergency services (casualty department)
+ Human resources development and management – personnel, salaries, allowances etc
+ Other support services – transport, laundry, grounds maintenance, physical assets management, etc
+ Training of health professionals
+ Utilities – water, electricity, telephone, etc.

The annual health sector plan is thus a consolidation of plans and budgets from rural health centers and clinics, mission institutions, district program plans (district office and district hospital), Provincial Medical Director's office (and the provincial hospital), central hospital plans, central MOH plans and plans from health related statutory bodies and institutions. Ideally, programs supported and/or implemented by NGOs are captured during the district planning process.

Is there a potential for a provider-purchaser split in Zimbabwe?

African countries that explicitly separated the provision of health services from policymaking and financing functions of the sector include Uganda, Ghana and Zambia. The Zambia National Health Services Act of 1995 established the Central Board of Health (CBoH) with responsibility for the provision of health services. The CBoH was responsible for monitoring, integrating and coordinating health service delivery by district and Hospital Management Boards throughout the country. The MOH assumed responsibilities for policy making, regulation, resource mobilization, external relations and conducting performance audits on the work of the CBoH. In essence the MOH contracted the CBoH to provide services on its behalf. However in 2006, after several years of implementation the Zambian government repealed the National Health Services Act and dissolved the Central Board of Health. This move effectively reversed a major health reform policy of the government. As a result the government had to make arrangements to reabsorb almost 25 000 health workers into the government pay roll. The Ghana Health Service was similarly established by an Act of Parliament in 1996 as a body responsible for implementing national health policies under the Minister of Health through the Ghana Health Service Council.

For Zimbabwe such an arrangement would mean that the Ministry of Health and Child Welfare (the Secretary for Health, support staff at HQ and the Provincial Medical Directors offices) on one hand become responsible for setting the strategic direction, human resources planning and projection, coordination of training functions within the sector, standards setting and monitoring, resource mobilization and allocation, policy development, international relations, stewardship and regulation of the sector. In fulfilling its regulatory role the MOHCW would continue to rely on the Health Professions Authority, the Medicines Control Authority of Zimbabwe including the establishment of an inspectorate within its unit responsible for Quality Assurance.

The other arm of the public health system would then be responsible for the implementation of national health policies including service delivery. The composition of this arm of the sector would consist of central hospitals (semi-autonomous), the Zimbabwe National Family Planning Council (ZNFPC) and other relevant service delivery statutory bodies, provincial hospitals and rural and urban local authorities which with decentralization would incorporate district and urban health systems respectively.

Figure 3.2: Possible functional relationships in a purchaser-provider split.

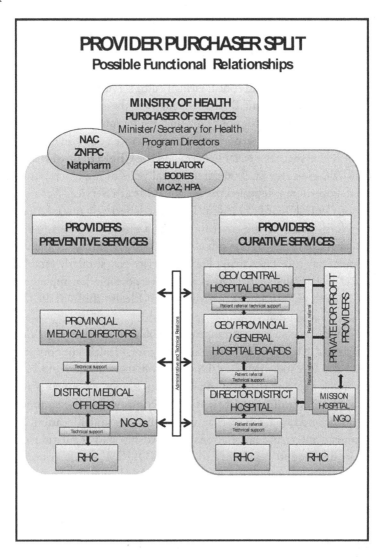

Possible configuration of a provider-purchaser split

The purchaser arm of the public health sector, as is the case in Ghana and Zambia, would consist of a national council or board appointed by the Minister of Health. Such a body would be accountable to the Minister of Health and headed by a Chief Executive or some such senior position supported by a number of directorates. Leadership for the sector would be provided by the Minister of Health and the office of the Secretary for Health as the Accounting Officer and Chief Health/Medical Officer. This implies that more functions would be de-concentrated from the center to the provincial and district levels in line with the overall decentralization policy of government. The office of the PMD would be expected to continue to play an intermediate role of technical support, supervision and the development of operational policies and guidelines and operating under the administrative direction of the provincial governor. For example, a provincial health directorate would be part of the office of the provincial governor, functionally and horizontally integrated with other departments at this level and sharing some resources such as administration and financial and/or transport management systems within the governor's office.

Similarly, at the operational level, devolution is possible at the Rural District Council level whereby the district health department is established within the Rural District Council administration. The health department would be headed by the District Medical Officer (or District Health Director) who is responsible to the District Administrator. Religious or mission institutions would continue to fall within the district health system. The risk of inadequate management and coordination capacity within local government structures remains a real potential obstacle to devolution.

A policy framework would have to be developed to ensure that semi-autonomous institutions such as provincial and central hospitals remain an integral part of a functioning referral system. Figure 3.2 illustrates a likely functional relationship within a possible provider-purchaser split.

Planning and budgeting within a provider-purchaser divide

One of the major responsibilities of the MOHCW is to mobilize and allocate resources from both the government and development partners to finance the work of the sector or to purchase health services on behalf of communities. Under this hypothetical structure the MOHCW would be accountable for public funds allocated by parliament for the provision of public health services irrespective of whether they are used by the provider or the purchaser of health services.

The MOHCW has the responsibility to coordinate the strategic planning process and setting national targets for the health sector. The provider arm would be responsible for operational planning and budgeting for service and program delivery. Under devolution, district and provincial plans are approved by the RDCs and subsequently by the office the Provincial

Development Committee (PDC). Sector ministries must ensure that provincial plans are in line with national policies, priorities and that their collective effort achieves agreed national targets. Management Boards at Central and Provincial hospitals have the responsibilities of planning, budgeting and implementing hospital business plans according to national policies and priorities.

The above processes should result in a consolidated health sector budget estimate which the MOHCW submits to Treasury. Budget negotiations between the MOHCW (purchaser) and Treasury should include representatives of providers of public health services; the PMDs, representatives of urban and rural local authorities, ZACH (representing mission institutions), the Health Services Board and semi-autonomous institutions. After the budget is approved the Ministry of Finance (and Economic Development) would allocate the funds, either directly to the providers of services and some to the MOHCW for its operations or allocate all the funds to the ministry of health to pass on to the service providers on a contractual basis. The preferred option would be to allocate the funds directly to each of the providers of services.

As with any change process, a restructuring exercise is bound to generate controversy and dissatisfaction to one party or the other. In the case of a provider – purchaser split there are likely to be relational problems of overlap and/or duplication of roles and/or functions between the MOHCW (the purchaser) and the providers of health services. A potential area of overlap is that of national policy development by the MOHCW versus that of operational policy development by the provider arm of the sector. Role clarity is as important as the need for reconciliation between technical accountability within the provider organization that is upwards and administrative accountability which is horizontal within the Rural District Councils. A clear framework that guides the functions of the referral system within the provider arm of the sector (consisting of missions, municipalities, the private sector and semi-autonomous institutions) must be defined. Responsibilities for recruitment, employment, professional development, promotion, continuing education, posting and transfer, discipline and dismissal of health staff require special attention, especially in a context of decentralization.

There are also opportunities to be exploited from such a restructuring process considering that the structure of the organization must allow for the realization of clear and distinct roles between the providers of services and the MOHCW as the purchaser and regulator of the sector.

Conclusions and the way forward

There have been two major restructuring phases of the MOHCW in Zimbabwe, with the rest of the exercises involving tampering with the organization at its periphery without any substantial changes to the structure. The first phase occurred soon after independence to address inequities in access to health care and to facilitate the implementation of Primary Health Care (PHC). The levels of the health delivery system were reviewed so as to emphasize the role of the health center and community levels and the establishment of offices of the Provincial Medical Directors and District Health Management Teams.

The second major phase was in the 1990s in the context of the country's ESAP, civil service reforms, health sector reforms and the Presidential Review Commission on Health. The main focus of this phase was on health sector reforms; the decentralization of health service delivery to RDCs, the establishment of semi-autonomous hospitals, the commercialization of some government departments and the introduction of contracting out of some government services.

Central to the reorganization of the internal structure of the MOHCW was the need to strengthen coordination and facilitate integration within the ministry. There was also the need to define the leadership role of the MOHCW within the sector through strengthening its strategic role and authority. To some extent this has been achieved through the establishment of distinct directorates and departments and the creation of bodies with consultative, advisory and representative responsibilities within the sector. The new structure has also made it possible for the MOHCW to assume leadership within the sector, to mobilize resources for the sector, to undertake strategic health planning, financial management and budgeting. The continued ability of the MOHCW to deliver its core functions will depend on continuous assessment of its staff requirements and their capacity to undertake these functions. It is however unlikely that existing staff redeployed as a result of the new structure will all have the necessary skills to fulfill their new roles. As a result the restructuring process must be underpinned by a capacity building process which is based on a robust staff development plan.

The challenge continues to be one of defining effective lines of authority within the MOHCW, especially the need to reconcile professional roles, leadership and authority with general management authority. There is also a need to harmonize professional hierarchical relations with the core functions and the overall structure of the MOHCW. The question is; to what extent is the MOHCW willing to go to accommodate professional lines of authority as a guiding framework for its structure? The organization has serious problems of dual authority where, for example, professional staff at the district or institutional level is required to report to local heads such as the District Medical Officer or institutional head, but also continue to report to program managers at the ministry headquarters. The other question concerns the ability of the structure of the MOHCW to facilitate career mobility for its staff? Does the structure allow those people that move upwards to the top of the organization's hierarchy to increase their authority, responsibility and potential within the organization? A well-designed structure in an effective organization should be able to address all, if not the majority of the issues discussed above.

Notwithstanding the desire for departments to have a clear separation of functions, it is also necessary that as the structure of an organization evolves it transforms the organization into a cohesive unit in which the different parts function in unison and in the same direction. This is possible where there is a common vision, common goals and values within an organization.

Changes to the structure of the MOHCW in themselves are not sufficient to ensure effectiveness. It is the degree of influence, the role and operations of the leadership, the executive and operational levels of the organization that count most. Hindsight indicates that positions created on the basis of core organizational functions usually pose a serious threat to the career mobility of professionals, especially those who are yet to acknowledge and accept that the world is no longer monolithic, hierarchical and bureaucratic but fleeting, fluid and flexible. It is partly the result of such misunderstandings of structural re-organizations that organizations undertake repeated cycles of organizational restructuring.

Review questions

1. Describe the process you would follow to undertake a functional analysis of a MOH you are familiar with.
2. What do you understand by the term 'strategic decision making body'?
3. Elaborate on the term 'provider-purchaser split' within the health sector. Give an example of a ministry of health that has implemented this type of reform objective.
4. Describe the lessons learnt from experiences in the implementation of Hospital Autonomy in Sub-Saharan Africa with respect to the following issues:
   - Funding mechanisms and sustainability
   - Management structures
   - Service role of autonomous hospitals
   - Equity issues
   - Legislative review in support of this initiative

4

HUMAN RESOURCES FOR HEALTH IN ZIMBABWE

Introduction

As the issue of human resources for health (HRH) takes the center stage globally, the World Health Organization (WHO) classified 57 developing countries, including Zimbabwe, as having a critical shortage of HRH. This group of countries is characterized by a health worker density of less than 2.5 per 1 000 population. On this scale Zimbabwe has a physician density of 0.16, a nurse density of 0.72 and an overall density of 1.23 health staff per 1 000 population, Table 4.1. According to the WHO, available statistics indicate that for Africa to achieve its MDGs it must achieve a health worker density of at least 250 doctors, nurses and midwives per 100 000 population as well as eliminate internal disparities in staff distribution. An important fact in this context is that the quality of health services, their efficacy, effectiveness and accessibility depend directly on the number of health workers, their deployment and working conditions. The UN Commission on Trade and Development estimates that each migrating African professional represents a loss of US$ 184 000 to Africa. Paradoxically Africa is estimated to spend US$ 4 billion a year on salaries of about 100 000 foreign experts.

Table 4.1:   Zimbabwe's health worker density (2002)

Staff category	Total number	Density/ 1 000 popn
Doctors	2 086	0.161
Nurses	9 357	0.724
Dentists/ Technicians	310	0.024
Pharmacist/ Technicians	883	0.068
Environmental Health Officers/ Technicians	1 803	0.139
Laboratory Scientists/Technicians	917	0.071
Other Health workers	743	0.057
Health Management and Support	581	0.045
Sum Total	16 680	1.290

Source: Human resources for health, Country Fact Sheet (2006), [Online] Available at: http://www.afro.who.int/home/countries/fact_sheets/Zimbabwe.pdf [Accessed on 25/03/2008]

Tables 4.2 (a) and 4.2 (b) provide information on the staff situation in the public health sector covering the year 2003 and the period December 2005 to June 2007 in Zimbabwe. It is however difficult to assess the implications or degree of impact on service delivery of the vacancy rates shown in these tables, mainly because the basis for determining the staff establishment is not clear. However, considering that the government has an interest in filling all the available posts and that it continues to train various health professionals, it is clear that the HRH situation is deteriorating rather than improving. The fact that there are more vacancies amongst management posts and those of program managers implies that more experienced and qualified staff are leaving the ministry compared to junior and inexperienced staff. The consequences of such a scenario are that the leadership and strategic role of the health sector is compromised. The high vacancy rates for medical doctors (53%), nurses (30%), radiographers (43%), pharmacists (39%) and laboratory staff (45%) means that the health delivery system has very serious capacity problems in delivering the right quantity and quality of health services. A vacancy rate of 83% for program managers means that public health programs do not have the necessary high level technical support and the necessary guidance to the operational level.

Table 4.2 (a): Ministry of Health and Child Welfare staff vacancy rates (2003)

Health professional	Establishment	In post	Vacancy	Vacancy rate
Doctors	1172	822	350	30%
Pharmacists	98	30	69	70%
Pharmacy technicians	167	107	60	36%
Nurses	17 214	12 554	4 660	28%
Radiographers	122	104	18	15%
Hospital equipment technicians	84	41	43	52%
Laboratory scientists	392	264	128	33%

Source: HERA Midterm reviews of the HSSP I and II Zimbabwe January 2004.

The root causes of the HRH crisis in developing countries have been well researched and can be summarized as follows:

- Capacity for HRH planning and development
  - absence of effective HRH policies
  - poor personnel information systems
  - delayed response to increasing attrition rates (out migration, HIV/AIDS)
- Training (production) capacity
  - lack of a training policy
  - inadequate investment in training institutions
  - donors not interested in supporting pre-service training
  - poor quality of training institutions
  - inadequate output of health professionals
  - poor remuneration of trainers
- Management of HRH
  - poor recruitment and deployment policies
  - inability of the sector to recruit additional staff
  - unmet health worker needs due to:
    - low salaries
    - excessive workload
    - inadequate support and supervision
    - inadequate pre-service training to prepare staff for actual practice
    - poor work environment
- Non health system issues
  - education system not producing enough qualified people to pursue careers in the health profession
  - unstable political and economic environment
  - inadequate investment in the health sector
  - active recruitment by developed countries who offer better conditions

Table 4.2 (b): Health workers in post and staff vacancy rates in the Ministry of Health and Child Welfare (2005 -2007)

Category	Establishment	Year					
		December 2005		December 2006		June 2007	
		Number in post	% vacancy rate	Number in post	% vacancy rate	Number in post	% vacancy rate
Top management posts	56	7	88%	13	77%	16	71%
Doctors	1562	668	57%	667	57%	738	53%
Nurses (all grades)	19290	13495	30%	14768	23%	13699	29%
Environmental health Officers/Technicians	2387	1293	46%	1220	49%	1157	52%
Pharmacists/Technicians	548	338	38%	318	42%	332	39%
Radiographers	456	158	65%	154	66%	261	43%
Physiotherapists/Assistants	457	374	18%	355	22%	368	19%
Nutritionists	1005	783	22%	761	24%	787	22%
Orthopedic Technicians	42	35	17%	33	21%	35	17%
Dentist/Dental Therapists	302	195	35%	192	36%	181	40%
Laboratory Scientists/Technicians	580	324	44%	320	45%	317	45%
Research Scientists	87	23	74%	21	76%	36	59%
Health Information officers/Statisticians	230	93	60%	100	57%	145	37%
Health Promotion Officers	62	41	34%	42	32%	38	39%
Hospital equipment technicians	155	78	50%	72	54%	85	45%
General Administration	7793	6708	14%	6207	20%	5879	25%
Program Managers	54	11	80%	8	85%	9	83%
Total all categories	35066	24624	30%	25251	28%	24083	31%

Source: Ministry of Health, 2006

Factors contributing to HRH shortages in Zimbabwe

Causes of staff attrition

Several factors have over the years contributed to the country's evolving human resources for health crisis in Zimbabwe. Notably, the situation got worse in the years soon after the country implemented its first Structural Adjustment Program (SAP) in the early 1990s. According to Chikanda, A (2005) the health sector in Zimbabwe has been significantly affected by the out migration of skilled workers mainly as a result of the consequences of the country's Structural Adjustment Programs. The brain drain in Zimbabwe has also been exacerbated by the deteriorating economic, social and political conditions with the health sector being the most affected.

It is also important to note that the Ministry of Health and Child Welfare has always lacked the capacity to plan for the development of human resources. The human resources department in the ministry has in the past operated as a personnel administration department with a capacity only to deal with the recruitment of staff, maintenance of discipline and handling complaints, without the ability to deal with the core issues of human resources planning and management. The health sector relied too much on the Public Service Commission which did not seem to appreciate the unique nature of managing human resources for health issues. Because of lack of capacity and foresight, the Ministry of Health has not been able to make accurate projections of national health workforce requirements. The ministry has relied on the fixed establishment model which is often determined without the benefit of objective evidence. A major contributing factor to the above problem has been the ministry's poor personnel information systems, which after being upgraded, there was no in house capacity to use the system.

As a result of some of these shortcomings the health sector has not been able to link workforce requirements to training capacity required to enable it to project HRH requirements into the future. There is a serious lack of analytic capacity to inform decisions that will ensure that professionals with the right skills are available in the right numbers and deployed to the right place at the right time. An example of a lack of foresight by the government is the decision taken in 1995 to abolish the training of State Certified Nurses (SCNs). This politically motivated blunder resulted in a 50% reduction in the number of nurses trained per annum in Zimbabwe. The consequences of this decision were exacerbated by the fact that it was extremely difficult to deploy Registered General Nurses (RGNs) to work in Rural Health Centers. As a result, many Rural Health Centers (RHCs) and RDC clinics were staffed by unqualified nurse aides.

The HIV epidemic has contributed significantly in increasing the natural attrition of staff in Zimbabwe, though not much work has been done to objectively quantify this in Zimbabwe's health sector. Loss of productivity and attrition result from absenteeism due to sickness leave and HIV related deaths across all categories of health staff. Projections made before the widespread use of ART on the proportion of healthcare providers who would die from AIDS each year indicated that in a country with a stable 15 percent HIV prevalence, as an example, it was expected that between 1.6 and 3.3 percent of its healthcare workers would die from AIDS annually. It was assumed then that the rate of HIV infection was constant and that it would take an average of 10 years from the time of infection to death.

Efforts to keep health workers on the job in the public sector in Zimbabwe have been both a challenge and a nightmare for the authorities. This has been partly the result of the central role played by the PSC in determining the conditions of service for all civil servants and the absence of a coherent human resources for health policy framework. Problems in this area have over the years proved to be intractable despite the fact that their causes are known; poor working conditions, poor remuneration, non-recognition of staff efforts and the perceived poor image of the health profession. The general tendency has been for institutions like the PSC and ministries of finance to subordinate efforts by the health sector to resolve HRH to macroeconomic factors such as the need to reduce the size of the civil service and the wage bill, Dusault, G and Dubois, C (2003).

Health professionals leave the public sector, indeed the country, in order to achieve personal and professional goals; to earn a living, to continue their education, to experience other cultures and to expand their professional experience, amongst many other reasons. Poor salaries and working conditions at home or the lure of better ones in other countries entice many to sacrifice and leave their homes. In some instances poor staff management practices have also contributed to the degree to which health professionals leave their places of work. The Ministry of Health and Child Welfare and the PSC, by and large, failed to resolve long standing problems related to salaries, working conditions, continuing education, staffing levels, job security and staff housing.

In her research document, Gaidzano, R (1999) adequately presents the plight of health workers in Zimbabwe when she states that doctors and nurses expressed frustrations which included; being over worked and underpaid, shortages of other support health professionals, exhaustion from moonlighting, acute drug shortages at the work place, lack of protective clothing and equipment which increased occupational safety concerns, poor supervision and support from specialist doctors and perceived corruption in the promotion processes within the nursing field. It is common knowledge that health staff and the public complain about chronic shortages of essential drugs and other supplies at public health institutions. Overcrowded hospitals and a frequent breakdown of equipment have made the work environment unsafe and exposed both patients and staff to hospital-acquired infections and ineffective diagnostic procedures and treatment practices.

Health workers have expressed concerns with regards unclear career development opportunities and the lack of recognition of their experience. Recruitment and staff management procedures of the Public Service Commission (PSC) often took too long to resolve personnel issues. On average it took between 3 to 6 months before newly recruited health workers received their first pay cheque. In some cases, if the MOHCW submitted proposals for a review of conditions of service for health workers, delays of up to 3 years were not an uncommon experience before there was any response from the PSC, if at all. Such delays often resulted in health workers taking decisions into their own hands and resorting to industrial action. Most episodes of industrial action by health workers have been the result of poor communication between the MOHCW and staff associations on one hand and between the MOHCW and the PSC. This resulted in both the MOHCW officials and the majority of health workers opting for de-linkage of the health staff from the PSC.

The attrition of health workers from the public health sector was initially to the local private medical sector as opportunities increased a result of its rapid growth. However, as a result of the rapidly deteriorating macro economic situation in the country the private medical sector also became less competitive and health professionals turned to the local NGO sector which offered better salaries than the private medical sector, and in some cases paid salaries in foreign currency. As time went by fewer patients could afford services offered by private general practitioners and specialists.

With local opportunities exhausted, health professionals preferred destinations beyond the country's borders such as neighboring and overseas countries which, in the main, included Botswana, South Africa, Namibia and the UK, Australia and New Zealand. Between 1999 and 2000 the number of nurses employed by the public sector in Zimbabwe decreased by 20% as a result of out-migration. According to Stilwell, et al. (2003) information from the Nursing and Midwifery Council of the UK indicated that in 1998/1999 a total of 52 nurses from Zimbabwe were registered in the UK, 221 in 1999/2000 and 382 in 2000/2001. A total of 2 346 work permits were issued for nurses from Zimbabwe by the UK in 2000. A study by Chatora, et al. (2003) on migration issues found that 68% of health workers in Zimbabwe intended to migrate. These reports indicate the potentially devastating prospects of out migration on Zimbabwe's health delivery system.

Strategies put in place by the government to stem the HRH crisis

The development of a well coordinated human resources policy and strategy has continued to be a challenge for the health sector in Zimbabwe. The development of a comprehensive human resources policy and strategy requires an all inclusive process involving all relevant stakeholders in the HRH area. Such local stakeholders include, at least, the Ministry of Health and Child Welfare, the Health Service Board, the Public Service Commission (PSC), the Ministry of Finance (MOF), health workers, professional associations, and members of academia, training institutions, NGOs and civil society groups. The most important issues to be considered in the policy process are:

+ Human resources planning and development issues
+ Training, recruitment and deployment
+ Geographic distribution
+ Review of staffing and staff establishment.
+ Skills mix.
+ Conditions of service
+ Performance management
+ Staff attrition
+ Monitoring and evaluation

Strengthening the Human Resources Department in the MOHCW

The Ministry of Health and Child Welfare has over the years worked closely with the PSC in its efforts to resolve long standing health workforce issues. The Ministry of Health has also implemented several health sector specific reforms which complemented government wide civil service and economic reforms. In seeking ways to improve efficiency, coordination and its capacity to achieve organizational objectives, the ministry embarked on and undertook a number of restructuring exercises. One reform which had an impact on the management of the health workforce is that which established semi-autonomous central hospitals. These institutions are managed by Hospital Management Boards who employ hospital managers on three year performance contracts as opposed to Health Service Board employment conditions or PSC conditions of service. It is also likely that in the future other staff at these institutions will be transferred from being employees of the Health Service Board to being direct employees of Hospital Management Boards. Hospital Management Boards will be guided by employment standards and general conditions of service set by the Health Services Board.

The role, structure, functions and staffing of the Human Resources Department of the MOHCW continues to be a cause for concern. At the central level the Human Resources Department has the responsibility to coordinate human resources planning and the development of policies and procedures that ensure order at the workplace. Considering the complex nature of a health care organization, the role of the ministry of health's Human Resources Department must go beyond dealing only with personnel administration to tackling human resources issues in a holistic manner. The department must rise to the occasion and organize its work to deal with Human Resources Planning, Human Resources Development, Human Resources Management and Human Resources Monitoring and Evaluation (Human Resources Information Systems).

These are highly specialized functions which are beyond the capabilities of clerical staff, the majority of whom have for a long time occupied key positions in the ministry's Human Resources Department. Though the MOHCW structure (as approved in July 2007) provides an opportunity for the department to deal with all these issues, staff in the department requires specialized training in these areas.

Training health professionals

Zimbabwe has a large number of training institutions for different categories of health professionals. These include Ministry of Health hospitals and multi-disciplinary training institutions, some private hospitals, universities and technical colleges, see tables 4.3 and 4.4. The absence of an overarching and comprehensive training policy on pre-service and in-service training of health professionals has been one major constraining factor. This has meant that there is no coordinated approach to the production of an adequate health workforce for the country. In the pursuit of quality and transparency in the training of health professionals, professional bodies have responsibilities to develop and/or approve curricula and examinations for their respective health professionals. For example, the Nurses and Midwifery Council of Zimbabwe sets and grades professional examinations for the nursing profession. Basic nurse training is undertaken mainly at Ministry of Health institutions, mission hospitals and, in some cases, private for profit hospitals. The medical school also undertakes basic nurse training at degree level. The curriculum for medical doctors in Zimbabwe has to be agreed to by the Schools of Medicine, the Health Professions Authority and the Ministry of Health and Child Welfare. The Health Professions Authority has the additional responsibility of inspecting and accrediting central hospitals in terms of their suitability to train medical doctors.

The 1999 Review Commission on Health recommended the establishment of a second medical school in Zimbabwe as well as a significant increase in the output of trained nurses. The medical school at the University of Zimbabwe has over the years increased its intake of medical students from 60 during the pre-independence era to the current 200. This is however below the target of 400 medical doctors proposed to be trained annually as of the year 2000. A second medical school was established at the National University of Science and Technology (NUST) which is located in the country's second largest city of Bulawayo. Its first intake of 18 medical students was admitted in February 2005 followed by another intake of 17 in August the same year. In 1982 the University of Zimbabwe established an Institute of Continuing Health Education (ICHE) to train post graduate medical specialists, table 4.4. In 1993 the Ministry of Health and Child Welfare collaborated with the Department of Community Medicine of the University of Zimbabwe and introduced a field based Masters program in Public Health. The initiative was supported by the Rockefeller Foundation under the concept of "Public Health Schools without Walls".

Virtually all the training institutions in Zimbabwe have been seriously affected by the human resources crisis in the country. The situation has been so severe that the medical post graduate programs which in 1997 had a combined annual enrolment of at least 51 trainees enrolled only 13 trainees in 2006. More disturbing are the 2006-07 statistics on the availability of lecturers. The overall vacancy rate at the medical school was 57% with the departments of physiology and anatomy with 95% and 96% vacancy rates, respectively. With an establishment of 8 lecturers, the department of histology had only one lecturer in post in 2007 and hematology had no lecturer.

Table 4.3:   Basic Training Programs for Human Resources for Health in Zimbabwe

Institution	Program	Duration	Qualification	Annual intake
Basic Degree Programs				
University of Zimbabwe	Medicine	5 Years	MBChB	200
	Dentistry	5 Years	DDS	20
	Pharmacy	3 Years	BPharm (Hons)	30
	Physiotherapy	4 Years	BSc (Physiotherapy)	20
	Occupational Therapy	4 Years	BSc (Occupational therapy)	20
	Nursing	3 Years	BSc (Nursing)	15
	Environmental Health	4 Years	BSc (Environment, Hons)	10
	Medical Laboratory	4 Years	BSc (Lab, Hons)	20
	Radiology	3 Years	BSc (Radiology)	10
Basic Diploma, Certificate Programs				
Nurse Training				
5 Central Hospitals	General Nursing	3 Years	Diploma in General Nursing	720
7 Provincial Hospitals	General Nursing	3 Years	Diploma in General Nursing	500
District /General Hospitals	General Nursing	3 Years	Diploma in General Nursing	290
District /Mission Hospitals	Primary Care Nurses	18 months	Certificate in Primary Care Nursing	600
Environmental Health Training				
Bulawayo Polytechnic College	Environmental Health Officers	3 Years	Diploma in Environmental Health & Food Inspection	8
3 Multi–Disciplinary Training Institutions	Environmental Health Technicians	3 Years	Certificate in Environmental Health	60
Radiography Training Programs				
2 Central Hospitals	Radiography	3 Years	Diploma: Diagnostic or Therapeutic Radiography	40
2 Provincial Hospitals	X-Ray Operators	1 Year	Certificate for X-Ray operators	20
Dental Training Programs				
Dental Training School	Dental Therapy	3 Years	Diploma Dental Therapy	20
	Dental Technician (Part 1)	2 Years	Certificate for Dental Technician	10
Pharmacy Training Programs				
2 Polytechnic Colleges	Pharmacy Technician Course	2 Years	Diploma in Pharmaceutical Technology	40
Rehabilitation Training Program				
Morondera Provincial Hospital	Rehabilitation Training Program	2 Years	Certificate in Rehabilitation	20
Hospital Domestic Supervisors Training Program				
Parirenyatwa Hospital	Hospital Domestic Supervisors Course	2 Years	Certificate for Hospital Domestic Supervisor	10
Medical Laboratory Technology Training Program				
University of Zimbabwe	Medical Laboratory Scientist (Technologist)	3 Years	Diploma in Medical Laboratory Technology (BSc)	30

Table 4.4: Post Basic and Post Graduate Training programs for Human Resources for Health in Zimbabwe

Post Graduate Diploma Courses

Institution	Program	Duration	Qualification	Annual Intake
University of Zimbabwe	Medicine	4 Years	M. Med Medicine	8
	Anesthetics	4 Years	M. Med Anesthetics	8
	Pediatric Surgery	4 Years	M. Med Pediatric Surgery	8
	Neurosurgery	4 Years	M. Med Neurosurgery	8
	Obstetrics and Gynecology	4 Years	M. Med Obstetrics & Gynecology	8
	Ophthalmology	4 Years	M. Med Ophthalmology	8
	Psychiatry	4 Years	M. Med Psychiatry	8
	Radiotherapy/Oncology	4 Years	M. Med Radiotherapy/Oncology	8

Post Graduate Diploma Courses

Institution	Program	Duration	Qualification	Annual Intake
University of Zimbabwe	Anesthetics	1 Year	Diploma in Anesthetics	8
	General Pathology	2 Years	Diploma in General Pathology	6
	Ophthalmology	1 Year	Diploma in Ophthalmology	8
	Psychiatry Health	1 Year	Diploma in Psychiatry Health	6
	Venereology	1 Year	Diploma in Venereology	5
	Nurse Education & Adult Education	2 Years	Diploma in Nurse/Adult Education	16
	Health Education & Adult Education	2 Years	Diploma in Health/Adult Education	15
	Specialist Laboratory Technology	2 Years	Spec Diploma in Laboratory Technology	25

Post Basic Nursing Diploma

Institution	Program	Duration	Qualification	Annual Intake
Central Hospitals	Midwifery	1 Year	Diploma in Midwifery	65
Provincial Hospitals	Midwifery	1 Year	Diploma in Midwifery	60
Mpilo Central Hospital	Advanced Clinical Officer course	2 Years	Diploma in Advanced Clinical Practice	8
Ingutsheni Psychiatry Hospital	Psychiatry Nursing	3 Years	Diploma in Psychiatry Nursing	20
	Nurse Anesthetist	1 Year	Nurse Anesthetist Diploma	10
Parirenyatwa Hospital	Intensive Care Nursing	1 Year	Diploma in Intensive Care Nursing	10
	Community Nursing	1 Year	Diploma in Community Nursing	30
	Nurse Administration	1 Year	Diploma in Nurse Administration	15
Avenues Private Hospital	Operating Theatre Nursing	1 Year	Diploma in Operating Theatre Nursing	10

Other Training Programs

Institution	Program	Duration	Qualification	Annual Intake
Parirenyatwa Hospital	Health Teacher Training	1 Year Dist Learning	Health Teacher Diploma	25
	Dental Technology (part 2)	2 Years	Diploma in Dental Technology	5

Health Administrator Training Program

Institution	Program	Duration	Qualification	Annual Intake
Harare Polytechnic	Health Services Administrator Course	3 Years	Diploma in Health Services Administration	15

Until 1998 the four urban based Central Hospitals were the only institutions that offered pre-service training for Registered General Nurses (RGN) at Diploma level in Zimbabwe, Table 4.5. In order to increase the output of nurses a major policy decision was made to decentralize the training of RGNs to the country's provincial and general hospitals. As a result of this decision the annual output of nurses increased from about 400 to nearly 1000 nurses, Table 4.7. However, because of the poor conditions of service prevailing in the public sector at one time, the MOHCW was only able to attract and employ about 30% of the output of nurses from its training institutions.

Table 4.5: Out-put of Registered General Nurses from nurse training institutions (1975-1998)

Year	Parirenyatwa	Harare	UBH *	Mpilo Central	Annual Total
1975	46	61	105	28	240
1976	69	48	72	54	243
1977	67	48	67	54	236
1978	66	80	75	43	264
1979	73	60	49	43	225
1980	97	67	56	46	266
1981	50	139	82	36	307
1982	77	122	96	57	352
1983	74	123	58	56	311
1984	115	116	77	45	353
1985	121	115	72	42	350
1986	97	121	62	54	334
1987	95	130	65	47	337
1988	121	116	75	47	359
1989	113	150	62	53	378
1990	105	150	51	46	352
1991	129	160	58	51	398
1992	119	149	53	58	379
1993	106	178	50	52	386
1994	109	125	51	46	331
1995	105	132	51	54	342
1996	Not available	140	49	53	(242)
1997	Not available	133	88	69	(290)
1998	Not available	90	104	40	(234)
Total	1954+ (2386)	2753	1628	1174	Data Incomplete

United Bulawayo Hospitals

Table 4.6: Registered General Nurse Training program intakes and outputs (2003-2009)

Name of Institution	INTAKES BY YEAR								OUTPUT PER YEAR						
	2003	2004	2005	2006	2007	2008	2009	Total	2003	2004	2005	2006	2007	2008	2009
Harare	159	159	205	196	180	195	180	1274	159	151	146	173	180	195	180
Parirenyatwa	167	162	141	184	180	180	188	1194	140	148	123	138	182	162	188
Chitungwiza	100	123	184	185	50	100	100	842	30	28	24	24	137	184	194
Mpilo	138	123	126	147	118	127	131	910	114	77	77	38	126	147	118
UBH	126	132	132	134	132	129	131	916	74	87	118	88	126	147	118
Masvingo	124	72	116	131	60	40	40	583	36	41	49	76	93	109	135
Marondera	60	40	40	43	40	40	40	303	23	42	36	42	35	41	41
Chinhoyi	164	85	64	41	41	80	80	555	54	52	47	129	95	64	46
Bindura	41	56	40	40	40	40	40	297	24	7	5	50	40	40	40
Mutare	127	101	50	0	80	80	0	438	17	48	46	112	50	48	0
Kwekwe	68	40	40	48	70	40	40	346	0	40	64	0	40	40	40
Gweru	68	83	102	72	90	90	90	595	66	29	0	43	102	102	72
Tsholotsho	0	20	19	20	20	20	20	119	17	20	27	18	15	21	22
Gwanda	81	73	79	81	0	40	80	434	21	75	11	25	93	82	76
Luisa Guidotti	0	24	24	0	48	24	0	120	0	0	19	0	19	20	0
Karanda	0	20	24	20	14	14	14	106	0	14	12	3	19	24	20
Muvonde	10	44	22	26	24	30	30	186	0	0	0	20	22	48	24
Bonda	30	0	31	33	32	30	30	186	0	20	0	28	30	30	30
St Annes Brunapeg	0	24	26	22	22	22	22	138	14	17	11	10	25	26	26
St Luke's	11	18	34	34	26	26	26	175	15	12	11	18	18	34	34
Gutu	0	30	30	30	30	30	30	180	0	0	0	0	30	30	30
St Theresa	0	0	0	30	30	30	30	120	0	0	0	0	0	0	30
Mashoko	0	0	30	30	30	30	30	150	0	0	0	0	0	0	30
Total	1474	1429	1559	1547	1357	1437	1364	10167	804	908	826	1035	1477	1594	1494
Primary Care Nurses	305	630	728	839	742	741	0	3985	0	270	608	743	728	839	742
Total									804	1178	1434	1778	2205	2433	2236

Table 4.7: Training out-put of nurses and allied professional categories (2000)

Profession	Type of Course	Training Program	Total Output
Nursing	Basic	Diploma in general Nursing	887
	Post Basic	Diploma in Midwifery	288
		Diploma in Community Nursing	14
		Diploma in Nursing Administration	24
		Diploma in Nurse Anesthetist	9
		Diploma in Intensive Care Nursing	26
		Diploma in Operating Theater Nursing	41
		Diploma in Psychiatric Nursing	22
		Diploma in Nursing Education (UZ)	3
		Diploma in Ophthalmic Nursing (Malawi)	5
		Master of Science in Nursing (UZ)	9
	SCN Upgrading Course	Diploma in General Nursing	396
Dentistry	Basic	Diploma in Dental Therapy	12
Radiography	Basic	Diploma in Radiography	20
Pharmacy	Basic	Pharmacy Technician	31
Environmental Health	Basic	Diploma in Environmental Health (EHT)	22
Rehabilitation	Basic	Certificate in Rehabilitation	21

Source: Report of the Secretary for Health and Child Welfare, 2000

To offset the decrease in the nurse training output resulting from a misguided political decision to discontinue the training of State Certified Nurses (SCNs) the MOHCW introduced the Primary Care Nurse (PCN). These nurses are trained at 18 institutions which have a combined annual output of more than 600. Between 2003 and July 2008 these institutions had trained a cumulative total of 3 830 PCNs, table 4.8. The PCN is professionally trained for a period of 18 months, after which they are registered with the Nurses and Midwifery Council of Zimbabwe at certificate level. The PCN is specifically trained to provide health services at health center level within the Zimbabwean health service delivery environment.

In 2008 the first group of PCNs who qualified in 2003 became eligible to apply for a 12 month post basic training in midwifery after which qualification the PCN attains a diploma certification status. Similar, but less rigorous efforts have been implemented to increase the availability of other health professionals such as dentists, dental therapists, advanced clinical officers, laboratory technicians, etc.

Improving the general conditions of service for health workers

The responsibility for improving the conditions of service for health workers has traditionally been that of the Public Service Commission (PSC). The PSC approves and controls the staff establishment, determines grades, salary scales, allowances, advancements and promotions for all government departments. The Ministry of Health had always been concerned with the seemingly half hearted manner in which the PSC responded to its work force issues. As an example, whenever the health sector submitted proposals to improve the conditions of service for health workers the PSC always took its time to respond, if at all, usually only to do so when there was a crisis. It was the view of the Ministry of Health that the PSC did not fully appreciate the complex nature of the health sector as it tended to resort to fragmented short term measures which did not address the fundamentals of HRH problems. It is a known and obvious fact that problems in the functioning of one group of health professionals have ripple effects on the effective function of other members of the health team. Industrial action by nurses in a hospital has a direct impact on the quality of work and function of medical doctors. The same applies to laboratory scientists, pharmacists and radiographers. This, however, did not seem to be that obvious to the PSC, which for example, resorted to resolving nurses' issues separately from those of doctors. The health sector had no other option except to call for "de-linkage" of the health sector from the PSC as part of its reform agenda. This was achieved when the Health Service Board was established in 2005 to take over health related functions of the PSC.

In terms of Section 4 of the Health Service Act the functions of the Health Service Board include:

♦ Appoint persons to offices, posts and grades in the Health Service, and

♦ Create grades in the Health Service and fix conditions of service for its members, and

+ Supervise and monitor health service employees, and
+ Inquire into and deal with complaints made by members of the Health Service;
+ Supervise, advise and monitor performance of Hospital Management Boards, and
+ Handle appeals in relation to disciplinary powers exercised by Hospital Management Boards over members of the Health Service employed in any government hospital; and
+ Assist in resource mobilization for the Health Service; and
+ Exercise any other function that may be imposed or conferred upon the Board in terms of this Act or any other enactment.

Between the two organizations, the PSC and the MOHCW, several attempts have in the past been made to improve the conditions of service for health workers in Zimbabwe. Comparative analyses of conditions of service for health professionals within the SADC region have also been undertaken. However, limited consultations with local stakeholders such as health professionals and/or their professional bodies were undertaken. As a result, whenever these two institutions made proposals, they invariably fell short of the expectations of health professionals. The PSC also watered down the MOHCWs proposals on the grounds that these would have contagion on demands by professionals in other ministries. At the end of it all the resolution of health sector workforce issues remained at the mercy of other sectors often resulting in frequent episodes of industrial action by either nurses and/or medical doctors.

The PSC invariably implemented salaries which were way below those received by health professionals in the SADC region, especially compared to South Africa, Namibia and Botswana. For example, in 1997 the annual salary of the Secretary for Health in Zimbabwe, who according to the Public Health Act has to be a medical doctor, was equivalent to US$ 13 347 compared to that of a junior medical doctor in Botswana who received about US$ 14 400. A nurse in Zimbabwe received a monthly salary equivalent to US$ 416 compared to a Botswana counterpart who received about US$ 1 000. In justifying this state of affairs the PSC claimed an inability to afford the proposed wage bill. The PSC has offered health personnel various combinations of housing allowances, soft loans for the purchase of vehicles, transport allowances, uniform allowances, rural allowances and cash in lieu of private practice which were largely non taxable.

Table: 4.8: Primary Care Nurse Training Program output in Zimbabwe (2003-2008)

Training School	Commencement Date Aug 03	Jan 04	July 04	Jan 05	July 05	Jan 06	July 06	Jan 07	July 07	Jan 08	July 08
1 Bonda	-	-	26	-	26	-	26	-	24	-	24
2 Howard	22	22	20	22	20	20	22	20	20	20	20
3 Inyathi	-	18	20	21	20	22	22	20	20	20	20
4 Maphisa	20	23	22	23	22	20	22	18	18	18	18
5 Mnene	46	39	41	42	39	40	34	38	38	38	38
6 Mt Selinda	22	19	22	20	20	22	22	20	20	20	20
7 Mt St Mary's	30	30	29	24	30	30	30	28	28	28	28
8 Murambinda	-	16	24	22	24	24	26	22	22	22	22
9 Mutambara	26	-	22	24	26	26	26	24	24	24	24
10 Nkayi	22	18	23	22	23	22	24	20	20	20	20
11 Nyadire	30	26	28	22	22	24	24	22	22	22	22
12 Sanyati	25	30	26	31	30	30	30	28	28	28	28
13 Silveira	31	-	22	22	21	21	24	22	22	22	22
14 St Theresa	-	20	-	24	14	-		Has stopped training PCNs			
15 Tshelanyemba	32	6	22	22	23	24	24	28	28	28	28
16 Gokwe	-	-	-	-	22	-	-	-	-	20	20
17 St Albert's	-	-	-	-	-	20	-	20	-	20	-
18 Mt Darwin	-	-	-	-	-	-	-	20	-	20	-
Totals	305	267	363	346	404	345	494	350	354	350	354
Completion dates	31-01-05	30-06-05	31-12-05	30-6-06	31-12-06	30-6-07	31-12-07	30-12-08	31-12-08	30-6-09	31-12-09
No. sitting exam	296	279	241	375 (347)	490	395	409				
Number passed	270	234	213	313	470	355	381				
Cumulative No	305	572	935	1281	1663	2008	2502	2830	3097	3402	3830

Source: MOHCW. All intakes from July 2005 output will be larger (± 10) due to the bridging course. Consisting of those candidates due to join in each intake that were not successful in the RGN program.

However, as the hyperinflationary environment worsened the purchasing power of these packages were quickly eroded, leading to more demands by health workers. By September 2008 the country's rate of inflation had reached a whopping 231 million percent. The purchasing power of salaries for civil servants became uncompetitive mainly because the cost of goods and services was pegged at the parallel foreign exchange rate of approximately US$ 1.00 to ZW$ 60 million (April 2008) whereas their salaries were pegged at an artificial official exchange rate of US$ 1.00 to ZW$30 000. Even though government opted to review the salaries of civil servants every six months and attempted to control the prices of essential commodities, government salaries were still not able to keep pace with the hyperinflation. It was a "dog chasing its own tail" with no end in sight.

The situation prevailing in terms of incomes of professionals in Zimbabwe could not have been better described than by the government's own mouthpiece, the weekly Sunday News of 13 July 2008. The article entitled *"Maids earn more than professionals"* stated that *"company executives barely made it to the ZW$ 100 billion margin"*. The same article also quotes a local employment agency for domestic employees as saying, *"we insist that our client pays them 100 Rands (South African currency) or 80 Pula (Botswana currency)*, which, based on the exchange rate prevailing at the time, was equivalent to ZW$ 1 trillion!

Incentives schemes for health workers

In 2006 the government started implementing a pilot staff retention incentive scheme in the health sector which benefitted staff in "vital posts" and working at selected districts in rural areas. The initiative was introduced with the assistance of the European Union (EU). These vital posts consisted of positions occupied by members of the District Health Executive (DHE) – the District Medical Officer (DMO), the District Nursing Officer (DNO), the District Health Services Administrator (DHSA), the District Environmental Health Officer (DEHO) and the District Pharmacist in the selected districts. The package which was modeled on the Zambia Health Workers Retention Scheme was implemented in three districts in each of the eight rural provinces of Zimbabwe. On instistance by the donor one of the three institutions or districts in each of the provinces had to belong to a faith based organization.

The first component of the incentives package targeted the District Medical Officer (DMO) and the Government Medical Officer (GMO) who were offered:

+ A "top up" rural hardship allowance, education allowance, on call allowance and non private practice allowance, paid in foreign currency.
+ An official vehicle for use by the DMO
+ Renovations to the DMO's house, as well as houses for other medical doctors.

The second component of the package targeted the rest of the DHE members and consisted of:
+ A service vehicle for use by the DHE
+ Upgrading of telecommunications systems
+ Electrification and water reticulation systems
+ Information technology for the institution
+ In-service training for DHE members
+ The purchase of household and recreational items

Health workers benefiting from the scheme were required to open foreign currency accounts into which their allowances were deposited. Funds for the rest of the DHE were deposited into an existing Health Service Fund (pool fund) account at district level. Health workers who benefited from the scheme were employed on a performance contract which has penalty clauses for any breach of the contract. The MOHCW also piloted another incentive scheme which was financed by the Global Fund and was selectively targeted at improving the conditions of service for laboratory staff. This scheme was part of support to Health Systems Strengthening by the Global Fund and was aimed at improving the quality of TB, Malaria and HIV/AIDS programs.

In the wake of the 2008 national elections the government of Zimbabwe unveiled yet another skills retention initiative which it referred to as the first phase of the Medical Sector Skills Retention Program. The program consisted of the allocation of a total of 510 vehicles for personal use by senior and middle level medical doctors, senior nurses and other health professionals; the distribution of 97 ambulances to public sector institutions and the distribution of 52 staff buses to central, provincial and district hospitals throughout the country.

Considering the extent and duration of the HRH crisis in the country it was the opinion of many analysts that the government should have adopted a more holistic approach as opposed to piloting initiatives in a fragmented manner. The principle behind these initiatives was not new though these incentives needed to benefit health professionals as a team as opposed to excluding other categories of health professionals. When such initiatives are supported by external funds or are implemented in an ad hoc manner, there is always the problem of sustainability. Sustainability can be guaranteed if such schemes are designed within the national macroeconomic framework which incorporates them within civil service salary and pay reforms.

Towards resolving HRH issues

There are several aspects of the human resources problem that can be targeted for possible resolution and these include:
+ The supply of personnel
+ Plan for adequate numbers of staff in the various workforce categories – projections
+ Training – different categories of staff with the necessary skills
  + Adapting curricula to policy objectives
  + Developing new teaching & learning methods
  + Monitoring training requirements
  + Developing training infrastructure
  + Training an adequate number of trainers
  + Regulating training institutions & programs

Work conditions – develop policy guidelines to address
+ Recruitment methods
+ Retention of staff
+ Career management
+ Staff deployment – equitable distribution of staff
+ Methods and levels of remuneration and incentives
+ Management of labor relations

Performance Management – to ensure that staff provides effective efficient & high quality services
+ Orientation of staff to the organization
+ Establishing and enforcing practice standards
+ Implementing appropriate payment methods – linked to productivity
+ Developing management practices tools
+ Implementing quality assurance frameworks
+ Developing evaluation and accountability mechanisms

Systems for monitoring and evaluation
  ◆ Developing indicators to monitor & evaluate HRH (HR information systems)

Most important of all is an engagement at the global level on international recruitment of health workers from developing countries by rich countries, without, of course infringing on health worker rights to mobility. Donor instruments must be redesigned so that they provide long term support to sustained HRH development and retention. The state must engage with non-state organizations (NGOs) who also contribute to increased internal brain drain by actively recruiting health workers from the public sector and offering better conditions of service. Cognizance of their contribution to the evolution of the HRH crisis in developing countries, in May 2008 NGOs developed a Code of Conduct on health systems strengthening in developing countries. NGOs pledged to adopt relevant practices that will not affect long term sustainability of public health systems by limiting their recruitment from the public sector. They pledged to support efforts to improve conditions of service in the public health sector so as to encourage workers to remain in the public sector and to support efforts to expand pre-service training.

Health sector reforms and HRH

The impact of macroeconomic reforms on human resources for health has been widely discussed in the literature. Major elements of health sector reforms address issues of cost reduction, improving performance, increasing equity, decentralization and public private collaboration. As is the case with SAPs, the implementation of health reforms has direct and indirect consequences on the development and management of HRH.

For those reforms in which one wishes to make cost savings in a health budget one must identify those items that are the major cost drivers for health expenditures. The health sector is a labor intensive industry with HRH costs which may contribute upwards of 60% to the recurrent health budget. Whilst SAPs have traditionally advocated for the downsizing of the civil service, health sector reforms on the other hand push for the right sizing of staff within the sector. This implies the application of rational methods of determining staff requirements, usually based on workload estimates as opposed to standard staff establishments which do not have any rational basis. Other reforms have advocated for improved skills mix and an increase in the number of assistants and technicians, the introduction of new categories of health workers and the modification of staff working conditions by carefully rationalizing methods of remuneration. The intention in this case is to broaden the base of the HRH triangle within the sector. A good example is the introduction of the PCN in Zimbabwe and the proposal to increase the role of the clinical nursing officers at district hospital level.

The introduction of performance appraisal systems for health professionals is aimed at linking remuneration to expected health worker performance. This however requires an extensive review of existing incentive systems and the improvement in work organization within government. In the same context, some institutions have resorted to employing staff on part time contracts and on a shift basis, depending on the workload experienced at any particular time. This has made it possible for the health sector to offer employment opportunities to some retired health professionals who are willing to work part time at public health facilities. In the same vein, private practitioners also provide part time services at government institutions.

The decentralization of service delivery and the transfer of additional responsibilities in decision making to the lower levels of the health system mean that appropriate capacity has to be developed at these levels. Additional staff with experience in the management of health services has to be deployed or employed at the same level. In some cases additional management posts have to be established to ensure that additional responsibilities are effectively executed.

Kolehmainen-Aitken RL (1998) has analyzed four HRH issues that arise from the decentralization of health services. Data on HRH is critical to any decision to reallocate staff that has previously been under the Public Service Commission to local government. Information on job positions, grades and job descriptions is usually not available or is outdated and only available at the central level. It should be acknowledged that with decentralization, the transfer of staff to local control is more complex than the handover of facilities and equipment and that there is usually a need to create a new organizational structure, positions and the revision of job descriptions. In order to achieve equity in access to health services it is necessary to develop a staff deployment policy and thus establish a more balanced distribution of health professionals throughout the country. This can be complemented by the development and implementation of innovative incentives and strategies to retain staff in rural and remote areas that are considered difficult to staff.

Conclusions and the way forward

In Zimbabwe de-linkage of health staff from the PSC was achieved through the establishment of an autonomous Health Services Board. The allocation of the operational budget of the Health Service Board through the MOHCW is however a matter of serious concern. Such a situation compromises the independence and objectivity of the Health Service Board in making decisions regarding the grading of health posts, determination of promotions and conditions of services for its "paymaster", the MOHCW. It is therefore not surprising that there have been anecdotal reports of situations where some ministry of health officials have attempted to use the budget as leverage to "encourage" the Health Services Board to make appointments outside the Board's due process. Considering that the Board is a legal entity in its own right, a decision must be made to ensure that it receives its budget allocation directly from the Treasury. The salary and wages budget for the MOHCW should be the result of financial estimates that arise from discussions between the Board and the MOHCW, in line with the ministry's planning and budget process. Lessons must be learnt from the difficult relationships that prevailed between the PSC and the MOHCW.

Furthermore, it is not appropriate for the Health Services Board to have been assigned the responsibility to "supervise... health service employees". This is the day to day responsibility of health institutions and the CEOs of semi-autonomous institutions. It is also inappropriate for the Health Services Board to supervise and monitor the performance of Hospital Management Boards. This task is well within the responsibilities of the office of the Minister of Health and Child Welfare.

Now that the health sector has developed its HRH Policy framework, the Ministry of Health must ensure that the actual implementation of the policy responds to the requirements of health service delivery and health needs. Coordination mechanisms must be developed to ensure harmony amongst the various HRH activities, including putting in place a monitoring and evaluation framework. All possible efforts must be made to mobilize enough resources to support the activities that are required to realize the objectives of the HRH policy. The potential for inadequate institutional capacity to implement the policy must be pre-empted. Due cognizance must be taken of the fact that the unavailability of adequate information on staff distribution is another potential impediment to evidence based policy implementation. Ultimately the government and its development partners must express their willingness and commitment to improving the HRH situation in the country. Chatora R, *et al* (2006) have developed simple guidelines which can assist countries in formulating, developing and reviewing their HRH situations, policies and plans. These guidelines are targeted at government departments, in particular ministries of health.

The total output of institutions responsible for training HRH must be increased in line with the projected needs of the national health system, both public and private. Where the government does not have adequate capacity to train, private institutions should be encouraged and contracted to train health professionals under the close scrutiny of professional bodies. This is to ensure that they produce acceptable quality health professionals. Development partners must commit to invest in additional support to complement government efforts to increase the capacity for pre-service training. Incentive schemes must also include the retention of trainers of health professionals.

There must be due cognizance of the fact that HRH issues are unique in their own right and that there is a serious HRH problem that needs to be resolved as a crisis. There must be a clear realization that it takes a very long time to rectify policy mistakes made in the HRH area. For example, a 10% rise in the number of medical school entrants only produces a 2% increase in the supply of doctors in a period of 10 years. Therefore, any attempts to scale up services, e.g. the ART roll out programs, must allow for the appropriate lead times needed to train and develop health professionals, (Dubois 2004).

The Health Services Board in Zimbabwe should be given the leeway and resources to develop and implement incentives and conditions of service that can attract and retain staff. The MOHCW should establish an effective human resources department staffed by well qualified human resources professionals. Appropriate indicators and a monitoring and evaluation framework must be developed to monitor progress towards the achievement of HRH objectives and targets.

To conclude, solutions to the HRH problem are complex and lie in:
+ Evidence based and effective workforce planning and rationalization
+ Shifting tasks from higher level professionals to lower level workers through the review of policies and licensing procedures.
+ Improving HR information systems to ensure accurate and up to date information

- Improving HRH management by strengthening HR departments, training staff in HR management, processes, practices, etc
- Developing incentive schemes to keep workers on the job; financial and non financial incentives; clear career structures; efficient recruitment, employment and transfer processes, policies and practices; safe work environment.
- Establishing partnerships to share the work load within the public sector.

At the end of it all, it is the responsibility of national governments, complemented by development partners, to increase health expenditures and allocate adequate amounts of resources to strengthen the area of HRH development, especially in improving their conditions of service, leadership development and strengthening HRH management within ministries of health.

Review questions

1. Identify the main factors contributing to the Human Resources for Health crises in Africa.
2. Describe the process you would follow in developing a HRH policy and plan for a ministry of health in a developing country.
3. Develop a framework that you can use to monitor and evaluate progress in the implementation of a HRH policy and plan.
4. What are the implications of the HRH crisis in the achievement of the MDGs?
5. What are the advantages and disadvantages of de-linking the ministry of health from the Public Service Commission or any similar body that determines salaries and conditions of service for all civil servants in a country?

5

DECENTRALIZATION OF HEALTH SERVICES

Introduction

Decentralization is common in almost all the African countries that are reforming their health sectors. There are several aspects to decentralization, namely; the devolution of authority and responsibility from central government to local government agencies, the deconcentration of functions from higher to lower levels within the administrative apparatus of government and the delegation of responsibilities and functions from central government units to other more autonomous or specialized government agencies such as research institutes, parastatals, reference laboratories etc.

The main objective of decentralization is to promote efficiency and public accountability. In this context the central organs of government are responsible for the establishment of equitable means of allocating resources and ensuring the existence of effective regulatory mechanisms in the sector as a whole. Each country identifies the appropriate balance between centralized and decentralized functions, responsibility and/or authority that best meet its own policy objectives.

The design of a decentralization policy requires the identification of the functions of the organization that are likely to benefit from such a policy direction. There are several functions that have the potential to benefit from decentralization within the health sector, Box 5.1. Within each of these functions it is necessary to determine the objectives that have to be achieved. For example, under human resources, does the ministry want the local agency to be able to hire and fire staff or to determine their conditions of service? In some cases decisions are best made at the central level rather than at the operational levels, e.g. human resources planning, resource allocation, policy formulation, etc. On the other hand other decisions require to be made at the operational level e.g. the development and application of exemption mechanisms, use of revenue from cost recovery, etc. In other situations decisions that would have otherwise been made at the decentralized level have to evolve in a phased manner in tandem with capacity building efforts.

It is important to realize that decentralization is a power game and as such there will always be conflicts and tensions during its implementation. The potential for and extent of such conflicts, possible losers and winners must be evaluated well in advance so that appropriate measures can be taken to mitigate their impact. It is helpful to develop a strategic plan for the decentralization process so as to accommodate any capacity building needs. A form of feedback mechanism and a monitoring system to keep the process of reform on track and to identify any corrections necessary along the way must be considered imperative.

Box 5.1 Decentralization and functions of the ministry of health

Functions of the MOH that can be decentralized
Planning
• Program design
Finance
• Revenue generation and sources
• Budgeting: revenue allocation
• Expenditure management and accounting
• Financial audit
Human Resources
• Staffing (hiring, firing, evaluation)
• Salaries and benefits
• Training
Service Delivery and Program Implementation
• Targeting service delivery
• Monitoring and oversight of service providers
• User participation
• Contracting
Operations and Maintenance
• Drugs and supplies (ordering, payment and inventory)
• Vehicles and equipment
• Facilities and infrastructure
Information Management
• Data collection, processing and analysis
• Dissemination of information to various stakeholders.

Decentralization policy in Zimbabwe

In December 1994 the Government of Zimbabwe (GOZ) reiterated its policy decision to implement decentralization through the transfer of responsibilities and functions from central government to field offices and local authorities in the form of Urban and Rural District Councils (RDCs).

Legislated roles of Urban and Rural District Councils

Local governance in Zimbabwe is based on sub-national institutions in the form of Urban and Rural District Councils in urban and rural areas of the country respectively. There are 28 Urban Councils established under the Urban Councils Act (Chapter 29:15) of which 6 are City Councils, and 58 Rural District Councils which are established under the Rural District Councils Act (Chapter 29:13).

Urban and RDCs have greater responsibilities for planning and development in their areas of jurisdiction. The delivery of health services was one of the major responsibilities of these councils. To facilitate this transition and the implementation of added responsibilities the Ministry of Local Government, Rural and Urban Development (MILGRUD) and the MOHCW developed guidelines to assist RDCs in the management of the delivery of their health services. The guidelines included those for staffing norms, standard plans for health facilities, criteria to guide RDCs in locating and designing new health facilities and guidelines to manage human resources.

RDCs have always owned and managed several static clinics which are staffed according to MOHCW norms and supervised by the District Nursing Officer or the Community Health Nurse. Staff salaries have also been paid by the MOHCW through a grant to the RDCs.

The roles and responsibilities of RDCs in the provision of public health services are outlined in the Public Health Act and the RDCs Act of 1988, as follows:

♦ To provide health services within their local authority or area of jurisdiction, including curative, preventive and rehabilitative services.
♦ To operate health facilities such as hospitals, clinics, health centers and mobile health services.
♦ To provide maternal and child health services including maternity and Family Planning services

♦ To operate ambulance services within their area and refer patients to the next level of health care when necessary

♦ To provide and prepare for disaster control in order to preserve life and property

♦ To provide safe water supplies and sanitation in their local authority areas

♦ To carry out disease and environmental health control activities which include:

    ♦ Inspection of premises.

    ♦ Air and water pollution and sanitation.

    ♦ Refuse disposal of both solid and liquid waste, including its treatment.

    ♦ Carrying out business and building inspections including monitoring building standards.

    ♦ Issuing licenses to institutions that meet health standards.

    ♦ Ensuring the provision of vermin and insect control measures.

    ♦ Carrying out inspections and ensuring that health regulations on food handling and sale on premises are met, (Lenneiye, 2000).

At the MOHCW headquarters level there is a section which deals with the administration of staffing and financing issues related to RDCs and missions, the Councils and Missions Section. The day-to-day operations of the health activities of RDCs are supported and coordinated by the DHMT under the guidance of the Provincial Medical Directors.

RDCs have always experienced problems in the running of their health services, some of which are:

♦ Inadequate funding

♦ Inadequate staffing levels

♦ Poorly maintained facilities

♦ Poor financial and health information systems

♦ Delays in payment of salaries for their staff

♦ Health facilities which do not meet the minimum standards set by the MOHCW.

Framework for decentralization in Zimbabwe

In 1994 the Government of Zimbabwe (GOZ) commissioned a needs analysis for capacity building within local government authorities. As a follow up to this analysis a strategic plan for building the capacity of RDCs was developed and adopted by government. The government established the Rural District Council Capacity Building Program (RDCCBP) which was wholly supported by a consortium of like-minded development partners.

During the same year the Minister of the Public Service, Labor and Social Welfare announced that *'government would transfer functions within central government hierarchy by shifting some responsibilities of ministries to field offices and local authorities through decentralization'* (Hansard, 1994). The implementation of the decentralization process was delegated to a Working Party of Permanent Secretaries which in turn was serviced by the Capacity Building Co-coordinating Committee (CBCC) responsible for the day-to-day co-coordination of the decentralization process.

The Ministerial Committee on decentralization which was established in 1996 adopted the following 13 Principles which form the basis for the decentralization process in Zimbabwe.

1. "That decentralization is necessary and desirable and is based on the clear understanding that it promotes and strengthens democracy and civic responsibility as citizens participate in their governance and development. It also helps in minimizing bureaucracy by reducing the levels of decision-making and thereby achieving greater efficiency of operations. However, it will not be taken as a strategy for dumping problems of sector ministries to Rural District Councils.

2. That decentralization be defined and understood to mean the legislated transfer of functions and authority from central government to local authorities such as the Rural District Councils (RDCs) on a permanent basis. Once provided for in law, such transfer of powers and functions can be reversed only on the basis of an amendment to the appropriate law.

3. That there is need for all ministries to use the same local institutions for the implementation and management of decentralized functions and not to create parallel or separate institutions. Where parallel institutions exist, these should be harmonized.

4. That decentralization is a process and not an event, as such; it should be implemented cautiously and progressively, having regard to the human, financial and material capacities of the local authorities to which the transfers would be made.

5. That in respect of those activities and projects to be undertaken by local authorities, sector ministries retain the power and authority to set standards, monitor performance and consistency to national policies and standards, and intervene appropriately to ensure

compliance. This means that local authorities will, in executing their legal powers and responsibilities, be required to comply with the requirements of national policies, laws and regulations.

6. That an inter-ministerial committee of Ministers to manage decentralization and capacity building be established. In this regard, the existing inter-ministerial Capacity Building Co-coordinating Committee (CBCC) will report to a Working Party of Heads of Ministries, who in turn will report to Ministers on policy issues.

7. That central government, in implementing decentralization, shall strengthen financial, human and material resource capacities of RDCs so as to make them effective institutions in the provision of the social and infrastructure services needed for sustainable local development.

8. That central government will continue to be responsible for the provision of trunk services which impact upon more than one local authority area or are of a national character. This refers to all social, infrastructure and economic projects that impact upon more than one local authority and call for more resources than can be mobilized by one local authority.

9. For this purpose, line ministries concerned will provide guidelines on which projects are to be undertaken by local authorities having regard to the social and economic impact of projects, the capital outlay required and the level of professional and technical expertise needed to execute the projects.

10. That the transfer of powers and functions by line ministries to RDCs be done by the line ministry concerned and that the Ministry of Local Government, Rural and Urban Development will co-ordinate and facilitate this effort.

11. That all monies for recurrent and capital expenditure sourced by line ministries and are earmarked for rural district councils be disbursed to the Rural District Councils soon after the promulgation of the Appropriation Act. Such grants will not pass through the Ministry of Local Government, Rural and Urban Development (MLGRUD).

12. That all loans to RDCs should be channeled through the MLGRUD except for those loans from the National Housing Fund administered by the Ministry of Public Construction and National Housing which will be disbursed direct to the

councils by that ministry. The Ministry of Public Construction and National Housing disburses the loans only after the local authority concerned has been granted borrowing powers by the MILGRUD.

13. That in Zimbabwe there be only two levels which collect taxes, levies, and other user charges namely central government and local authorities. Thus RDCs should collect such taxes, levies, fees and user charges for those services they should provide in terms of any appropriate law or regulation".

The Public Service Commission would manage the transfer of personnel from central government to RDCs where this happens as part of decentralization.

Theoretical concepts of decentralization

Decentralization involves the transfer of authority, or the dispersal of power from central institutions to specialized functional units which then assume responsibilities for public planning, management and decision-making, resource mobilization and allocation at local government level (Fersler, 1965). There are several forms and degrees of decentralization, namely; deconcentration, delegation and devolution. Minis and Rondinelli (1989) distinguish between three types of decentralization:

Administrative decentralization

This is defined as the transfer of responsibility for planning, management, and the raising and allocation of resources from central government and its agencies to field units of government agencies, operational units or levels of government, semi-autonomous public institutions or corporations, area-wide, regional or functional authorities, or non-governmental private or voluntary organizations. This type of decentralization can be subdivided into three categories: devolution, deconcentration and delegation.

Devolution to Local Government

This entails the creation of units of government which are to a great extent autonomous and consisting of distinct legal entities from central government. Authority is transferred to elected local governments and central government retains some authority to control or oversee the activities of such units. Local governments have the power to raise revenue and make expenditures on local programs and projects. They have the power to make decisions independent of central government.

Deconcentration

Facilities or functions are dispersed from central government to local units with the objective of improving effectiveness and efficiency of delivery systems. Central directives can however be adjusted to suit local conditions within guidelines set by the central level. This type of reorganization is financed through grants from the central authority to provincial, district or local administrative units. Deconcentration is an important intermediate step, which can improve the managerial process as a temporary option where a shortage of staff and skills limits full decentralization. Terms like functional and integrated deconcentration have sometimes been used where such entities share resources such as administrative costs or finances across sectors.

Delegation

Managerial responsibilities for defined functions are transferred to lower levels of government, which are not within the regular bureaucratic structure, lower units such as public corporations, semi-autonomous institutions and various parastatals or quasi-government organizations and institutions. In the health field delegation has been used in the management of teaching hospitals in some African countries (Mills, 1990) in the name of improving efficiency in the management of public sector enterprises.

In each of these forms of decentralization significant authority and responsibility usually remains at the center. In some cases this shift redefines the functional responsibilities so that the center retains policy making and monitoring roles and the periphery gains operational responsibility for the day-to-day administration.

Decentralization can enhance community empowerment, participation and provide a greater opportunity for the responsiveness of governments to local needs. The application of decentralization in the health sector reflects recognition of both the need to move resources to the neglected poor and to facilitate community participation. The reallocation of authority and resources is a major issue that affects internal power relationships within the public sector and the access of social groups to the decision-making process and state resources. This transfer is however not absolute.

Whilst privatization has been considered by some as a form of decentralization, Collins and Green (1994) are of the view that privatization and decentralization are essentially two different phenomena. One reallocates within the system and the other reallocates between systems. They further argue that if privatization is to be justified for developing countries it should be on the basis of its own arguments and not those of decentralization.

Proponents of decentralization further argue that a centralized bureaucracy suffers from inflexibility, excessive administrative levels and an inability to provide services which are responsive to the needs of different types of clients. Many countries have pursued this policy as a solution to the delays which are caused by long and winding channels of administration and communication.

Various models of decentralization will have differing effects on equity. As an example, the decentralization of revenue generation and resource allocation are likely to bring with them difficulties in the preservation of equity based policies. Richer districts would naturally be able to generate more funds locally. With retention and local use of such resources, inter-community inequities would arise. Equalization grants to poor districts from central government would become a disincentive for any community willing to raise finances locally.

The decentralization of health services in Zimbabwe

The proposed role of the central Ministry of Health in a decentralized system

In many instances of decentralization the administrative role of national health departments seems to have decreased considerably. The truth of the matter is that decentralization can only be effective '*if the center develops its strategic role, allowing the periphery to be the major operational arm of the health sector*' (Cheema, et al, 1983).

In its decentralization concept paper the MOHCW envisages the role of the central MOHCW to be confined to but not limited to the following:

- ♦ Health policy formulation
- ♦ Mobilization and allocation of resources, public health budget analysis and formulation
- ♦ Human resources planning, development and national deployment of personnel
- ♦ Provision of a regulatory environment to facilitate the operation of all providers of health

+ Epidemiological surveillance, monitoring and evaluation of the health status of the nation
+ Liaison with international health organizations and aid agencies
+ Setting standards and monitoring adherence to such standards

The effective implementation of decentralization policies has often proven to be difficult because of:

+ Reluctance of central ministries to transfer the power that matters i.e. resources to the local level
+ Lack of the right mix of skills at local level
+ Lack of accompanying changes or supporting roles that are needed at central level e.g. capacity to monitor
+ Powerful interest groups such as civil servants who, because they may not be willing to be employed by local government, tend to undermine attempts to decentralize decision-making to the districts (Sikosana, et al. 1997)

There is the general view that there are some areas of decision-making powers that should not be decentralized, namely:

+ General provisions concerning health policy as this is considered a fundamental preserve of the state
+ Strategic decisions on the development of health resources, including human resources development and deployment, accreditation and licensing, major capital developments, sourcing expensive equipment and development of the national research agenda
+ Regulation of the health sector to protect the public interest in the areas of professional practice, quality of drugs and standards setting
+ Monitoring, assessment and analysis of the health of the population particularly monitoring equity between different geographical regions and social strata (Saltman, (Eds) 1999)

The form of decentralization proposed for and adopted by the Zimbabwe health delivery system is a hybrid of administrative decentralization characterized by a combination of deconcentration to the district level and devolution to Rural District Councils and semi-autonomous public health institutions.

Decentralization has in the past few years become central to the MO-HCW's health reform agenda which started in the mid 1990s (MOHCW, 1995). The concept paper on decentralization developed by the MOHCW proposes the transfer of the management of RHCs and district hospitals to RDCs, the establishment of Hospital Management Boards (HMB) at provincial and central hospitals as well as the establishment of District Health Management Boards (DHMB).

The government wide decentralization process coordinated by the Capacity Building Coordinating Committee (CBCC) specified that the RDCs would be responsible for the following:

+ *The procurement and management of ambulances.*
+ *The hiring of all staff and decentralization of their conditions of service including salaries and allowances.*
+ *The provision of sanitary services including effluent treatment and disposal.*
+ *The provision of child welfare and nutrition services.*
+ *The provision of environmental health services including health and hygiene promotion.*

In addition to the above:

+ *The funds for these activities sourced by the Ministry of Health and Child Welfare will be disbursed direct to the councils and all assets, movable and immovable such as buildings, vehicles, plant and equipment belonging to the government should be transferred to the RDCs.*
+ *The transfer of further responsibilities should be cautious and gradual, taking cognizance of the councils' capabilities to absorb and manage the new responsibilities.*
+ *The agency through which monitoring and supervision of district health functions will be the Provincial Health Executive'.*

The MOHCW also proposed that RHCs and district hospitals be transferred to and be managed by RDCs. The above list complements the health responsibilities of RDCs outlined in the Public Health Act.

An outline of the decentralization process in the MOHCW

In 1999 a study was conducted to review how the process of decentralization in the MOHCW had been conceived and to determine the extent to which it had been implemented since the adoption of the decentralization policy framework in 1994. The study covered several areas which include the policy formulation process within the MOHCW, the extent of implementation and the impact of decentralization on the health delivery system. The following sections outline some of the findings from the study.

The rationale and objectives of decentralization

The generic rationale behind decentralization is to facilitate the implementation of more flexible and adaptable management practices, inter-sectoral co-ordination and community participation. Decentralization also claims to provide a framework for greater responsiveness of government policies to the needs of local populations.

During the course of the study it was not possible to find any explicit statement on why the MOHCW chose to embark on the process of decentralization. A statement in the concept document states that 'In line with international trends, it is proposed that district health services be owned by Rural District Councils...to ensure efficiency and responsiveness to local needs' (MOHCW, 1995).

A review document by the Danish International Development Agency (DANIDA) states that the goals of decentralization in the Zimbabwe health sector were:

+ 'To make health services more responsive to user needs and preferences by bringing the planning and management of services closer to the point at which they are delivered, and

+ To delegate decision making to the appropriate levels of management so that operational matters are decided by those responsible for providing the service' (DANIDA: Zimbabwe, 1997)

From the point of view of central government, decentralization is aimed at contributing to the attainment of *the political, administrative and economic objectives of government*. The objectives of which have been stated as:

+ To promote democracy, public participation and civic responsibility;

+ To increase efficiency and effectiveness in government and therefore enhance service delivery;

+ To reduce the role and cost of central government administration' (GOZ/CBCC, May 1998)

The objectives of the Public Service Commission (PSC) in the decentralization process have been expressed in the context of Civil Service Reforms as being: *'to facilitate speedy and efficient decision-making when providing government services to the public....'* (GOZ/PSC, May 1998).

The consensus building process

Records show that the Ministry of Health and Child Welfare began its consultative process on decentralization in 1994. There is evidence that consultations involved policy makers within the health ministry and MOHCW representatives from the district, provincial and central levels. There is however no conclusive evidence that civil society and other government departments were fully involved in these consultations. Documents show that the outcome of the consultation process on decentralization and other reforms was presented and adopted at a national workshop of stakeholders which was held in Harare in February 1996. Records of the meeting indicate that some NGOs and development partners attended the feedback meeting which represented the end stage of the process to develop a decentralization strategy for the health sector.

Information collected through interviews with health workers shows that the majority believe that the consultation process on the decentralization of health services was inadequate. Only 11% (CI: 7.6-15.9) of those interviewed had personally participated in the policy and strategy formulation processes. This result may however reflect the high turnover of staff within the MOHCW.

From the CBCC report of June 1998 there were some concerns expressed by provincial heads of government ministries as to the lack of consultation and information dissemination about the decentralization process. It was stated that, *"There was a lack of consultation before the enactment of the decentralization policy and a subsequent lack of dissemination of the policy within some ministries. Decentralization has been kept as a secret for head offices alone".*

Community groups under the umbrella of the Community Working Group on Health (CWGH) expressed a similar view on the decentralization process, that, *'it is perhaps yet another example of "thinking for" rather than "thinking with"'* (CWGH, 1998).

This same study referred to above did not find any documented evidence which suggested that donors had explicitly brought pressure to bear on the government to pursue the policy of decentralization. However, a record of the minutes of a special CBCC meeting held on the 29th August

1997 states that this particular meeting had voiced its concerns as to the role of donors in the decentralization process; *'there was a strong feeling that there was donor competition in the decentralization exercise and the CBCC needed to be careful in making decisions that would not embroil them in donor politics.'*

Pilot versus full-scale decentralization

An earlier version of the ministry's concept document on Health Sector Reforms (MOHCW, 1995) stated that *'Given the difficulties of successfully managing the process of decentralization, adequate attention needs to be paid to the political and economic context in which implementation is taking place... It is strongly recommended that the proposed form of decentralization be piloted in one province with a potential for an adequate supply side response'.*

It appears that this position was subsequently abandoned in-line with the government framework for decentralization which involved all the administrative districts of the country. Reference to piloting decentralization does not appear in the final version of the ministry's concept document.

Rather than adopt a radical approach to health reforms the ministry of health opted for an incremental approach to its reforms. This approach is in line with principle (4) of the government's 13 Principles on decentralization.

The institutional framework to support decentralization

By 1997 an institutional framework to support the decentralization process in government had been agreed to and consisted of:
- A Cabinet Committee of Ministers on Decentralization
- A Working Party of Permanent Secretaries
- A Capacity Building Coordinating Committee (CBCC)
- Provincial Development Committees (PDC)
- District Development Committees (DDC)

On its part the MOHCW established a Strategic Development Unit to co-ordinate its health reform program. DANIDA and the EU provided technical advisors who were attached to this unit.

Legislative changes to support health sector reforms

There has been an assumption that because the Rural District Councils Act (1988) allows RDCs to undertake up to 64 separate functions, this provision automatically provides the legal framework for the implementation of decentralization. Despite this assumption proposals were made to review the Rural District Councils Act so that it could explicitly provide for the processes, roles and responsibilities of the various parties within a decentralized governance system.

The promulgation of the Health Professions Act (1999) established the Health Professions Authority of Zimbabwe (HPA), as the successor organization to the Health Professions Council (HPC) of Zimbabwe. The Health Professions Authority, as established, is an independent regulatory body that monitors the quality of professional practice in Zimbabwe on behalf of the Ministry of Health and Child Welfare.

The amendment to the Drugs and Allied Substances Control Act (No 1) of 1996 paved the way for the establishment of the Medicines Control Authority of Zimbabwe (MCAZ) as a semi-autonomous organization replacing and taking over the functions of the Drugs Control Council (DCC) of Zimbabwe. The responsibilities of the MCAZ include the registration and control of prescription, sale, dispensing and storage of drugs by both the private and public sectors. Amongst other responsibilities this organization monitors the quality of all medicines registered for prescription in the country and ensures that there is ethical practice within the pharmaceutical industry. In this same area of managing public sector pharmaceuticals another Act of Parliament was enacted to commercialize the MOHCW owned Government Medical Stores. In its place a government owned, not-for-profit commercial company managed by a Board of Directors was established.

The Medical Services Act (1998) provides the legal framework to guide the establishment and operation of health establishments by public and private providers and for the first time, in Zimbabwe, the regulation of medical insurance schemes. Under this Act the Minister of Health seeks to:

+ Regulate the establishment of private hospital development.
+ Regulate access to both private and public hospitals.
+ Regulate the operations of the Association of Healthcare Funders of Zimbabwe (AHFoZ), formerly known as Medical Aid Societies, (private or voluntary health insurance schemes).
+ Monitor the quality of care in private and public health institutions.
+ Establish Hospital Management Boards.

In terms of Section 30 of the Audit and Exchequer Act [Chapter 22.03] and an Act of Parliament of 1996 the MOHCW established a Health Services Fund (HSF) which allows all government hospitals, the MOHCW headquarters, provincial and district offices to operate separate bank accounts for this fund. This account facilitated the deposit, pooling and local use of revenue from user fees, funds from some donors and other donations. The main objective was to provide flexibility in the local management and use of both donor and GOZ funds allocated to the provinces and districts.

Capacity building to support decentralization

Successful initiatives to decentralize authority have almost always been accompanied by management strengthening at the central, regional and district levels. There has always been a deliberate focus to improve the capacity of local government, amongst other things, in tendering, contracting, supervision procedures and the training of local contractors in bidding and project implementation.

As central and regional staff shift from exercising control as supervisors to emphasizing policy formulation, strategy development, resource mobilization and technical backstopping, they must receive appropriate training in these areas.

In Zimbabwe there was some concern about the absence of linkages between decentralization in sector ministries and the RDCCBP at national level. Sector ministries did not know how to achieve this link and to relate their internal capacity building efforts to those of the CBCC. This situation has been attributed to a structural problem whereby central government is structured and operates on a sectoral basis yet the development of linkages between capacity building and decentralization demands an inter-sectoral approach.

The mindset of sector ministries remains focused on the demands of their individual sectors and not on a common or integrating environment created by the capacity building program. An impression was thus created that the capacity building and decentralization programs were largely creations of top-level managers.

The RDC capacity building program had 3 components to it:
♦ Capital funding which provided financial resources
♦ The institutional development component for organizational development
♦ The Human Resources Development component to address basic deficiencies in administrative, financial and technical skills

The MOHCW established a Management Strengthening Project as early in the process as 1990. The project focused on the development of a management competence framework for managers in the Zimbabwe health system. It formed the basis upon which the Executive Management Development Program was developed. The objective of the program was to develop a critical mass of skilled managers at the national, district and provincial levels. The study results indicate that this program did not reach most of the intended groups of people within the MOHCW as only 17% (CI: 12.6-22.4) of those interviewed had taken part in the capacity building program.

Public participation and decentralization

Guaranteeing public participation in decision-making through the involvement of communities and their representatives is one of the major objectives of decentralization. In Zimbabwe evidence shows that over the years community participation continued to be weak. This is because communities expected and believed that the government would continue to provide free health care and that their role was merely to consume it. As a result communities were never exposed to experiences in local planning, resource mobilization and the monitoring of their own health services and health status.

The development of priorities at local level requires the input of a variety of skills. Communities must be able to clearly articulate what their priorities are, the professionals must say what is feasible and possible and administrators to oversee the process. The involvement of local communities in decision-making must be real with a balance between professional input and popular will. Information gathered must be such that it helps individuals to act effectively with respect to their own destiny in health.

Since the early 1980s the government of Zimbabwe developed participatory and local governance structures through which the public and local communities could participate in decision-making processes at the local level. Some of these structures are shown in Figure 5.1:

- ◆ Village Development Committees (VIDCO)
- ◆ Health Centre Committees
- ◆ Ward Health Teams
- ◆ District Development Committees (DDC)

There are several operational problems which the committees depicted in Figure 5.1 have been faced with. The main problem has been that of little or no participation from the members. This has been attributed to few or no incentives for the members to attend these meetings. In some cases there are feelings of frustration because these committees often do not have any meaningful influence or authority over the operations of health staff at the local level (Lowenson et al., 1999). In other instances local leaders are held back from participating by illiteracy, lack of knowledge of government procedures and low awareness of their rights (UNDP, 2000).

Figure 5.1   Structures for local participation in Zimbabwe

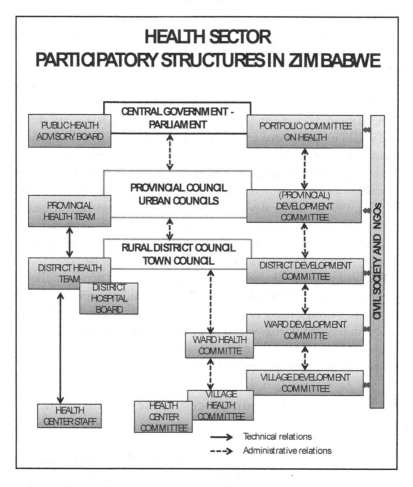

In 1997 the Strategic Development Unit (SDU) of the MOHCW developed planning guidelines to strengthen the planning process within the MOHCW in preparation for the devolution process. The plans would be developed within the framework of the National Health Strategy and in line with the Medium Term Expenditure Framework (MTEF) of government. This meant that the plans would be rolled over three years and implemented on the basis of annual plans at the various levels of the health system. With the subsequent restructuring of the MOHCW the SDU was abolished and replaced by a Planning Unit within the Policy and Planning Division.

Management structures at the local level

In proposing the establishment of Hospital Management Boards (HMB) the MOHCW also proposed that the board members be appointed by the Minister of Health and Child Welfare. This suggestion did not go down well with the Community Working Group on Health (CWGH) who felt that a board appointed in this manner would not carry the mandate of interest groups. In order to reduce this democratic deficit the CWGH proposed that the appointments be transparent and include elected and nominated representatives from civil society groups.

It was further proposed that such representatives should have access to information and education needed for them to make informed decisions (CWGH, 1999). Similar views were expressed by focus group discussants in the study on decentralization who suggested that the composition of Hospital Management Boards needed to be *'flexible and include qualified persons of integrity who live within the catchment area of the facility'.*

The final position adopted on the composition and accountability of Hospital Management Boards at central and provincial hospitals was that they would be responsible to the Minister of Health and Child Welfare. Membership to the boards would be by appointment by the Minister of Health and Child Welfare from nominations from civil society, professional and other groups as specified in the Medical Services Act.

Has the decentralization process achieved the intended results?

A study conducted in Botswana (Leuglo and Molutsi, 1994) states that decentralization did not achieve the goals of equity as had been expected. Instead the process resulted in increased bureaucratic barriers to decision making. The authors conclude in their article that there was little evidence of increased community participation or inter-sectoral co-ordination as a result of the decentralization process in that country.

The assumption underlying decentralization is that decentralized units will spend resources efficiently and provide higher quality services. It is expected that there will be improved staff motivation and satisfaction leading to an increase in their responsiveness to local needs.

A study conducted to determine the outcome and impact of decentralization in Zimbabwe showed that changes which could be directly attributed to decentralization were in the main confined to processes of policy formulation and structural organizational changes.

Financial Management

There was strong evidence that managers at the provincial, district and institutional levels were now making financial decisions and transactions much more quickly, especially in the use of resources in the HSF. It is no longer necessary for cost centers to ask for permission each time they have to spend money. What is required is for the DHMT to make sure that they stay within the set budget, stick to the approved plans and account for the expenditures in line with their program of work. However cost centers have continued being unable to transfer funds between budget items without authorization from the central level to do so. Overall the operation of the HSF has to a great extent allowed the DHMT the flexibility and "freedom" they needed to utilize funds at this level.

Staff Motivation

There was no evidence that the implementation of decentralization had brought about job satisfaction, higher morale and increased motivation amongst staff as had been expected. Instead staff demonstrated, in both overt and subtle ways, their resentment to the decentralization process, especially the proposed staff transfer to RDCs. This was probably due to uncertainty as to the future of their careers and an expression of their unwillingness to be employed by RDCs. Staff were convinced that the MOHCW was merely dumping its responsibilities for managing health services to RDCs who had never demonstrated the capacity to manage health services.

Determination of conditions of service for employees

The responsibility for determining conditions of services for permanent staff within the public health sector was not transferred to local management bodies. However, a Health Service Board was established to take over the responsibilities of the PSC with respect to determining conditions of service for health workers. The Zimbabwe National Family Planning Council (ZNFPC) and the National AIDS Council (NAC) of Zimbabwe determine conditions of service for their staff outside the PSC and Health Service Board. Organizations that attained a commercialized status, such as the National Pharmaceutical Supplies Company (Natpharm) and the Medicines Control Authority of Zimbabwe (MCAZ) have the full authority to determine the salary levels and conditions of service for their staff. However, conditions of service for the CEO require approval by the Management Board and concurrence by the Minister of Health and Child Welfare.

The MOHCW is not a direct employer of health workers and as such cannot discipline, hire or fire staff without recourse to the Health Services Board. It is expected that in the future staff working at provincial and central hospitals will be employees of the respective Hospital Management Boards who will determine their conditions of service. District staff is expected to be employees of RDCs.

Equity and access to services

Exemption mechanisms for patient eligibility to 'free' medical services at public health facilities have been in place for some time in Zimbabwe. These have however been centrally determined. In some cases patients earning less than a stipulated salary per month or those that are considered poor are identified by community leaders and given letters of exemption from paying fees at local health facilities. In urban areas and district centers officers from the social welfare department undertake these responsibilities. Practical experience has demonstrated that this is a mammoth task that is beyond the capacity of this department. District Medical Officers and Medical Superintendents of provincial and central hospitals have delegated powers to exempt deserving patients from paying hospital fees.

A major problem experienced in implementing the user fee policy has been that some RDCs and mission institutions continue to charge user fees in rural areas. This practice is against the prevailing policy of government. Resolution of this malpractice requires both dialogue and the enforcement of legislation that empowers the MOHCW to regulate user fees across all providers, especially those that receive state assistance.

Autonomy in decision-making

Table 5.1 demonstrates how the decision-space approach draws on the principal agent analysis framework. This framework describes the range of effective choices that central authorities can permit decentralized units to exercise in their day-to-day operations. The table also provides an overview of the functions which decentralized units have discretion over in decision making. Increasing flexibility in local decision-making on human resources management, for example, allowing managers greater ability to discipline, hire and fire staff, has the potential to increase efficiency and quality of services.

The following observations can be deduced from Table 5.1:

+ Salary levels of staff at provincial and central hospitals are defined by the Health Services Board though local authorities and some management boards are allowed to "top-up" salaries to the extent that each of their different budgets will permit them to do so.
+ The hiring and firing of staff is severely restricted by the Health Services Board. Such powers can and must be provided for within the governance rules of hospital boards.

The current situation is that whilst the MOHCW is the principal agent within the health sector it was severely restricted by the PSC (now the Health Services Board) and the MOFED in exercising full control over the management of human resources. It is clear that the MOHCW's ability to determine incentives and sanctions will continue to be restricted by the decisions of the Health Services Board. The MOHCW thus has no final decision making powers on staff disciplinary matters and it cannot provide incentives to staff without reverting to the Health Services Board. These restrictions have adversely affected the overall performance of the whole organization.

Table 5.1 Decentralization and autonomy in decision-making

Category	Measure	Range of Choice
Revenue Sources. 1. Allocation of Expenditures 2. Fees	1. % of funds from central level. 2. Ability of local management to set fee levels.	1. 100% for public sector institutions. 1. 0% for Autonomous institutions like the MCAZ. 1. 100% grant for autonomous hospitals though they retain revenues from user fees. 2. Moderate: autonomous hospitals, private hospitals and national Pharmaceutical Company need approval from Minister to set fees.
Service Delivery 1. Hospital Autonomy. 2. Program Choices. 3. Contracts with Private providers of services.	1. Choice and range of services for autonomous hospitals. 2. Norms for local programs.	2. Narrow: within prescribed package of services by level of delivery. 2. Narrow: all levels implement nationally defined programs and nationally agreed targets. Local epidemiology taken into account. 3. Moderate: nationally recommended services to subcontract. 3. Wide: for procurement of supplies but within national procurement procedures.
Human Resources. 1. Conditions of service. 2. Contracts 3. Civil Service Staff 4. Staff-Mix	Determination of salary levels. Contracts for non-permanent staff. Hiring and Firing. Types and Number	1. Wide: for urban local authorities as they set their own salary scales. 1. Wide: for autonomous institutions who determine salaries outside the Health Service Board. 1. Narrow: MOHCW Headquarters and the district level whose salaries are determined by the Health Service Board. 2. Narrow: MOHCW institutions can employ part time unskilled labor and professionals – but budget held centrally. 3. Narrow: restricted by the Health Service Board. 3. Narrow: MOHCWW Staff levels must be by the Health Service Board and ministry of finance. 4. Autonomous institutions determine own staffing levels.
Access Rules. Targeting.	Exemption mechanisms.	Narrow, as exemption mechanisms are set nationally. Moderate for central hospitals as heads of hospital institutions have some prerogative to exempt some patients from paying fees.
Governance Rules 1. Management Boards. 2. Community participation.	Size and composition. Composition and role of community participation.	1. Narrow: set by statutory instruments. 2. Narrow: composition and roles determined by legal statutes – but elected locally.

The way forward

Decentralization is a means to an end and not an end in itself. Whilst decentralization is a very popular policy within the health sector in African countries, it should not be taken as a universal panacea to all flaws in the health system. From the above analysis, not all changes in the performance of a decentralizing health system can be attributed to the decentralization process as there is the potential that these may also be the result of other political and economic factors and processes.

Decentralization is a complex issue of a political nature which involves changes in power relations, especially power transfer to lower levels of government. It must therefore not be taken for granted that everybody will embrace decentralization wholeheartedly and that the outcome of decentralization will always be positive.

The outcome of the Knowledge, Attitudes and Practices (KAP) study on decentralization in the health sector which was undertaken in Zimbabwe confirms the hypothesis that there will always be those who want to maintain the status quo. Such people as would rather perpetuate the role of bureaucracy in the decision-making process or those with entrenched doubts about the capacity of local level administration to undertake new responsibilities will always be there. The more local the level, the more likely that dilemmas will arise over the scarcity of management skills as well as the potential for fragmentation in the provision of health services.

Where there is staff resistance, this can be managed through training and education programs that enlighten and change their negative mindset. Local government weaknesses should be dealt with through targeting the concerns identified rather than resorting to despondency and resignation.

Without perpetuating a centralist culture and tradition, there are four main domains in which decision-making powers should continue to be the responsibility of the central level, namely:

♦ Health policy
♦ Strategic decisions on the mobilization and allocation of resources
♦ Regulation
♦ Monitoring, evaluation and surveillance

Regular evaluation of the decentralization process is an essential component to the understanding of its costs and benefits, to formulating better and effective processes of change and in assessing its impact on health delivery systems.

Decentralization of health services to RDCs

The primary objective was to decentralize health service delivery at the district level to RDCs as these are the main local administrative authorities. In delegating responsibilities for health delivery to RDCs the MOHCW had expected that the RDCs would be required to deliver the district core health service package in terms of an agreed service contract. The PMD would be expected to provide professional and technical support to the district as the implementation level. At the horizontal level, the DMO or district health director and the DHMT would be part of RDC structures. The DMO being expected to provide professional leadership, advice and to be the professional link between health policy and implementation. The DMO would assist the RDC health (sub) committee or indeed District Health Management Boards to appreciate and deploy specialist skills in an appropriate and rational manner within the district. The process of de-centralization of health service delivery at district level never progressed beyond the conceptualization stages.

Planning for health service delivery

Should the decentralization process continue to its logical conclusion, planning for the delivery of health services in Zimbabwe is expected to continue to be guided by a national health strategic framework or any other agreed framework that the MOHCW will agree with its partners in health. The implementation of the strategy will also be on the basis of three year (medium term) plans, annual (operational) rolling plans and in synchrony with government's Medium Term Expenditure Framework (MTEF). Several and successive cycles of annual plans will be rolled out until the end of the plan period of the strategy. The planning process is ex-pected to be all-inclusive, a mix of top-down and bottom up strategies and involve all stakeholders in health, including communities. National criteria will continue to guide the establishment of facilities, staffing norms and service quality.

The RDCs would be expected to set their own service or program tar-gets in collaboration with the Provincial Medical Directors. In practical terms this means the adoption of medium term planning complement-ed by operational plans at the district level, the setting of local priorities, objectives and targets for each RDC, which when combined will achieve national health objectives and targets. The PMD is expected to provide technical inputs into the local health planning process. Councilors are expected to show interest in health issues beyond their obsession with the construction of new health facilities at every opportunity. There must therefore be a deliberate effort to ensure that councilors are made aware of health issues in their districts, national health policies and any other relevant information. This will ensure that the decisions they take are well considered and informed rather than being based on personal priorities and patronage.

In the event that a RDC is unable to discharge its duties in accordance with the terms of the contract it is expected that the Minister of Health and Child Welfare or delegated authority shall be empowered to put in place alternative arrangements for the provision of services for those communities serviced by the particular RDC. In such situations the PMD could be the interim health authority to ensure an uninterrupted provision of health services to affected communities.

Any agreement between the RDCs and the PMD will include performance targets to be achieved during the course of the contract period. Performance parameters should cover areas of quality, adherence to national policies, processes, procedures, procurement of adequate program inputs and the delivery of agreed outputs, outcomes and impact.

Management structures

In terms of the Local Government Act and the Public Health Act each RDC is required to provide specified health services and programs, other social services and related tasks. With decentralization, the RDCs will be expected to establish health (sub)-committees or District Health Management Boards as part of their administrative structures. The functions and responsibilities of these committees will be of a management nature. It is expected that the health services committee will incorporate as part of its membership, some of the members of the DHMT, in particular the District Medical Officer and/or the Health Services Administrator.

The District Health Executive will be accountable, administratively first and foremost to the RDC for its day-to-day functions. From a technical point of view the DMO is responsible to the PMD whose role is to provide technical support to the DHMTs. Such support will include monitoring and evaluating adherence to government health policy, quality of care issues, monitoring of equity issues, accountability and the achievement of locally agreed health targets.

In terms of the Medical Services Act all district hospitals are required to establish Community Health Councils whose terms of reference are defined in Statutory Instrument 208 of 2001.

Financial flows to the district level.

This is a matter of serious concern to the RDCs as most of them do not have any reliable sources of finance to enable them to provide adequate social and other services to their communities. RDCs are expected to mobilize financial resources for the delivery of health services from any of the following sources:

+ Government allocation: from general taxation, channeled through the MOHCW or direct disbursement from treasury.
+ Local Government taxes
+ Revenue from cost recovery (as per health financing policies of government)
+ Donor Funds (directly or through MOHCW)
+ Health Insurance Schemes
+ Donations from well wishers
+ Borrowing
+ Returns from investment

It is proposed that overall financing for health service delivery continues to be the responsibility of the MOHCW. The MOHCW is expected to allocate block grants to RDCs on the basis of an agreed resource allocation formula. The frequency of transfer of funds to the RDCs health account should be based on an agreed regular schedule of disbursements, probably quarterly or bi-annually and subject to agreed conditions being fulfilled:

+ Approval of (quarterly/bi-annual) plans and budgets for the next plan period
+ Submission of a report on the implementation of activities of the previous plan period
+ Expenditure reports on funds allocated for the previous plan period

Once there is mutual confidence in the financial management systems of RDCs, it should be possible in the long term for RDCs to receive their health allocation on an annual basis. It is envisaged that a simple contract specifying the core health service package as the basis for service delivery by the RDC will be signed between the RDC and the MOHCW. RDCs are expected to allocate additional resources for health service delivery from their own revenue base. Donor funds are expected to continue to be allocated through the MOFED (to be captured on budget) to the RDCs or from the MOFED through the MOHCW to the RDCs, depending on the agreed framework.

Accountability

The RDCs have always been required to adhere to the basic tenets of accountability in resource management and will be expected to continue to do so. It is also anticipated that RDCs will prioritize health service delivery in their plans, allocate the necessary resources and allow the DMO adequate flexibility in the management of resources meant for health within the RDC. Inputs meant for health service delivery such as personnel, finance, information and transport. It is also expected that RDCs will not reallocate resources meant for health services delivery to other council programs. In the initial stages of the decentralization process funds meant for the delivery of health services within the RDCs will be ring fenced so as to protect them from being diverted to other council activities.

Implementation of user fee policies

Rural District Councils and semi-autonomous hospitals are expected to adhere to prevailing government policies on cost recovery. Services provided by RDCs are public goods meant to complement government efforts to improve equity in access to health services. In the event that RDCs are allowed to charge user fees they will be expected to invest the revenue accruing from such fees in the provision of health services within the district. RDCs are encouraged to actively source finances from third parties such as the Association of Healthcare Funders of Zimbabwe.

Referral of patients

Provincial and central hospitals will continue to offer referral and specialist services for patients referred from district and provincial hospitals respectively. It is necessary that someone or some authority pays for or purchases referral services on behalf of those patients who are not able to pay. Those patients who are not entitled to 'free' health care will pay for their own referral care or have it paid for by third parties. The following paragraphs describe some of the modalities which are available for the payment of referral services.

The district hospital can pay the Hospital Management Board (HMB) of a central or provincial hospital an agreed amount of money in advance (capitation) to cover referral services. Such a payment is expected to cover the costs of the referral of indigent patients. This option avoids the problems of billing and arguments over numbers and diagnostic categories. The danger with such an arrangement is that referral hospitals may be tempted to under-service patients in order to make savings on their advance payments.

District hospitals can opt to pay for referred patients on a case by case (per capita) basis. This arrangement requires the establishment of an efficient billing system and verification mechanisms for services rendered. The disadvantage of this option is that the administrative costs of such a system are very high. The system also requires improved capacity for billing and financial management at both the referring and receiving centers.

Other options must recognize that the resources allocated to provincial and central hospitals are primarily meant to cover the costs of referral services and that these institutions were established for the sole purposes of delivering referral services. Additional payment for referral services could be interpreted as duplication in the payment for such services.

The Health Services Fund

RDCs and semi-autonomous hospitals are required to operate local bank accounts in terms of the Act that governs the Health Services Fund. It is also proposed that expenditures from the RDC health accounts be approved only on the basis of two or more signatories consisting of at least one member from the DHE (DMO or Senior Accountant) and the other from the RDCs general administration. The MOHCW is expected to deposit its grant allocation to the RDC health account at agreed intervals and on time.

Employment of professional staff

MOHCW staff may be transferred from the MOHCW or the PSC to RDCs. In this light it is important to note that RDCs already employ health staff whose salaries are paid through a grant administered by the MOHCW. There are four options to consider in transferring staff to RDCs:

♦ Direct transfer of health staff to RDC institutions (with their consent)
♦ Redeployment within the public service, for those not willing to be transferred

♦ Abolition of office, where there are no vacancies for redeployment within the service.

♦ Secondment of MOHCW staff for an initial period, of say 2 years, after which period staff can remain with the RDCs or opt for abolition of office

In the event that the process of transfer of staff to the RDCs actually takes place, the councils must have the powers to hire, fire and discipline such staff as well as determine their conditions of service. These powers may be subject to general guidelines set by the Health Service Board. RDCs will be expected to employ and deploy professional health staff in accordance with the provisions of the Health Professions Authority of Zimbabwe and under the direction of the DMO and his/her professional staff. Some RDCs may not be able to compete and attract professional staff. Such a situation is likely to adversely affect equity and the quality of health service provision across different RDCs. The MOHCW may have to strike a balance between maintaining a central institution for personnel deployment and allowing individual RDCs to be innovative enough to put in place incentives to attract and retain health staff on their own.

Review questions

1. Even with the implementation of decentralization there are some functions which only the central level should take responsibility for. Discuss these functions and why they must continue to be exercised as central level responsibilities.

2. A decentralized health system functions more efficiently than a centralized bureaucracy. Discuss this statement in the context of practical experiences.

3. In the context of decentralization and restructuring of the health system, define and discuss the concepts of strategic and operational capacity.

4. The implementation of decentralization policies has the potential to affect equity, efficiency and sustainability. Discuss the above statement on the basis of evidence from countries that have decentralized their health systems.

6

HEALTH FINANCING

Introduction

Health financing refers to the manner in which financial resources are mobilized to fund the health sector and has major equity implications for health status and risk protection for people. It is the provision of funds by health care purchasers to acquire health care coverage and/or health services. The following are some of the modalities for health financing found in Africa:

- Public financing sources
  - General taxation
  - Income from sale of natural resources
  - User fees
  - Grant assistance
  - Social Insurance
  - Borrowing
  - Efficiency gains in use of existing funds
- Private financing sources
  - Private insurance
  - Out of pocket expenses
  - Community Insurance
  - Grant assistance
  - Borrowing
  - Charitable contributions

Despite the fact that African countries rely on a variety of sources to finance their health services they still do not spend enough resources on health. There are only a few countries in the region that have comprehensive financing strategies for their health sectors. The major problem in most of them is the severe shortage of government resources to support the provision of an adequate package of quality health services. This situation usually manifests itself in the deterioration of the quality of services provided at public health delivery institutions. This is further exacerbated by inefficient and inequitable allocation of resources within the sector. The concept of efficiency has two aspects to it, namely allocative and technical. Technical efficiency refers to "doing things right" by producing a specific health outcome, intervention or service at lowest cost. Allocative efficiency on the other hand refers to "doing the right things" by purchasing the most cost effective mix of outcomes. Countries have tended to spend most of their health resources on large hospitals which are located in urban areas where they serve the already privileged members of society at the expense of the poor. Poor systems of budgeting, purchasing and monitoring often result in inefficient resource utilization within the health sectors of these countries.

Weaknesses in systems of accountability within government lead to resources being spent on the wrong priorities. In some cases the resources do not reach the intended beneficiaries at the health center or hospital. Where resources actually reach the providers of health services or health center, health workers may not be motivated enough to put them to good use. In other instances households do not take the opportunity to utilize available services. In terms of the proportion of their income, poor households spend much more on health care than households that are well off.

Sources of health finance

In most African countries interactions between suppliers (providers) and consumers of health services consist of interactions between patients, the government, Non-Governmental Organizations (NGOs), the private for profit sector, faith based organizations and in some cases payers who include insurers. As a result health financing policies must be able to regulate the roles of all the above actors. In this context this chapter explores the reforms that the MOHCW in Zimbabwe introduced as part of its health care financing options and its desire to achieve and maintain equity and efficiency in resource allocation and utilization.

Financing reforms in Zimbabwe have focused mainly on the mobilization of additional resources and the optimization of the use of existing resources. This objective was pursued largely through the implementation of reforms in the areas of tax revenues, government borrowing, user fees, and formal insurance schemes, donor financing and strengthening partnerships with the private sector.

The main sources of health sector financing in Zimbabwe are, Figure 6.1:

+ Budget allocations from treasury to the MOHCW (tax revenue)
+ Budget allocations to other government departments such as the ministry of education, local authorities, the uniformed forces etc. (tax revenue)
+ Budgets of local government departments (urban authorities and RDCs) from local revenue sources
+ Contributions from development partners
+ Contributions from local and international NGOs
+ Donations from overseas to the Zimbabwe Association of Church Related Hospitals (ZACH)
+ Employer contributions
+ Individuals, through out-of-pocket payments and private health insurance
+ Ear marked taxes e.g. the HIV/AIDS Trust Fund.
+ Lotteries and other well-wishers

Countries that operate a "national health service" model of delivering health services rely heavily on tax revenue for financing their public health system. Such systems are credited with being politically acceptable, transparent and are geared towards achieving equity in access to health care. The other features of this model are that it provides health coverage for the whole population mainly through a network of public providers. The problem with reliance on tax based revenue to support the delivery of social services in developing countries has always been that these economies are too small to raise adequate resources to sustain such services. As a result of limited fiscal space, most of these countries do not have the capacity to generate enough resources to fund the recurrent costs of their health needs, to fund the full costs of their economies, the incremental costs associated with new investments, and the servicing and repayment of external debts.

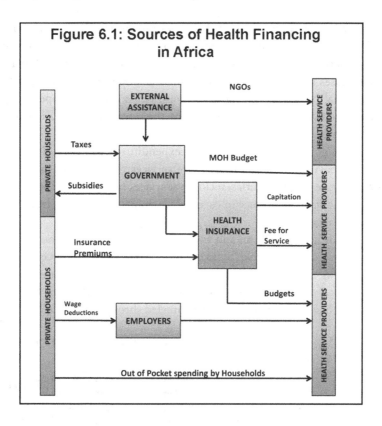

Figure 6.1: Sources of Health Financing in Africa

The Zimbabwe Ministry of Finance and Economic Development (MOFED) has over the years been the major source of health financing for the public sector. Funds for health and health related activities from the Ministry of Finance and Economic Development have been channeled through the MOHCW, the Ministry of Defense, Ministry of Home Affairs, Ministry of Justice, Legal and Parliamentary Affairs and the Ministry of the Public Service, Labor and Social Welfare and other quasi governmental departments like the Zimbabwe National Family Planning Council.

Donors in Zimbabwe traditionally channeled funds destined for support to the health sector through Vote of Credit (VOC) transfers. With the establishment of a Health Services Fund (HSF) in 1999 some donors disbursed funds to the MOHCW through the HSF. This process involved the MOHCW submitting regular requests for specific amounts of donor funds which the Central Bank then transferred to the National Development Fund (NDF) in the MOFED. The MOFED immediately transferred these funds to the MOHCW headquarters' HSF account. The MOHCW would then disburse appropriate amounts of funds to the operational level on a quarterly basis, based on agreed quarterly work plans. In some cases donors provided direct financial support to some local and international NGOs operating in the country. As more developed countries reduced direct financial support to the government of Zimbabwe more and more aid has been channeled through NGOs.

Households contribute to health expenditures through direct out of pocket payments for the health care services they consume at public and/or private sector facilities, including services provided by Traditional Health Practitioners. Households also contribute to voluntary health insurance schemes.

Local Authorities (urban and rural) allocate resources for the delivery of health services within their areas of jurisdiction. These resources are derived from local tax revenues, user fees and grants allocated by the central government. Health grants from central government and meant for local authorities have over the years been channeled through the MOHCW.

Table 6.1 Government allocation (%) to the health sector (2001-2004)

		Revised budget estimates	Revised budget estimates	Budget proposal
	2001	**2002**	**2003**	**2004**
% allocation to health				
Total MOHCW expenditures/ total GOZ	5.4	5.2	8.8	8.0
Total MOHCW expenditures /GOZ non-statutory & non-constitutional	10.2	9.0	10.7	9.5
Growth in real terms (%)				
Total expenditures	-21.6	-3.3	-24.0	-9.2
Non-salary	-	0.9	-16.3	-14.6
Salary	-	-7.6	-32.8	-1.5

Source: HERA Mid-term review of the Health Sector Support Programs I & II, January 2004

Employers in the private sector contribute to health financing through contributing to employee benefit health insurance schemes. In some cases employers have established their own health facilities which are used exclusively by their employees and immediate family members. Employers also make direct payments to other providers of health services, including public health facilities, who are consulted by their employees.

Intermediary organizations such as the MOHCW act as conduits for health resources by reallocating funds they receive from different sources to other providers of health such as missions, local NGOs, Rural District Councils and municipalities.

Structure of the MOHCW budget

The budget structure of the MOHCW has traditionally consisted of four Sub-Heads namely:

- ♦ *Administration and General:* - for financing the operations of the MOHCW headquarters activities (about 3% of MOHCW budget).
- ♦ *Medical Care Services:* - for supporting service delivery operations of central, provincial, district hospitals and health centers, including the procurement of drugs and other essential supplies. Some elements of Preventive Services are also supported from this item. On average this item constituted about 84.3% of the sector budget, about 40% of this budget item went to salaries, wages and allowances and 25% to the procurement of essential inputs for the delivery of health care.
- ♦ *Preventive Services:* - the eight Provincial Medical Directors and program managers at central level are responsible for coordinating the implementation of public health programs which are financed from this budget item,(12% of the sector budget, about 35% of this allocation went to salaries, wages and allowances and 50% to field operations). Field operations have traditionally included the following program activities:
  - ♦ Disease control (mainly tuberculosis, HIV, STI, malaria and other epidemic diseases).
  - ♦ Environmental health activities.
  - ♦ Expanded Program of Immunization (including the purchase of all MOHCW vaccine requirements).
  - ♦ Health education.
  - ♦ The Government Analyst Laboratory.
  - ♦ Integrated Management of Childhood Illnesses.

- National Program of Action on Children. (NPA).
- Nutrition activities.
- Reproductive health programs.
- The Village Health Worker Program.
- *Research*: (about 1.5% of health sector budget).

Examples of health insurance schemes in Zimbabwe whose funds flow from households and employers include:
- The Work-mans' Compensation Insurance Fund
- The National Pensions Scheme
- The National Social Security (Fund) Agency
- Health Care Funders - under the Association of Health Care Funders of Zimbabwe

Private Voluntary Organizations mainly receive funding from donors directly and disburse them to "not for profit" private providers or utilize them in the direct provision of health services. A few Voluntary Organizations also receive subventions from the government, especially those that deal with the elderly and people with disabilities.

The best example of earmarked taxes in Zimbabwe is the AIDS Levy which was introduced in 1999 as surtax on employee and corporate incomes. This fund supports the multi-sectoral national response to HIV/AIDS. In its first 12 months of operation the levy accumulated revenue equivalent to US$20 million. The fund is administered as an AIDS Trust Fund by the Board of Directors of the National AIDS Council (NAC). Of the 2001 tax based allocation to the MOHCW 4% came from this fund.

Proceeds from this fund are disbursed to private organizations, community based organizations, organizations for people living with HIV/AIDS, communities, civil society groups, NGOs and public sector organizations that deal with HIV/AIDS prevention, control and the mitigation of its socio-economic impact. Some of the funds are used to pay school fees for children orphaned by AIDS. Both internal and external auditors audit the fund. When Zimbabwe introduced the AIDS fund in 1999 it was probably the only country that taxed its citizens to raise funds to support its national response to HIV/AIDS.

The National Health Accounts (NHA) conducted in 1994 and 1999 show that compared to the levels soon after independence in 1980 the private sector has become a major contributor to total national health expenditures, Table 6.3. According to the 1999 National Health Accounts

(NHA), total national health expenditures constituted 7.8% of the GDP. Private sector health spending accounted for 4.1% of the GDP (US$ 18.68 per capita) compared to public expenditures which accounted for 3.7% of GDP (US$13.73 per capita). Donor contributions accounted for 0.9% of the GDP (US$4.84 per capita) in the same year. Overall, in 1999 private spending constituted 50.1% of total national health expenditures compared to 34.6% in 1987. The public sector, including donors, contributed 36.9% and 13% respectively to total national health expenditures in 1999.

According to the 2001 National Health Accounts, the private sector contributed 54.6% of national health expenditures compared to 45.4% by the public sector. Donors contributed 5.4 % to national health expenditures and only about 1% of MOHCW expenditures. In previous years development partners have contributed up to 30% of total MOHCW expenditures.

Table: 6.2 Health budget as a percentage of total national budget (2000-2006)

Budget Year	% of Total National Budget
2000	9.2
2001	11.5
2002	9.5
2003	12.7
2004	9.5
2005	11
2006	9.33

Source: Zimbabwe Budget estimates, 2000 -2006

Table 6.3 National Health Accounts (1987, 1994-95, 1999 and 2001)

Public Sector	1987	1994/95	1999	2001
MOHCW	42.3%	29.0%	27.7%	35.9
Other ministries Local Govt.	10.4%	10.0%	9.2%	4.1
Donors	12.7%	12.2%	13.0%	5.4
Total Public Sector	65.4%	51.2%	49.9%	45.4
Private Sector				
Individual Direct payment	10.0%	30.5%	23.0%	29.5
Health Insurance	16.5%	11.8%	20.1%	11.1
Employer based Care	8.0%	5.7%	7.0%	14.0
Missions and NGOs	1.1%	0.9%	-	-
Total Private Sector	34.6%	48.8%	50.1%	54.6
Total	**100%**	**100%**	**100%**	**100%**

In 1996 the total cost of delivering Primary Health Care services in Zimbabwe was estimated to be Z$46 (US$ 5.0) per capita. Government expenditures contributed Z$25 (US$ 2.7) per capita to this amount. This translated to a financing gap of Z$ 19 (US$ 2.3) per capita per year for the provision of PHC services. In the same year, out of an estimated requirement of Z$134 (US$ 14.7) per capita per year, Z$119 (US$ 13) per capita was available to finance hospital services (Social Health Insurance, 1996).

Out of pocket payment by individuals or households constitutes a significant proportion of total health care financing in Zimbabwe. The NHA studies for 1999 and 2001 showed that out-of-pocket payments in Zimbabwe accounted for 23% and 29% of national health expenditures, respectively. This proportion is very significant at the household level, considering the ever increasing levels of extreme poverty in Zimbabwe and indeed in the African region. Such payments are extremely regressive, as they constitute a very large proportion of the income of poor households who tend to fall sick more often than the rich. One objective of a financing policy must be to ensure that households do not become poor because of paying for the use of health services. As a rule of thumb, where out of pocket health spending is less than 15% of total health spending, very few households face catastrophic health spending.

User fees

User fees are paid by clients or patients at the point and time of consumption of health care services. They usually differ by patient group (wealthy and poor), services received (preventive, curative or chronic illness) or between facilities (such as between public and private facilities or primary level and hospital level care) and may cover all or part of the actual cost of the service. The rationale given for the introduction of user fees is usually that there is a need to generate additional revenue in order to improve the quality of health care, and consequently to increase the demand for quality services. Some people have argued that user fees promote more efficient consumption patterns by reducing over use of health services. Available evidence has since proved otherwise as improvements in the quality of services have rarely materialized, the revenue generation potential largely marginal and fees have deterred the poor from utilizing health services.

The history of user fees in Zimbabwe dates back to the pre-independence era when fees were levied at all levels of the health delivery system. When the new government took over power in 1980 they initially abolished user fees for primary health care at all public health facilities. User fees however continued to be levied as a disincentive to patients who bypassed the referral system. All patients who had an income of less than Z$150 (US$ 100) per month were exempt from paying user fees at public health institutions, unless they did not follow the referral system.

The policy move to abolish user fees is estimated to have resulted in a loss of government revenue from user fees amounting to US$ 3 million in 1980. The government expected that the move to abolish government subsidies to the private medical sector at government institutions would offset the above loss in revenue.

Over the years the government policy on user fees has proved to be very erratic both in its formulation and implementation, Table 6.4. The huge hike in user fees introduced by government in January 1994 was an attempt to reflect the economic costs of providing health care in the public health sector. The new fees were based on the Relative Value Schedule

(RVS) used by the private sector. At the time the MOHCW published a fee policy which was more comprehensive and explicit in its content than the previous ones had been. The policy was geared more towards revenue generation than had previously been admitted by the MOHCW. Previously the position of the MOHCW was that the aim of user fees was more to improve the referral system than to raise revenue.

There is evidence that if user fees are associated with improvements in the quality of care they may encourage increased utilization of health services. The introduction of an efficient exemption mechanism has the potential to protect the poor from paying fees that they usually cannot afford. Such exemption mechanisms should also ensure that those who are able to pay for health services actually pay for the services they consume.

However, if user fees deter the poor from using health services when they need them, equity in utilization is compromised. This must be interpreted to mean that relative to what they are able to pay, the poor should not pay more than those who are able to do so! For example, the reintroduction of user fees in Zimbabwe in June 1993 resulted in a 30% decline in the utilization of services at Rural Health Centers (Zigora, et al, 1997, personal communication). There were several reasons cited for this phenomenon, including the inability of patients to pay, ineffective exemption mechanisms and criteria which had not been widely disseminated to communities. The process of assessing the income levels of patients presented health workers with an ethical dilemma. It was very difficult for them to reconcile decisions to deny medical treatment to patients who deserved it but were not able to prove that they were eligible for 'free' health services. The fee waiver system proved to be unworkable especially at the health center level where there are no clerical staffs to manage the fee structure.

The administration of the fee structure at RHCs became prohibitive because clerical staff from the district offices had to travel long distances to health centers to collect revenue which in most cases was far less than the transport costs incurred. Most of the health centers did not have adequate security for the safe keeping of monies raised from user fees. Poor and inefficient billing systems at some hospitals also led to huge losses of potential revenue. In cases where corrupt officials diverted funds to their own use such cases often remained undetected for very long periods of time.

Table 6.4 Policies on user fees over the years in Zimbabwe

Time period	User Fee Policy
September 1980	Abolition of all user fees (except Parirenyatwa Hospital).
1991	User fees reinforced by GOZ – exemption letters from local councilors and Social Welfare Officers required.
November 1992	Threshold for exemption from paying user fees increased from Z$ 150 (US$ 22.0) monthly salary to Z$ 400 (US$ 59.0). Patients earning Z$ 400 or more to pay user fees.
January 1993	All Fees abolished at rural health centers and clinics in rural areas. Some RDCs and missions however continue to charge fees in defiance of this policy.
June 1993	User fees reintroduced in rural areas.
January 1994	User fees at public health facilities increased by more than 2.5 times – based on the Relative Value Schedule used by the private sector.
March 1995	Fees at rural health centers and clinics abolished except those at clinics owned by urban local authorities.
May 1996	Upward adjustment of fees by more than 50%.
January 2002	*A comprehensive user fee policy for public health facilities:* No fees to be charged at Government RHC and RDC clinics. No fees charged for maternity services (ANC, Delivery and Post natal care). Free health services for children under the age of five years. Free TB treatment-public and private sector. Free treatment for psychiatric patients. Free treatment for pensioners (alternatively Health Insurance Schemes to pay, if they are members. Fees to be automatically reviewed in line with changes in the Relative Value Schedule used by the private Sector. Urban local authorities not bound by fee levels in the public sector but would require ministerial approval to adopt any revised fee structures. Urban local authorities and central hospitals to be reimbursed the loss of revenue resulting from implementing exemption mechanisms. Reimbursements from the Social Dimension Fund (SDF) or other safety-net mechanisms.

In order to reduce the number and impact of fraudulent activities and to improve efficiency in the management of user fees at public health institutions Vogel (1998) suggested the following measures to be put in place:

+ To clearly define entrance points for the hospital
+ To issue receipts with duplicate copies to serve as evidence for payment
+ To rigorously enforce a system to determine those clients who are eligible for exemption
+ To conduct periodic spot checks to ensure that all staff are following the above recommendations
+ To conduct regular audits of financial transactions and flow of funds

For a user fee scheme to be sustainable the following issues need to be addressed:

+ Ensuring that the fee structure is simple and easy to administer.
+ Reviewing fee levels on a regular basis, annually if possible.
+ Developing simple exemption mechanisms in conjunction with local communities or their representatives.
+ Basing the fee structure on uniform principles across all the levels of the health system and across the country, taking into consideration the types of services provided.
+ Developing guidelines on financial management, control practices and how the revenue collected will be used.
+ Putting in place mechanisms to monitor the socioeconomic impact of the fee policies.
+ Ensuring that the introduction of user fees result in improvements in all aspects of quality of care – (drug availability, positive staff attitudes and increased staff morale).
+ Ensuring the availability of reliable and safe local banking facilities.

Non-governmental institutions like missions, self-governing hospitals, urban local authorities who are required to implement government exemption policies must be monitored and compensated for revenues lost as a result of implementing government user fee and exemption policies.

Considerations in abolishing user fees

The MOHCW has had several policy positions on the subject of user fees, including abolishing them for specific levels of the health system, for specific services as well as implementing targeted exemptions from the payment of such fees. The problem has been the haphazard manner in which such policy shifts have been adopted and implemented. There is however a rational process which organizations can follow in effecting such policy changes.

Consideration of the legal framework for user fees

The RDCs Act and the Health Services Act provide the legal basis for the collection of revenue in the form of user fees and taxes for services provided by RDCs and other health providers. Furthermore, the MOHCW has formulated policies that govern the collection and administration of user fees by health providers in both the public and private sectors, including Faith Based Organizations and other NGOs. The policy objective is to harmonize user fee charging practices across public health facilities as well as to ensure that the implementation of user fees guarantees government's constitutional obligations to universal access to health. The laws also imply that emergency treatment cannot be withheld on the grounds of failure to pay and that the fee levels are subject to regular review and revision. The legal framework provides for the revenue to be used to support operational costs at facility level. Exemptions are provided for in cases of care associated with child birth, treatment of minors, pensioners, the unemployed, etc. There is also provision for the exemption of specific disease conditions.

Implications of abolishing user fees

The ministry of health must consider the implications of any policy change to both the organization and intended beneficiaries. The user fee policy has both positive and negative aspects to it. On the positive side user fees provide additional revenue that facilities can use to improve some aspects in the quality of health services they provide at institutional level. Such resources can be used to supplement government allocations to purchase medicines, hire temporary staff and undertake minor repairs to health facilities. Such revenue has a much more significant impact if retained and utilized at facility level as opposed to being collected by the treasury.

Negative aspects of user fees include the potential to deter would be users from accessing health care if they are not able to pay. This usually affects the poor more than those with the ability to pay for health services. User fees are an additional burden on out of pocket payments which include transport and other opportunity costs. In some cases the collection and management of revenue from user fees are a huge administrative burden on health workers, especially where there is no clerical staff and there is a shortage of health workers to attend to patients.

Policy intentions to abolish user fees

The government may develop a policy intention to abolish user fees as a deliberate move to ensure adherence to the country's constitutional provisions on the right of all citizens to universal access to (primary) health care. Such provisions can usually be achieved through the removal of economic barriers that limit access to health care services, especially by the most vulnerable groups. Such a policy move also ensures that the health sector effectively contributes to human capital development and national efforts to reduce poverty. The policy move is usually intended to promote increased utilization of primary health care services and to encourage timely and early use of health facilities, thus avoiding unnecessary delays in patients consulting service providers. Considering that households in the majority of countries in Sub-Saharan Africa already incur significant out of pocket payments which, in some cases, amount to more than 70% of health spending, such a policy aims to alleviate this burden from poor households.

Strategies to consider in abolition user fees

The health sector must effectively plan for a substantial and sustained increase in the utilization of health services likely to result from a policy to abolish user fees. Experience from elsewhere shows that the resulting increase in the utilization of health services can lead to drug shortages, deterioration in the quality of services and an increase in the workload of health staff. The sector must thus plan for a potential increase in drug supply requirements and, in selected cases, additional staff to deal with the increased workload.

The sector must thus develop strategies to mobilize additional resources to maintain and/or improve the quality of health services delivered and to compensate for the loss of revenue arising from the abolition of user fees. Options in this area include increasing the allocation of domestic finances to the health sector, to at least 15% of total government expenditures, in line with the Abuja Declaration and/or mobilizing donors to support efforts to increase tax revenues allocated to the public health sector. The health sector should also consider the establishment of a special fund (health facility fund) to finance those activities that were supported from revenue derived from user fees such as; the employment of temporary staff, the purchase of supplementary essential supplies/medicines and minor repairs to health infrastructure. Such a fund could be allocated to health facilities on the basis of the lost revenue. Where the utilization of user fee revenue was decided at local level, this could continue. Such an arrangement would ensure that facility managers do not feel deprived of potentially useful resources which they had directly controlled.

There must be a well orchestrated communication strategy developed as a means of dialogue to inform health staff about the specific policy change, its advantages, disadvantages and any untoward consequences and how they will be dealt with. Most importantly, as beneficiaries, the general public must be directly informed of the abolishment of user fees-, the effective date, at what levels of the system these will occur, who are eligible, what services are affected, what to do if health staff charge them for services provided, and so forth.

Health insurance in Zimbabwe

Health insurance schemes rely on the concept of solidarity which is based on the transfer of resources from those who can afford insurance to the poor. Health insurance is a means of offsetting catastrophic financial losses associated with severe illness or injury through risk pooling among many people. Such schemes can be compulsory and cover a whole segment of a population, e.g. Social Health Insurance funds, or they may be limited to those in formal employment. Insurance schemes may be voluntary as in private commercial or non-profit schemes.

There are several policy objectives to the introduction of health insurance, namely:

♦ Mobilization of additional non-government sources of funds
♦ Improving access to care by reducing barriers to access
♦ In some cases checking the rapid growth in government expenditures
♦ Improving technical efficiency by introducing competitive mechanisms into the health sector

Other stakeholders such as professional bodies, formal employment workers and employers perceive the objectives or benefits from health insurance in a different light. Providers see this as an opportunity to improve their earnings and increase access to new technologies that improve the quality of health care. The insured see this as an opportunity to expand the benefits they get from their insurers.

Where insurance coverage is universal and there is cost recovery, this potentially eliminates financial barriers to access to health care. In most African countries the majority of the population is in informal employment where it is difficult to organize the collection of premiums. One way of increasing insurance coverage for those in the formal sector is for the government to put in place compulsory coverage through a social health insurance scheme funded through tax. The other way is for the government to provide incentives for employers and individuals to purchase insurance through tax rebates on contributions to health insurance.

According to Griffin and Shaw (1995) the following conditions are necessary for a health insurance scheme to be able to operate, i.e. operational user fees, a large pool of people to be insured, the possibility of keeping premiums low and an adequate information base on health spending and utilization.

At some point in its policy development process the GOZ considered the establishment of community based insurance schemes. The concept was however never pursued. Despite the consensus reached by African Ministers of Health at the World Health Organization Regional Office for Africa (WHO/AFRO) Committee meetings, the MOHCW has never pursued or implemented the Bamako Initiative. This type of initiative is a voluntary scheme in which lump sum payments are made by households for services that are provided at local public health facilities, NGO facilities or private for profit facilities which charge user fees. Payment is usually in cash but may also be in kind and a package of benefits and conditions are clearly defined for those who have contributed to the fund. The communities themselves usually manage the fund locally.

By definition Community Based Health Insurance (CBHI) schemes involve pre-payment for health care and are controlled and managed by the community. Membership is voluntary with risk sharing from members of the community that are considered to be well off to those that are classified as poor. Such schemes complement rather than substitute for the NHS and SHI. However, because of their small size their capacity to achieve social protection is limited. The financial sustainability of most of these schemes is questionable. Voluntary and private insurance schemes have been operating in Zimbabwe for a very long time. In 1993 the World Bank estimated that 5.6% of the population in Zimbabwe was covered by private insurance schemes. This figure is estimated to have increased to 20% of the population or 1 million individuals by 1997. In the same year it was estimated that there were 27 Medical Aid Societies, (now referred to as Healthcare Funders), operating in Zimbabwe under the then National Association of Medical Aid Societies (NAMAS), now referred to as the Association of Healthcare Funders of Zimbabwe, as the umbrella body.

Voluntary health insurance is any insurance scheme that is paid for by voluntary contributions. Voluntary insurance is considered inequitable if there is no public intervention to subsidize the contributions or to regulate benefits and price. This type of insurance scheme requires a strong regulatory framework and a vibrant market economy.

These voluntary schemes consist of contributions based on a percentage of the salary of the individual who is a member. The employer and employee contribute at a ratio of 50:50. These contributions are usually tax deductible in order to promote the establishment of medical aid societies and to encourage people to join them. The current view on these rebates is that the government is unnecessarily subsidizing the private sector at the expense of public sector services which rely heavily on tax revenue for their sustainability.

In Zimbabwe insured individuals have the freedom to access health care services from either the private for profit, private not for profit or the public sector. Consultations from traditional health practitioners are however not covered by any insurance scheme.

The majority of people living in rural areas receive free health services from public health facilities, others opt to receive care on a cash or barter basis from traditional healers and yet others in the same category pay for health services at public and private facilities. At the dawn of the new millennium it was estimated that in Zimbabwe 15-20% of the population had no access to formal health sector services.

Social health Insurance (SHI) is characterized by a publicly mandated system that covers designated groups and is financed through compulsory payroll contributions and is administered by a semi autonomous body. Benefits can be accessed through public and private institutions. In 1984 the government of Zimbabwe made overtures to the effect that at some point the national health service would be funded through a compulsory

National Health Insurance scheme which would form part of a National Social Security System (GOZ/MOH, 1984). Such a scheme would be complemented by existing medical aid schemes already operating in the country.

There are however conditions that must be in place before any social health insurance scheme becomes fully operational. Adequate capacity must be developed to manage the scheme so as to keep administrative costs to a minimum. Mechanisms to collect premiums, pay claims and monitor providers must be in place as early as possible during the development process of the scheme. There must be full details of the economic costs of providing health services in public health facilities so that reimbursement rates are accurately set in order to recover the full costs of providing the services. Finally, there must be political commitment to use the establishment of the SHI as a means to increase government resources to the sector and not to substitute them. (SHI, 1996).

Since the proposal was made, the only visible step that has taken place with regards the SHI is a feasibility study which was conducted by the MOHCW in 1996. This study concluded that there was a potential for the establishment of a Social Health Insurance scheme in Zimbabwe though the administrative costs of operating such a scheme were likely to be prohibitive.

Individuals at community level who were interviewed during the course of this study indicated that they had no confidence in a health insurance scheme that is managed by officials of government. They instead preferred the establishment of a locally managed insurance scheme (SHI, 1996).

From the time the results of the study were disseminated in 1996 the Ministry of the Public Service, Labor and Social Welfare has been given the responsibility of coordinating the process of establishing a SHI in Zimbabwe. The task of bringing together employers, trade unions, the health profession, government ministries and representatives of civil society to discuss the matter has proven to be a daunting one for the ministry. Such a consultative process is crucial if there has to be broad based consensus and a guarantee of adequate safeguards on transparency and public accountability.

One of the weaknesses of a SHI is that it is not as progressive as financing health through tax based systems. The contribution rates are often a flat percentage of salaries or income with a ceiling on the income used to calculate the premiums. Those who earn above the ceiling pay an increasingly lower proportion of their total income.

The model that has been proposed for SHI in Zimbabwe is based on the principles of universal coverage and builds on the existing private, industry and employer based health insurance schemes. The objective is to cover the whole population, starting with those in formal employment. It is proposed that premiums will be based on payroll deductions for those in formal employment. Health benefits will be based on the Core Health Service Package as defined by the MOHCW in 1995. In terms of the Medical Services Act this package forms the minimum benefit package for all insurance schemes, including those in the private sector. Patients will have a free choice of health providers who will be reimbursed on a per capita grant system. Those wishing to access additional benefits beyond the basic package will either join other schemes or contribute an additional premium to complement the basic package.

The scheme will be funded through contributions from both employers and employees. Compulsory contributions of formal sector workers will be a proportion of members' earnings, plus set rates for dependents based on actuarial estimates. Those in informal employment will be able to voluntarily enroll in the SHI by paying into the fund.

The government is expected to contribute to the fund to cover the indigent and those who are unemployed or unable to pay for themselves. A carefully designed means testing is proposed to ensure that only those without the ability to pay are granted "free" access to health services. A certification system to identify those individuals who are not able to contribute to such insurance schemes has been proposed.

MOHCW facilities will continue to retain revenue from the user fees they charge. It is not yet clear how the operation of the SHI will impact on the allocation of the health budget to the MOHCW. However, since revenue from third party payments will be managed on the basis of the HSF, theoretically this arrangement should not negatively affect the MOHCW's allocation from the Treasury. The SHI should thus complement treasury allocations to the MOHCW rather than substitute them.

Since insurance usually encourages the overuse of health services (moral hazard) insurance companies often design measures to manage this phenomenon, some of which are cost sharing, limits to benefits and the need for frequent renewal of insurance. Some Healthcare Funders in Zimbabwe have introduced co-payment which consists of a flat fee that a beneficiary must pay for each service used. In other instances patients are required to pay some stipulated amount in out-of-pocket expenses before any benefits of insurance become accessible.

Risk selection is another phenomenon in insurance whereby individuals who are much sicker than average individuals tend to enroll in health insurance schemes. This behavior distorts the insurance markets by increasing the premiums, especially when healthier individuals avoid joining such schemes. Insurers tend to protect themselves from such phenomenon by putting in place stringent screening measures which may include requirement for medical examinations, review of claims history of prospective members, having a waiting period before benefits can be accessed by new members, exclusion of preexisting conditions from coverage and in some extreme cases refusing to provide coverage.

At one time medical aid societies in Zimbabwe excluded Family Planning methods from the benefits they covered. Under such exclusion clauses individuals are liable to pay the full costs or cost over and above what the scheme covers. Some schemes go to the extent of establishing a price list for therapeutically comparable drugs and establish a maximum reimbursement level per item prescribed. Since its introduction, the Essential Drugs List for Zimbabwe (EDLIZ) that is based on generic prescription has been used by Healthcare Funders of Zimbabwe for such purposes. The system makes patients financially liable if more expensive drugs are prescribed.

Supplier induced demand is a potential problem in cases where providers are retrospectively reimbursed as they usually tend to respond by increasing the volume or intensity (number of items of service per contact by over servicing individual patients) of treatment in order to maintain their volume of income levels.

Public and private sector collaboration in Zimbabwe

Public-private collaboration is a formal or informal cooperation between the public and private (voluntary and for profit) sectors in the provision and/or financing of health care services. This is considered to be an alternative way of making the best use of available resources by tapping into the relative strengths of the private sector.

In Zimbabwe such cooperation has been in place for a long time between missions, some private hospitals, general practitioners and the government. It has however taken a very long time for the government to realize that the private sector can play a significant role in improving equity and that emulating it could improve efficiency in resource utilization.

The private for profit sector

In Zimbabwe the viability of the private for profit sector has been guaranteed by a strong presence of employer based health insurance schemes. The shortage of government resources to support the delivery of quality public health services fuelled the rapid growth of the private sector as an alternative source of health care for those who could afford it. Theoretically this frees public sector resources so that they can be used to provide health care for the poor and most needy.

The growth of the private for profit sector has prompted the government to create an environment that enables collaboration between the public and the private sectors. The starting point is to establish a framework which ensures that market failures are identified and managed, issues of quality of care are addressed, and modalities for the licensing, accreditation and registration of both private and public institutions are put in place. The legislation enacted by the government of Zimbabwe also provides for the regulation of health insurance schemes operating in the country. Details of the regulatory framework are described in chapter 9 of this book.

In the early 1980s the government of Zimbabwe stated that whilst it accepted the historical reality of the existence of the private sector it had a duty to control it in the public interest (GOZ/MOH, 1984). The GOZ also stated that private practice for full time government employees would be phased out and that private hospital beds in government institutions would remain available to those private patients who could pay the full costs of the services. To date government hospitals have maintained private beds to allow medical doctors to admit and manage private patients.

General practitioners were given authority to undertake hospital sessions at public hospitals in order to improve clinical cover and to relieve hard pressed government medical officers. Central hospitals have since the early 1980s continued to offer specialists in the private sector the privilege to undertake sessions in exchange for the right to admit their private patients into government hospitals. These specialists received payment for each (two and half hour) session of clinical services they provided at government institutions. Because the level of payment for sessional consultants was not being reviewed on a regular basis and for a very long time, in line with prevailing rates of inflation, very few consultants have continued to undertake such sessions at government hospitals.

In some cases the MOHCW provides free vaccines and cold chain equipment (including refrigerators) to general practitioners in private practice who provide childhood immunization services. The proviso for such an offer being that the practitioners should not charge clients for the cost of the vaccines. Private hospitals that are allowed to treat tuberculosis patients receive free TB drugs from the state. Such hospitals only charge TB patients consultation and hotel fees but not for the cost of the TB drugs. The MOHCW, general practitioners, professional associations and the medical school collaborate in continuing education programs such as rational prescription practices, the introduction of new treatment policies and regimens, e.g. for Tuberculosis, STI, HIV/AIDS and malaria.

The MOHCW has over the years afforded government employees the privilege to engage in private practice after their official hours of work. Under these privileges government employed specialists are allowed to engage in private practice during one afternoon of their working hours per week. They are also allowed to admit their private patients into government private hospital wards at central hospitals including having the privilege to use government facilities to perform surgery or special procedures on these private patients.

District health executive teams have also been given the option to allow private practitioners who operate within the district hospital's catchment area, admission rights for their private patients at district hospitals. The revenue, other than that related to direct consultation and other doctors' fees accrues to the hospital's HSF. A major problem in the management of this process has been that of government inadvertently subsidizing the cost of health care provided to private patients admitted by private doctors in its institutions. This is mainly due to poor financial management and billing systems in most government health institutions.

The privilege to admit private patients into government hospitals had originally been restricted to specialists and consultants. With time this was extended to include generalist medical officers operating in the private sector who hold an open practicing certificate issued by the Health Professions Authority. Government employed medical officers (who are not specialists) are only permitted to undertake private practice during their own free time and outside official hours of work. Government employed general duty medical officers do not have the privilege to admit their private patients into government facilities. Government employed medical officers and general medical practitioners working in private practice are however allowed to do locum duties at government facilities as and when shortages of staff arise. To qualify to do locums in government institutions government employed doctors must be off duty or on leave. Most locum duties take place in emergency and accident departments of hospitals and are performed on a shift basis.

Junior doctors who are doing their internship are not allowed to do locum duties or to engage in private practice at all. This category of doctor is issued with a restricted practicing certificate which only allows him or her to practice at designated government institutions. Designated institutions include all the 5 central hospitals (teaching), Ingutsheni Mental Hospital and Hwange Colliery Hospital, which is a private hospital. The Ministry of Health and Child Welfare, the Faculty of Medicine and the Health Professions Authority of Zimbabwe are responsible for the designation of such institutions which they monitor on a regular basis to determine their continued suitability as teaching hospitals.

The problem has been that some medical doctors employed by the state have abused the privilege granted to them to do private practice. Some spend more time at their private surgeries than they do at their places of work and yet continue to draw full salaries and allowances from the government. In some cases some senior doctors employ junior doctors with restricted practicing certificates to work at their surgeries, even when they are supposed to be on official duty. These junior doctors prefer to abscond from their official duties. A few of these senior doctors have had to appear before the disciplinary committee of the Health Professions Authority for these and other offences. Some specialists use their positions of employment in government hospitals to recruit and refer patients to their private surgeries, where they treat them for a fee. In other cases they use government hospital facilities to admit their private patients as non paying patients yet recover fees from them.

The privilege to undertake private practice is not restricted to medical doctors. Nurses, laboratory technicians and radiologists are granted similar privileges under similar conditions. In the late 1990s when the public health sector began to experience serious shortages of nursing personnel the MOHCW and the PSC agreed to allow nurses employed in the public sector to do locum duties at government institutions, including at those institutions they were employed at. More opportunities were created for retired nurses or those employed in the private sector to be engaged on a part time basis at government hospitals.

The MOHCW also explored additional ways of collaborating with the private sector in the training of health professionals. An agreement was entered into with the Hwange Colliery hospital (a private hospital facility) to train Registered General Nurses. Another private hospital in Harare was granted approval by the Health Professions Authority to train nurses in post basic specialist areas such as Theater and Intensive Care nursing for both the private and public sectors. Mission hospitals have for a long time collaborated with the MOHCW in both the provision of health services and the training of nurses.

In the area of public health training the MOHCW developed a field based Masters in Public Health (MPH) degree program with the assistance of the Rockefeller Foundation and in collaboration with the University of Zimbabwe. Lecturers in this course are from both the University of Zimbabwe and the MOHCW.

The MOHCW has long standing collaborative arrangements with the private sector in the area of disease prevention and control, especially the prevention and control of malaria. The hospitality industry has conducted vector control activities in collaboration with the MOHCW in areas where tourism is the main industry. Drug and pesticide companies offer free training to MOHCW field staff in the use and maintenance of spraying equipment including the supply of such equipment free of charge. Some companies have joined hands with the MOHCW in conducting awareness campaigns on malaria and HIV/AIDS. In some cases the private commercial sector has adopted and supported hospital wards or departments by either renovating or equipping them.

The private not for profit sector

Collaboration with the private not for profit sector has generally been between the MOHCW and religious missions represented by the Zimbabwe Association of Church Related Hospitals (ZACH). This long time association has always been informal with no legally binding framework or contract. Details of the working arrangements are described in Chapter 8 of this book.

The government has a history of supporting local NGOs such as the Jairos Jiri Association for the disabled and nursing homes for the aged. The MOHCW provides financial assistance to these organizations to run their health services, mainly to support staff salaries and in other cases in the form of per capita grants to run nursing homes. Several other organizations complement the work of the MOHCW, for example, the Kidney Association of Zimbabwe supports renal dialysis programs in government institutions and Rotary International works with government in its efforts to eradicate Polio.

The framework of collaboration between the MOHCW and the not for profit sector generally requires that NGOs be registered with the government before they can start operating in the country. In Zimbabwe registration of NGOs is the responsibility of the Ministry of the Public Service, Labor and Social Welfare in line with the prescribed legislation. NGOs are required to deliver services that complement existing government priorities and within the country's health policies. Experience to date shows poor coordination of the NGO sector, both amongst themselves and in their working relationships with the MOHCW. For example, the MOHCW in Zimbabwe has a user fee policy which stipulates that no user fees should be charged for primary care services provided at health center level in rural areas. ZACH institutions have however continued to charge user fees in defiance of this policy, despite the fact that they receive health grants from government. The main reason being that the health grant from government was not adequate enough to support the health services they provided. One way to resolve this matter would be for the MOHCW to enter into a formal contractual agreement in which the MOHCW pays ZACH the full cost of delivering the core health service package. These institutions would in turn be required to deliver the package of services free of charge at the point of delivery. Several factors would need to be taken into account in determining the level of payment to ZACH institutions, namely; the salary grant currently being paid, the duty free status these institutions enjoy in importing their goods, subsidized drug purchases, charity funds and material donations their receive from abroad.

Table 6.5 is a summary of some of the incentives which governments, including the government of Zimbabwe, in the Sub-Saharan region have put in place to encourage collaboration with the private not for profit sector.

Table 6.5 Incentives for not-for-profit providers in selected countries in Africa

Incentives	Country
Provision of a Grant ·	Ethiopia, Malawi, Namibia, Tanzania, Uganda, Zambia, Zimbabwe,
Staff secondment	Ethiopia, Ghana, *Kenya, Malawi, Tanzania, Swaziland, Uganda, Zambia, Zimbabwe
Payment of salaries by Government.	Ethiopia, Ghana, Malawi, Namibia, Nigeria, Tanzania, Zimbabwe
Exemption of duty on imports of equipment and drugs.	Ethiopia, Ghana, Nigeria, Tanzania, Uganda, Zambia, Zimbabwe.
Purchase of Drugs from government drugs stores.	Ethiopia, Ghana, *Kenya, Malawi, Tanzania, Uganda, Zambia, Zimbabwe

*Based on: WHO/ARA/CC/97.2; *Proposal: Kenya, NHSS II*

Methods of Provider Payment in Zimbabwe

One of the main objectives of the Medical Services Act is to ensure the provision of quality health care across all providers of care and to provide incentives to keep the costs of health care under control. For example, the Act requires all health provider institutions, health professionals and training institutions to be registered and accredited before they can operate. Additional measures include regulation of cost sharing requirements, supply restrictions and increased use of medically appropriate care and practices such as the use generic prescriptions, adherence to standard treatment protocols and continuing education for practicing professionals.

Payment mechanisms for providers of care

Public sector providers receive an annual *line budget* from the Ministry of Finance to cover all the services provided by individual institutions during the course of the year. This mode of payment applies to all MOHCW facilities, parastatal bodies, local authorities and religious institutions that provide health services. Apart from being perennially inadequate to cover the needs of public sector facilities the line item budget limits the ability of hospital authorities to operate efficiently and to react to local circumstances as they cannot reallocate across budget categories. This type of payment promotes inefficiency and waste.

Public health facilities also derive some revenue from user fee payments which they are now able to retain for use at local level. Some of this revenue is from direct out of pocket payment by members of the public at the point of service delivery. The other revenue comes from the reimbursement of fees by third party insurance schemes. The Department of Social Welfare also reimburses central hospitals and urban local authorities monies for having provided free treatment to vulnerable groups who are eligible for free treatment in terms of the government user fee policy. The amount claimed for reimbursement by these institutions is on a per capita basis. Unfortunately, this type of payment provides incentives for institutions to inflate the number of patients they have attended to, especially considering that the Department of Social Welfare often has limited capacity to monitor any abuse of this system.

The majority of health professionals employed in the public health sector are paid monthly salaries and allowances. The level of public sector salaries is based on government salary grades which are partly determined on the basis of the profession, professional experience, qualifications, settings and responsibilities of the health professional. To some extent the public sector allows for negotiations to take place between the government (as the employer) and professional associations on the adjustment of salaries. Those health professionals who are engaged on a part time or shift basis are paid *pro rata*.

Private sector health facilities are paid user fees as direct out of pocket payment by patients or through third party payers. Private practitioners charge a fee for each consultation (or procedure) performed based on the Relative Value Schedule (RVS). If a private practitioner admits a patient in a private hospital the practitioner charges the patient for each visit, patient contact and any procedure performed. The admitting hospital charges the patient daily hotel (admission) fees as well as for each item used in the treatment of the patient. Semi-autonomous central hospitals have over the years also adopted a similar mode of charging patients, especially those that admit patients to private wards.

Practitioners using this type of payment have the potential to over-prescribe treatment and/or submit fraudulent/inflated claims to health insurers. The hyperinflationary environment experienced in Zimbabwe often makes it difficult for both providers and payers to determine the real costs of providing medical care in the country. As a result during the period of economic decline the pricing structure of medical services disintegrated to an extent that patients were left at the mercy of private practitioners who charged arbitrary and exorbitant fees without a consensus with health insurers.

Managed care has not been a common phenomenon in Zimbabwe. This system of provider payment involves the integration of health financing with the delivery of contractually defined health services to members. Members are provided with incentives to use a network of selected providers such as health facilities, general practitioners, laboratories and pharmacies. The next best example of managed care in Zimbabwe is that of the Premier Service Medical Aid Society (PSMAS) which employs and/or contracts medical doctors (general practitioners), manages diagnostic and health care facilities and has entered into formal agreements with some pharmacies to provide services to its members at pre-negotiated rates.

The MOHCW at one time entered into contractual arrangements in which private hospitals had to provide health services to surrounding rural communities where the government did not provide such services. A good example is the contract entered into between the MOHCW and a mine hospital which was required to treat patients referred from government district hospitals within one province, free of charge. The private hospital billed the MOHCW the total amount of treating individual patients based on the full costs of attending to each patient (per capita). The arrangement was difficult to monitor and had no incentive for cost containment. There was thus a potential for the hospital to over treat individual patients as well as inflating the number of patients treated.

The Health Services Fund

In 1997 the MOHCW established a Health Services Fund (HSF) under Section 30 of the Audit and Exchequer Act (Chapter 22:03). The main objective of establishing the HSF was to facilitate the collection and administration of revenue accruing from user fees. Revenue collected from user fees was intended to supplement government recurrent and capital budget allocations. This included the development and maintenance of health services, programs and related activities approved by the Secretary for Health. Funds flowing into the HSF consisted of revenue from user fees, interest earned from investment and funds donated or granted and accepted by the Secretary for Health to further the objectives of the HSF. Development partners channeled some of their funds directly into the HSF for use at the various levels of the MOHCW. The HSF was conceived as a mechanism to enable resources from various sources, including those from the government and development partners, to be pooled together in a manner that encouraged flexibility in their utilization. The HSF started operating in earnest in 1998.

Expenditures from the Health Services Fund were managed based on systems and procedures agreed between the government and participating partners, in this case DANIDA and the European Union (EU). At the initial stages of its establishment the utilization of the HSF was governed by strict rules and procedures which meant that the HSF could not be used to fund expenditure items such as advances, travel and subsistence; salaries and wages and capital investments. These funds were disbursed to MOHCW, RDCs and mission institutions on a quarterly basis against approved and costed plans or work programs. Subsequent fund releases were made contingent upon the complete liquidation of expenditures for the previous plan period, the submission of activity reports from the previous plan period and a costed program of work for the next plan period.

In order to improve transparency and accountability in the use of the HSF the MOHCW developed an Accounts Handbook and an Operational Manual for the HSF with full collaboration and approval by the Ministry of Finance (MOFED). The guidelines assisted MOHCW accounting staff to maintain acceptable internal control systems in managing the HSF. The operational manual detailed how the HSF assets were to be managed, the reporting requirements and policy guidance. By 2000 all districts in Zimbabwe had opened local HSF bank accounts to manage the HSF. This fund has continued to be managed by Hospital Committees and District Health Executive Committees assisted by two members of Community Health Councils, who represent the interests of local communities.

The establishment of the HSF initially experienced problems which involved delays in the completion of the manual meant to guide staff in the day to day management of the fund. Because members of the DHMTs and hospital executives did not receive training on the HSF guidelines on time they were not very clear as to what the funds in the HSF could or could not be used for. Some of the rules and regulations that governed the use of the HSF were too restrictive and in some cases conflicted with existing Treasury Instructions. MOHCW accounting staffs were not familiar with commercial accounting procedures that were adopted for the management of the HSF. Because of the poor planning capacity at the district level it was difficult to monitor expenditures against submitted plans.

District Health Executive members complained that despite the good intentions of the HSF it continued to be difficult for them to respond rapidly to local disease outbreaks using the HSF. For example it was not possible for them to undertake minor works such as repairing broken windows, furniture etc. In order to resolve some of the problems identified a review of the operations of the HSF was commissioned.

The review concluded that the rules and procedures of the HSF were not flexible enough and that they needed to be relaxed. As a result of the relaxation in the use of the HSF it was possible, for example, for the DHMTs to engage and pay the wages and allowances for temporary staff to undertake field activities in the prevention and control of epidemics. Hospitals were also able to use funds from the HSF to purchase drugs from the private sector. Private suppliers of goods and services had for some time stopped accepting government requisitions because it took too long for them to be honored. The advantage with the HSF was that it operated as a current account from which bank certified cheques were issued and quickly honored.

In order to get their orders settled quickly DHMTs and hospitals tended to use the HSF to pay for items that would normally have been charged to the regular MOHCW budget. However, where such payments had been made, the DHMTs were required to reimburse the HSF account with the same amount of money from the appropriate MOHCW budget item. Because MOHCW accounting staff were not used to handling current accounts they often overspent on the HSF current account and thus committing government to illegal bank overdrafts. As the use of the HSF became more liberalized a capital fund was introduced within this account. The objective of the capital fund was to facilitate, for example, the replacement of essential basic equipment, rehabilitation of infrastructure and the purchase of vehicles. Such capital projects were implemented only if they were part of an *approved* operational plan of the district.

In order to ensure that local communities were actively involved in the planning and budgeting process at the Rural Health Center level, it was agreed that a specified amount of resources in the HSF be allocated to this level. 40% of the HSF allocation (from both the government and development partners) was earmarked to support health center and community level activities. Financial accountability and management arrangements were to be based on existing local participatory structures such as health center and village development committee structures. The introduction of the HSF resulted in a significant increase in the revenue collected from user fees at institutional level. The MOHCW's recovery rate for revenue from user fees had been very poor, at best never exceeding 3.5% of the ministry's total recurrent budget. In contrast urban local authorities often collected up to 40% of their health service costs from user fees. For example, the Bulawayo City Council's health department recovered 30% of its health service costs from user fees and other related charges in 1994. Between the period 1999 and 2000 when the HSF had established itself and was up and running the revenue collected by the MOHCW from user fees increased by 125%.

Table 6.6 Revenue (millions Z$) collected from user fees (1996 - 2002)

Type of hospital	1996/97	1997/98	1999	2000	2001	*2002
Central hospitals				Z$102 (US$0.81)	Z$175 (US$0.21)	Z$356 (US$0.43)
Other hospitals				Z$128 (US$2.3)	Z$168 (US$0.17)	Z$368 (US$0.45)
Total	Z$34.8 (US$3.3)	Z$50 (US$3.0)	Z$99 (US$2.7)	Z$230 (US$4.18)	Z$343 (US$0.42)	Z$724 (US$0.88)
Debtors	Z$19.6 (US$1.9)	Z$62 (US$3.7)	Z$141 (US$3.9)	Z$341 (US$6.2)	Z$581 (US$0.71)	-

Fees abolished at RHCs

Several lessons arise from the ministry's experiences with implementing the HSF. The HSF was an incentive for increased user fee revenue collection at local level. Within a period of 9 months some of the HSF accounts had accumulated up to Z$1 million (US$ 18 000) at institutional level. In most cases this represented more than a five-fold increase in local revenue generation. Some institutions however became overzealous in collecting user fees to the extent that they disregarded exemption mechanisms prescribed by the government to cushion the poor. This made it difficult for the poor to access health services at central and provincial hospitals. The HSF made it possible to channel finances directly to the operational level in a more efficient manner which maximized opportunities for local priority setting. Previously all finances from the treasury went first to the central MOHCW and then to the provincial level before eventually reaching the district. The HSF formed the basis for the establishment of a flexible "common fund" which pooled finances from the government, revenue from user fees and donor funds. It also provided the DHMT with greater flexibility in financial management and direct control of local expenditures. The HSF has become an appropriate vehicle and mechanism for the decentralization of financial management within the MOHCW, which was a major step towards the devolution of financial management to the RDCs. In terms of the Medical Services Act hospitals that have attained semi-autonomous status are required to manage their grants and revenue from user fees using their HSF accounts.

Donor financing

Donor financing became a significant source of health financing in Zimbabwe soon after independence in the early 1980s. In 1994 it was estimated that total donor assistance to the health sector in Zimbabwe accounted for about 31% of public health expenditures and 12% of total expenditures on health. Traditional development partners and contributors to the health sector in Zimbabwe have been the World Bank, the Department for International Development (DFID) UK, United States International Development Agency (USAID), Japanese International Development Agency (JICA), DANIDA, United Nations Children's Emergency Fund (UNICEF), WHO, NORAD and the European Union (EU). In 1999 about 38% of development assistance to Zimbabwe came from the EU. Other development partners included the Netherlands government, the Swedish International Development Agency (SIDA), the Canadian Development Agency (CIDA), UNDP, Cooperazione Italiana, GTZ and UNFPA. A significant proportion of this development assistance was channeled through a number of projects some of which were implemented by international and local NGOs. The World Bank established a project implementation unit within the MOHCW whilst other donors like the EU and DANIDA seconded advisors to the MOHCW.

In 1996 when the MOHCW started the process of developing its National Health Strategy (NHS) (1997-2007) the sector increasingly assumed an active leadership role and initiated a systematic process of engagement with its development partners through regular meetings. Though at the beginning the strategic planning process did not actively involve a wide spectrum of development partners and stakeholders within the health sector, the process later became inclusive of civil society, professional bodies, church related institutions and NGOs. Whilst in the past interactions among stakeholders in the health sector consisted of briefing meetings, these were later broadened into more focused biannual meetings. One meeting focused on setting and agreeing on sector priorities, indicative health sector budget ceilings from government and donor commitments for the coming plan period. Progress in implementing the previous plan period was also evaluated. However, because the budgeting cycles for donors were different from those of the government it was not possible for development partners to provide firm commitments for the next plan period. This made it very difficult for the MOHCW to prepare a comprehensive sectoral plan ahead of the next plan period. The other meeting focused on monitoring progress in the implementation of the annual program and plan of work.

The management of development assistance in Zimbabwe has always been a challenge for the health sector, mainly because of the number of health projects that operated in the country. This challenge was compounded by the fact that each of these projects was funded by different donors with each donor conducting their own review missions and requiring separate reporting formats. These review missions were conducted at different times and all of them required the involvement of MOHCW staff. The ultimate result of this uncoordinated approach was an increase in transaction costs for both the donors and the MOHCW.

The MOHCW and DANIDA developed a framework for cooperation in the health sector, the Health Sector Program Support (HSPS 1 and 2). The implementation of the HSPS was an integral part of the implementation of the National Health Strategic Plan and thus its programming was coterminous with the annual rolling plans of the ministry. Funds from DANIDA were channeled and managed through the Health Services Fund (HSF) and were later to be pooled with those from the European Union and those from the government budget.

The HSF allowed MOHCW headquarters, District Health Management Teams and Hospital Administrators the flexibility and management control to utilize these funds to support a variety of activities in a timely manner. The management of HSPS funds through the HSF eliminated some of the bottlenecks and transaction costs related to separate monitoring and reporting mechanisms. The HSPS relied on the generation of MOHCW reports and the biannual joint meetings.

The evolution of a political and economic crisis in Zimbabwe heralded a period of uncertainty with regard the future of development assistance to the country. The Netherlands government and SIDA were the first Western countries to react to the crisis by terminating their development assistance to the government of Zimbabwe. These decisions to terminate development assistance to the health sector in Zimbabwe by these countries were unilateral, politically motivated and a reaction to the manner in which the land reform program was being implemented in Zimbabwe. DANIDA terminated its development assistance program to Zimbabwe in 2000 by suspending the HSPS valued at US$ 29.7 million followed by SIDA which suspended its program valued at US$ 6.4 million. Subsequent to all these events other development partners followed suit and either reduced or terminated their development assistance to the health sector in Zimbabwe. Those who continued with development assistance opted to channel it through non state actors such as local and international NGOs, mainly targeting pro-poor social programs. As a result there was a significant decline in development assistance to the health sector from an estimated 31% of public health expenditures and 12% of total health expenditures in 1994 to about 5.4% and 1% respectively in 2001.

One of the aid management tools that were evolving at the time (1997) included the Sector Wide Approach (SWAp) to health development. At the time the MOHCW resisted pressure from the World Bank and European Union to adopt the SWAp as a tool for managing development assistance to the health sector in Zimbabwe. The MOHCW objected because the number of health donors and the volume of aid flows were on the decline, whilst on the other hand relations between the government and the majority of its development partners were deteriorating. Considering that the main objective of a SWAp is to improve the management of development assistance based on some Memorandum of Understanding, it was the MOHCW's view that there was no conceivable way such a MoU could be entered into. The MOHCW was convinced that it was already conducting its business on the basis of sector wide thinking.

In restructuring the organization the MOHCW had abolished the project unit that managed the World Bank supported Family Health Project in the MOHCW. A single national health strategic framework (1997-2007) and a national health plan had been developed on the basis of an all inclusive consultative process. There were biannual joint consultative meetings, one of which focused on evaluating progress in implementing the previous year's health plan, resource mobilization for the coming plan period, prioritization and program planning. The other meeting focused on joint monitoring of midterm progress in the current plan period. To the extent possible, vertical funds were channeled to support programs in line with priories of the national health strategic plan, the three year and annual rolling plans and medium term resource ceilings.

A lot of challenges have remained in the management of donor assistance locally, of which the SWAp would only be a small part to any solution. Working relations between the government of Zimbabwe, NGOs and civil society groups continued to deteriorate mainly as a result of poor governance within the institutions of government. Access to development assistance continued to deteriorate with Zimbabwe being denied access to international finance from the Breton Woods and related institutions through the enactment of the Zimbabwe Democracy Economic Recovery Act (2001) by the United States Government. The EU also imposed sanctions which suspended some of the development aid previously earmarked for the health sector in Zimbabwe.

Calls for improved aid effectiveness

Recipient and donor countries have for a long time called for more effective management of development assistance in order to produce tangible results at the local level. One of the initiatives responding to such calls is the Paris Declaration (2005) on Aid Effectiveness. The Paris Declaration advocates for country ownership, harmonization, alignment, management for results and mutual accountability in the management of development assistance. Most such initiatives emphasize the need for developing countries to improve on their governance and to manage for results in order to accelerate progress towards the achievement of the MDGs. As a result several aid management instruments have been developed which include the Sector Wide Approach (SWAp), Poverty Reduction Strategy Papers (PRSPs), Poverty Reduction Support Credit (PRSC), Poverty Reduction Growth Facility (PRGFs) and the Medium Term Expenditure Framework (MTEF) process.

The implications of these initiatives are that donors must establish coherent policies at the global level and agree to strengthen and use government systems as a basis for common financial management and reporting procedures. Whilst developing countries must exercise effective leadership over their development policies and strategies and manage resources responsibly, development partners on the other hand must base their support on the country's national priorities, development strategies, institutions and procedures. The donors must harmonize their policies and approaches on global issues and allocate responsibilities amongst themselves at the global and country levels.

Challenges of increasing overseas development assistance include:
 ♦ The lack of global policy coherence and coordination of donors

- Lack of predictability in donor funding due to conditionalities, different donor disbursement cycles which frustrate macroeconomic management and program planning
- The growing "verticalization" of aid as a result of the GFATM, PEPFAR, GAVI, etc
- Increasing number of aid management instruments such as SWAps, PRSPs, (PRSCs), (PRGFs) and MTEFs which have created coordination, management and planning nightmares at global and country levels
- Inadequacy of monitoring and evaluation systems required to link resources to achievements and to provide an accountability framework for both the donors and the government.
- Significant amounts of development aid being "off budget" and not captured in the balance of payment or government budget.

The MDG approach highlights the links between health, education, water, sanitation, poverty reduction and socio-economic growth. Estimates indicated that a total of US$50 billion was required on an annual basis to achieve MDGs across all sectors and of this amount an estimated US$15-30 billion was required for the health sector annually. The health sector however faces several challenges in this area which include the human resources for health crisis, barriers to physical access to health care and weaknesses in the function of health systems. There is a need to build the capacity to estimate the financial requirements for health systems strengthening that will result in the delivery of the MDGs. (Schieber, G (2007).

Conclusions and the way forward

Financial reforms in most African countries have focused on the mobilization of additional resources for the sector, the optimization of existing resources and the achievement of sustainable health financing. The commonest strategies adopted include the implementation of user fees, formal health insurance schemes, partnerships with the private sector and re-prioritization in the use of public health resources. In other cases health systems have developed and implemented mechanisms for local accountability, hospital efficiency and improved the coordination of development partners within the health sector.

Legal reforms have been implemented to facilitate retention and local use of revenue generated from user fees at public health institutions. Some of this revenue has been earmarked to improve the quality of services at facility level. Policies have also been developed and implemented to ensure that those who are able to pay for health services actually do so. Experience has however demonstrated that on its own revenue generated from user fees in the public health sector is unlikely to be enough to address the growing health financing gap. If user fees are to contribute significantly to revenue generation then public health institutions must be allowed to charge fees that reflect the economic costs of producing and delivering health services. Such fee levels must be supported by appropriate safety-net mechanisms that are well publicized and can protect the poor and other vulnerable members of society.

Successful private-public collaboration dependents on many factors which include; the capacity to negotiate, construct and monitor contracts; effective financial management and accounting systems; reliable information systems and an effective regulatory environment. An effective and competitive contracting out process requires an adequate pool of partners to enter into contract with as well as a competitive free market environment. In most developing countries subcontracting has been confined to urban areas where there is a large pool of companies that can compete. The dilemma for policy makers and implementers is that the majority of district hospitals, the level at which these reforms matter most, are located in rural areas.

Efficiencies in resource utilization can be achieved through the introduction of cost effective essential health care packages as a means of rationing and prioritizing services. The development of core health service packages has often made it easier for ministries of health to monitor the quality and quantity of services, facilities and financial resources required to serve a particular segment of the population. Some countries have put in place measures that streamline expenditures on tertiary and central hospitals whilst others have gone a step further and increased the autonomy of these hospitals with the view to improving technical and allocative efficiencies.

Decentralization has been implemented as a means to improve accountability at the district level by allowing local decision making authority on budgeting, planning and monitoring of expenditures at this level. This has made it possible for districts to assume direct control over major budget items, revenue generation, its retention and utilization at local level.

The above measures require the development of coherent health financing policies for the countries' health sectors which must deal with some of the following issues:

+ Criteria for allocating financial resources to RDCs, urban local authorities and religious missions that provide health services
+ Modalities for the flow of donor funds to the district level
+ How to deal with earmarked funds such as resources from global initiatives, especially those that require the setting up of separate management and procurement systems
+ Legal reforms to support proposals to ring fence financial allocations to local authorities to deliver health services
+ The ideal proportions of financing curative versus preventive services
+ The role of the government and the private sector in financing health services in the country
+ Whether revenue collected from user fees at institutional level complements government allocations or not

Such policies provide a framework within which the role of the state in health financing is clearly defined to ensure that the health sector is adequately and sustainably financed. These policies must also ensure that available resources are equitably allocated, efficiently and effectively utilized on nationally agreed priorities. The state has an obligation to implement measures to correct any market failures that arise within the sector by exploring risk pooling strategies. A health financing policy must further define the total package of services the sector will provide, define services that will be provided free of charge and at what levels of the health system and provide clear eligibility criteria for exemptions. It must be clear how existing fee structures were determined in both the private and public sectors. Where there is a core health service package this must be costed so that the cost of delivering each intervention is available for each level of the health delivery system.

Such a policy framework must deal with decisions that affect the choices of services to be delivered, the roles of the various stakeholders, the structures and systems through which these services are delivered and the nature and management processes for the resources needed to operate the entire health system. The MOHCW needs to be clear as to the proportion of resources that are spent by different providers country wide. In this context it will be necessary to institutionalize National Health Accounts and to ensure that the ministry of health leads this process. Information from the NHA is crucial to the development of complementary policies required to deal with issues of poverty alleviation and social safety nets for the poor.

The same policy framework must define the roles and responsibilities of the private for profit sector, the development of more formal financing mechanisms between the MOHCW and local authorities, religious missions and RDCs. A formal financing agreement between the above parties can easily be based on the delivery of a costed package of core health services. It should also be clear to both parties what the government will or will not pay for in terms of contracted service delivery by these institutions.

All stakeholders must agree on the minimum acceptable levels of health financing for the health sector. The starting point could be the Abuja Declaration which stipulated that at least 15% of total government expenditures should be spent on health. The other parameter to use as an objective baseline is the recommendations of the CMH for at least between US$ 34 to US$ 40 per capita to be spent on a health package delivered in a developing country setting. Such a consensus position must consider health expenditures by the private sector and ensure that the two complement each other. According to Scheiber G, (2007) the monitoring of health expenditure performance must take into account the following parameters:

Local currency measures
  ♦ Total health spending
  ♦ Health expenditures as share of GDP
  ♦ Public versus Private expenditures
  ♦ Public health share of all public expenditures
  ♦ Share of administrative expenses
  ♦ Expenditure by type of service
  ♦ Capital versus recurrent budgets
  ♦ Nominal per capita expenditures
Numeraire currency
  ♦ Exchange rates
  ♦ Purchasing power parities

Many countries continue to allocate large proportions of their health sector budgets to curative services. It is thus necessary for a consensus position to be reached as to the best way to strike a balance between expenditures on curative services, without compromising the quality of services, and those on preventive services. Additional efficiency gains can be achieved through making rational decisions regarding the proportion of expenditures at the district and community levels versus expenditures at the central level.

Weaknesses in financial management and accounting systems are yet another area of concern which requires detailed appraisal in terms of available capacity at the national and district levels. Modalities of the flow of government and donor funds to the district levels need further scrutiny in order to ensure efficient and effective allocation and utilization of the resources at these levels of the system.

For Zimbabwe a combination of viable user fee policies, voluntary and social health insurance schemes and an efficiently operating Health Services Fund form a credible basis for sustainable health financing for semi-autonomous hospitals. If these institutions were allowed to charge economic fees based on the real costs of providing health care and they have efficient billing and accounting systems, only then can they be assured of some sustainable revenue base. It is probably overly ambitious to expect these institutions, especially provincial hospitals, to sustain all their operations on revenue accruing from user fees. Additional measures would have to be instituted to reimburse semi-autonomous hospitals the revenue they lose by adhering to government imposed exemption policies.

Furthermore macroeconomic policy can be designed and implemented in a way that facilitates the development of an efficient health sector, e.g. through hypothecated taxes on personal and corporate income, such as is the case with the AIDS Tax in Zimbabwe. Fiscal policy can be used to improve the allocation and utilization of funds, e.g. a lower rate of inflation has a disproportionately high positive impact on the poor through relatively larger real income than a higher rate. Good governance has the potential to reduce misallocation of resources through corrupt tendencies and encourages responsible utilization of resources.

Review questions

1. In introducing user fees some countries adopted the policy position that user fees are purely to improve the efficiency of the referral system and not to raise revenue. In your view how does such a policy achieve the said objectives?

2. The introduction of user fees has been associated with reduced utilization of health services by the poor. Such outcomes have been attributed to poor management and administration of user fee schemes. How can these and other adverse consequences of user fees be managed or prevented?

3. Several countries in Africa have for a long time had plans to introduce Social Health Insurance schemes. The majority of these plans have not seen the light of day. You are a consultant on health financing and you have been contracted to assist one of these countries to establish such a scheme. Submit a summary report of possible findings and recommendations to the authorities.

4. Previously, revenue collected from user fees in the public sector reverted to central government coffers. Describe the process which the MOH in your country must go through in order to be able to legally retain revenue collected from user fees at its institutions.

7

THE CONCEPT OF A CORE HEALTH SERVICE PACKAGE

Introduction

According to the Commission on Macroeconomics and Health (CMH) a basic package or core package of health services for a developing country must at least include those essential interventions that the state is willing to guarantee universal coverage through public (including donors) financing. The following criteria have been proposed to guide the choice of interventions to be included in the package:

♦ Technically efficacious and capable of being delivered successfully

♦ The targeted diseases should be those that impose a heavy burden on society (taking into consideration individual illness and social spillovers)

♦ Social benefits should exceed the costs of interventions.

♦ The needs of the poor should be stressed

♦ Should be covered universally and funded by public and donor funds

♦ According to the CMH the per capita cost should be in the order of between US$34 and US$40 per year

♦ Existing capacity must be able to deliver the package

♦ There must be linkages across services at different levels of the system

The process of defining and developing an essential health package is normally very time consuming, usually preceded by a complex process of determining the country's burden of disease. This process is then followed by the selection of interventions of proven cost effectiveness within the local context. In an environment where there is paucity of information on the burden of disease and where it is not possible to undertake a burden of disease study, the package can be defined based on information from reviews of literature and data from countries with similar epidemiological and demographic characteristics. The selection of services to be provided must take into consideration the existing epidemiological situation as well as the country's potential epidemiological transition to chronic and non-communicable diseases.

The World Health Organization (WHO) recommends that a minimum package for both low and middle income countries must be comprehensive enough to include HIV/AIDS prevention and treatment, family planning, the treatment of Sexually Transmitted Infections (STI), prenatal and delivery care. There has been concern that the burden of reproductive health problems has not been fully estimated or costed, especially the screening for cancer of the cervix. Whilst communicable diseases such as the control of tuberculosis and malaria are high on this agenda, non-communicable conditions must increasingly form an integral part of an essential package of health services. It is routine to include health support systems strengthening as part of the essential health package in the areas of diagnostic laboratory and radiological services, pharmaceuticals and procurement processes, management information systems, health financing and financial management systems, human resources for health development, infrastructure development, and supervision, planning and budgeting.

Systems must be developed or strengthened so as to effectively deliver the agreed interventions at the various levels of the health delivery system i.e. at the community level, health center level and hospital level. The package can however not be delivered in isolation of the rest of the health system. To achieve a continuum of care and a seamless health care delivery system it is necessary to also include some of the interventions not considered to be an integral part of the basic package of health services. Such services should form part of the referral system in the hierarchy of service delivery. Package interventions delivered at health center level should be able to receive prompt referral to the next level of the health system. The point of discussion is usually that of prioritizing between services provided at central hospitals and those provided at the primary health care level of the system. The referral hierarchy must include support by general hospitals and some specialist services.

Rationale behind an essential package of health services

Because resources are never enough to satisfy all the needs and demands for health care, rationing cannot be altogether avoided. The adoption of an essential package of health services is arguably one form of rationing or prioritization of health services by the government. An essential health package improves technical and allocative efficiency in the delivery of health care, facilitates the achievement of universal coverage of health services and guarantees access to cost-effective interventions that have the potential to deal with the main causes of the country's burden of disease. It is not a package for the poor but a package of services that satisfies the needs and expectations of the people and a package that is affordable to both the government and its partners to provide based on the principle of universal access and social protection.

The targeting of resources to a package enables the government to move closer towards achieving its objective of universal and equitable access to health services, especially by vulnerable groups. According to Bobadilla (1995) the concept of a package of services brings together interventions that can be delivered with the same level of technological sophistication through the same facility or level of the health delivery system.

Prioritization as a form of rationing health services

The setting of priorities involves making trade-offs between comprehensiveness, universality, equity, health gain and choice. Unfortunately this may involve individual preferences being sacrificed for the greater good. Arguments against explicit rationing in health care revolve more on how decisions to allocate health care budgets to particular forms of treatments are arrived at. The other view is that services must be prioritized from the point of view of communities, the effectiveness of interventions and their ability to be delivered efficiently. Yet others have argued that the cost efficiency principle must be given low priority.

Prioritization is likely to be accepted if it is transparent and enables different interests to contribute to decision making. Though it is possible to continue providing some of the services that are outside a defined package of care through public financing, it has also been argued that public financing should discontinue and access to such services be limited to those that can pay for them. The other option is for the services to be provided through privately financed insurance schemes. Such considerations may however go against the wishes and expectations of the people, the principles of universal access and guaranteed social protection. The government of Zimbabwe formally adopted a core health service package in 1995. Ever since the country attained its independence, health services have always been delivered at four levels, namely, the primary level consisting of community based services and those provided at the health center, the secondary or district level, the provincial or tertiary level and the central or quaternary (hospital) level.

Details of the Core Health Service Package for Zimbabwe are available in the MOHCW document, "The Zimbabwe Core Health Services Package (1995) and in Appendix 1. The following is a summary of the 1995 Zimbabwe core health service package:

♦ *Reproductive health – Safe motherhood initiatives and reduction of maternal mortality*
  ♦ Antenatal care.
  ♦ Delivery.
  ♦ Post partum care.
  ♦ Family Planning.
  ♦ Care of the new born.
  ♦ Micronutrient supplementation.
♦ *Child Health and Immunization*
  ♦ EPI services (outreach and static facilities).
  ♦ Integrated Management of Childhood Illnesses including ARI and CDD.
  ♦ Growth Monitoring (at static facilities and community based).
♦ *Preventive services and control of Communicable Diseases*
  ♦ Prevention and control of HIV/AIDS (PMTCT, VCT).
  ♦ Prevention and control of Tuberculosis (DOTS).
  ♦ Management of STIs (Syndromic).
  ♦ Management of opportunistic Infections.
  ♦ Prevention and control of Malaria.
♦ *Other diseases with a potential for epidemics – cholera, diarrhea, plague, etc.*
♦ *Water and sanitation*
♦ *Nutrition*
  ♦ Growth Monitoring – facility and community based.
  ♦ Micronutrient supplementation and surveillance – vitamin A, Iron and Iodine.
  ♦ Supplementary feeding program.
♦ *Rehabilitation services*
  ♦ Surveillance for disabled children – community based.
  ♦ Physiotherapy.

♦ *Pain alleviation, minor trauma and infection*
♦ *Essential Drugs supply*
   ♦ Essential Drugs List for Zimbabwe (EDLIZ).
   ♦ Drug supplies for community health workers.

In addition to the service delivery interventions outlined above the package includes the following health support services and systems:
   ♦ Drug procurement, distribution and management
   ♦ Laboratory services
   ♦ Information, Education and Communication (IEC)
   ♦ Support and supervision
   ♦ Human Resources Development
   ♦ Infrastructure development
   ♦ Planning, budgeting and management systems
   ♦ Monitoring and evaluation

The MOHCW in Zimbabwe did not specifically cost its package of health services because the World Bank had already costed a similar package of interventions to be US$22.00 per capita per annum. This package was at the time referred to as an essential health service package for middle and low income countries (World Bank, 1994). An updated package of essential services proposed by the CMH has an estimated per capita cost of between US$ 34.00 and US$ 40.00 per annum.

Costing and financing the health package

The cost of delivering a package of health services usually takes into account several parameters which include:
   ♦ The expected number of participants or users of the intervention at facility level
   ♦ The expected number of participants in turn depends on the intended coverage (%) for the intervention.
   ♦ The number of potential intervention users in turn depends on the target disease's epidemiological and demographic profiles.

In costing the package it is also necessary to consider inputs such as drugs and supplies, the quantities of which can be determined from existing or proposed clinical and treatment guidelines. Cost calculations assume no prior budget constraints as the intention is to determine the per capita costs which will result from delivering the full package of interventions. In addition to the above, inputs such as labor costs and the use of fixed capital equipment and buildings are included (Bobadilla, 1995).

Factors such as wages, the availability of infrastructure, the amount of inefficiently used infrastructure, the availability of hard currency and the quality of care ultimately alter the cost-effectiveness of any given intervention or package. The prevailing prices of goods and services purchased from the private sector, subsidies for other public services and the size and distribution of the population play a significant part in the ultimate costs of the package. From an economist point of view it is advisable to make cost efficiency adjustments, by assuming that all health service costs are 20% or 30% higher than calculated due to losses, waste, misdiagnoses, etc. (irrespective of the health intervention). The factor depends on whether the country is in the middle (20%) or low-income (30%) bracket. As a result input costs are multiplied by 1.2 or 1.3 to account for such efficiency losses.

The resulting costs are crude in terms of accuracy and order of magnitude and must be taken to be country specific as they are influenced by the prevailing disease patterns, demographic patterns and the economic situation, particularly with respect to inputs that depend on foreign currency which may be scarce in some countries. Salary inputs will vary significantly depending on the country's level of development and state of the economy.

As earlier indicated the MOHCW in Zimbabwe pegged the cost of its core health service package at US$22 per capita, in line with the estimates by the World Bank (1994). At the time the cost did not include inputs related to the use of Anti-Retroviral Therapy (ART), Voluntary Counseling and Testing (VCT) services and the Prevention of Mother to Child Transmission (PMTCT) of HIV. These services had not been fully developed at the time.

As the package is an integral part of the country's national health service the sources of finance include resources from the government complemented by contributions from development partners and the private sector. Additional sources in this area include priority based reallocation of existing resources, more efficient utilization of existing resources, cost recovery with appropriate safety net mechanisms and the introduction of a Social Health Insurance Scheme.

Up until the year 2000 the estimates of expenditure for the health sector in Zimbabwe were based on an estimated annual per capita cost of US$22. This meant that for a population of 12 million people the sector required approximately US$ 264 million per annum to deliver the package. However, as previously intimated, this estimate excluded the costs occasioned by advancements in the management of HIV/AIDS. Based on the recommendations of the Commission on Microeconomics and Health (CMH) the estimated per capita cost of providing an essential package of health services in a developing country is between US$ 34 and US$ 40. Based on these figures Zimbabwe would require at least between US$ 445 and US$ 524 per annum to deliver the package to a population of 13.1 million (UNDP: HDR, 2007-2008). This is the amount of money that the country would require to deliver the primary care package, assuming a population coverage of 100%. Due to inherent weaknesses in the country's health delivery system, it is unlikely that service delivery coverage of 100% can be achieved. Furthermore, it is important to take into consideration that the above cost estimates of the package do not include the provision of referral services at tertiary and central hospital levels.. There are also demand side considerations in this equation where some population segments may not be willing to utilize available services for several reasons.

Decentralization and the delivery of an essential health package

The decentralization process is expected to result in part of the health budget being allocated directly to the (DHMT) district level and, with time, to Rural District Councils (RDCs). Under such a scenario the DHMT becomes accountable to RDCs for any operational decisions on health expenditures. A costed package of health services would form the basis upon which health grants are allocated to RDCs depending on agreed targets on population coverage. In addition to these targets it is necessary to set norms and standards that will determine the quality of services expected to be delivered. Such standards provide a framework to monitor and ensure national consistency in the quality of health services across the various RDCs. The number of health staff assigned to a particular RDC will depend on the staff required to deliver the specific package at each level of the health system and the anticipated workload.

Table 7.1 Factors to consider in adopting a package of core health services

Developing the package	Comprehensiveness of the interventions Epidemiological profile and transition Involvement of beneficiaries in selection of interventions
Societal considerations	Responsiveness to societal needs and expectations Social justice, protection and universal coverage Participatory dialogue, accountability involving the people.
Financing the package of core health services.	There must be sustained and reliable government funds supplemented by external funding. The budget should be part of the MTEF process. It is necessary to consider pro-poor budget versus potential cost recovery. The role of social and private health insurance must be considered. Audit and accountability systems must be in place.
Strategy to introduce the package.	As a pilot or phased program. Nested within the existing public, NGO, private for profit organizations. Consideration of equity.
Essential supplies.	Integrated within existing drug distribution system (public/private). Developing or strengthening procurement and distribution systems which must be rapidly responsive. Improving stock management at the local level. Putting in place rational prescription practices (generic prescription). Developing and implementing a quality assurance program and regulating the pharmaceutical industry.
Human resources.	Ensuring there is an appropriate skills mix to deliver the package at each level. Assessing pre- and in-service training requirements. Putting in place incentives to attract and retain staff in remote areas and the public sector. There must be a possibility of interchangeability of functions. Job descriptions must be reviewed in light of the package.

Strategies to deliver an essential package of health services

To maintain their cost effectiveness, interventions within an essential health package must be delivered in an integrated manner. Integration implies that otherwise independent administrative structures and functions and attitudes of health workers must be brought together in such a way as to combine them. Because of synergistic interactions the effectiveness of the package of services as a whole is greater than any of the single components. Patients with little time to use the range of services available to them can take advantage of services delivered as a package. However, some critics feel that delivering a whole package of services may divert personnel time away from other services and render them less effective.

The integration of service tasks can be achieved through integrating service functions at health facility level through implementing the supermarket approach to service delivery using multi-skilled health workers. Such an approach ensures that patients and clients are able to access the full range of services on any day of the week at any time they visit a health facility. For example, a mother visiting a health center will receive her post natal care and her baby and child under the age of five years can also receive immunizations and their growth monitored, if these are due. Such an arrangement reduces the occurrence of missed opportunities in service delivery.

Whereas vertical approaches are disease specific in their focus, horizontal approaches are more holistic and focus on a particular level of the service delivery system providing the necessary linkages with the rest of the components of the health delivery system.

The integration of management and support functions emphasizes the inter-sectoral nature of planning and linkages in the implementation of multipurpose programs such as IMCI, STI, etc. In integrated systems budgeting and financial management processes allocate resources to multipurpose programs as opposed to disease specific "projects" or programs which use earmarked funds. The Health Service Fund (HSF) established in the MOHCW in Zimbabwe is a good example of the pooling of funds from different sources with minimal attribution to the sources or targeting of specific diseases at the operational level. The health information system is also geared towards collecting and analyzing data from several programs and services. The monitoring system is supported by an integrated supervision framework that uses an integrated checklist spanning across several programs and systems. Any qualified member of the DHMT can use the integrated checklist to monitor the performance of staff across all the interventions of the health package. Different training sessions conducted by different program managers or trainers is inefficient in terms of the utilization of financial resources and time. Staff is taken away from their work stations to attend several training workshops organized by different programs at different times whereas if an integrated approach where to be adopted such a move would result in efficiency gains.

Delivering the essential health package at each level of the health system

The essential health package in Zimbabwe facilitated horizontal and vertical integration of service delivery at all levels of the health system. At the primary level the continuum of care involved the establishment of linkages in service delivery between the community level and the health center. The concept resulted in a seamless and integrated delivery of health promotion, preventive, curative and rehabilitation services at the various levels of the system. The community level focuses on advocacy, promotion of use of health care services (improved demand), the treatment of minor conditions and referral of complicated cases to the health center. At this level the Village Health Workers (VHW), Farm Health Workers (FHW), CBDs, Traditional Midwives (TMs) and Traditional Healers (THs) complement each other in providing services. Traditional Healers are regulated through the Traditional Health Practitioners Act which is administered by the Minister of Health. In 2008 the MOHCW approved an organizational structure which includes a unit specifically established to coordinate Traditional Medicine.

The range of services provided at this level also includes the mobilization of communities and individuals to create an enabling environment for communities to take responsibility for their own health. Curative services are limited to the treatment of common and mild ailments which are locally endemic. Home-based care for chronically ill patients has increasingly become a major component of services delivered at this level. Community health workers identify and refer serious or complicated cases to the health center, distribute contraceptives, condoms and supply micronutrients such as vitamin A and iron. Traditional Midwives have over the years been trained on safe and hygienic deliveries, encouraged to refer complicated deliveries and to participate in the DOTS strategy.

The health center provides the first point of contact between communities and the formal health delivery system. The health center focuses on those patients referred from the community level by employing a team of multi-skilled health workers capable of providing the full package collectively and individually. Services provided by health center staff include primary level curative services, outreach services, and support and supervision to community based health workers such as Community Based Distributors (CBDs) and Village Health Workers (VHWs). More serious cases which are beyond the skills and technology found at the health center level are evaluated, stabilized and referred to the district hospital for further treatment. Referral criteria are built into the treatment guidelines for each intervention within the package. Staff development and in-service training are an ongoing process as staff is trained in using treatment protocols which guide the diagnosis and management of interventions in the package.

The design of the health center in Zimbabwe is based on a standard national prototype that has the capability to deliver a comprehensive package of core health services. This design is supported by agreed staffing norms of at least two nurses, one of whom is a midwife, a nursing aid, an Environmental Health Technician and a general hand. Staffing levels are increasing being determined by the levels of workload at a particular health facility. According to government policy the recommended catchment population for a health center is between 8 000 and 10 000 persons.

At the district level the District Health Management Team (DHMT) is responsible for coordinating the planning and budgeting process and the implementation, monitoring and evaluation of service and program delivery within the district. The DHMT provides regular support and supervision to a network of health facilities within the administrative district. It is an accepted fact that a well functioning health center combined with a first referral (district) hospital can effectively deal with more than 90 per cent of health care demands and reduce the burden of disease by up to 30 percent. The district hospital thus provides generalist clinical services to support referrals from RHC s, clinics and mission institutions. The majority of conditions managed at this level require more sophisticated medical and surgical interventions. These mainly include emergency surgical, gynecological and obstetric cases and complicated clinical cases. Services provided at this level rely on health teams whose skills are complemented by those of a medical doctor. Ideally all district hospitals should have radio or telephone communications with their RHC s, clinics and mission institutions in order to effectively fulfill their roles as referral institutions. Functional motorized transport is also an essential part of their inventory. At the tertiary level health services are coordinated by the office of the Provincial Medical Director (PMD) which is responsible for coordinating the planning and budgeting processes, program implementation and monitoring and evaluation within the province. The PMD also ensures that health delivery is conducted within the government health policy framework as well as providing technical and logistics support to DHMTs.

Clinical services that support the district health package are delivered at the provincial hospital. Though provincial hospitals are earmarked for semi-autonomous status, the full implementation of this policy is likely to take very long. Except for a few, provincial hospitals are understaffed relative to their service responsibilities. They also have poor infrastructure and do not have the capacity to raise revenue to sustain their operations. In terms of support to the delivery of the essential health service package, the provincial hospital provides general clinical care and selected specialist services in support of the district level. Specialist services supposed to be provided at the provincial hospital include internal medicine, pediatrics, obstetrics and gynecology and general surgery.

Central hospitals are at the top of the country's referral system and provide specialist referral support to the district level through general and provincial hospitals. Central hospitals also play a significant role in "inadvertently" providing primary care services to the urban population. This situation has arisen because urban areas, in which central hospitals are traditionally located, do not have gate keeping institutions such as district hospitals to deal with uncomplicated cases. Unfortunately, primary care services delivered at central hospitals are much more expensive than when provided at the district or health center levels, making this arrangement an extremely inefficient way of utilizing scarce resources. This has made it important for government to plan for the provision of intermediate facilities that will deal with primary care patients in urban areas. One option is to upgrade some health facilities in urban areas to the functional level of district hospitals. The other is a more expensive alternative of constructing new district hospitals in each of the major urban areas.

The establishment of central hospitals as semi-autonomous institutions calls for additional policy consideration to ensure that patients referred from district and mission (ZAC H) hospitals continue to have access to specialist referral services at these facilities. Simply stated, referred patients should not become a financial burden to the operations of central hospitals. Any such policy must take into consideration that in fulfilling their roles as semi-autonomous institutions these hospitals are required to develop their own admission policies, implement sustainable cost recovery policies, generate a major portion of their operational costs from user fees and become self-financing in the long term.

In the absence of the above measures being implemented, semi-autonomous hospitals are likely to restrict "free" access to referral and specialist services by the poor. The state must fulfill its obligation to guarantee the poor unimpeded access to specialist and referral services since these institutions are part of the national health system. As long as user fees remain a legitimate source of revenue for semi-autonomous hospitals user fee policies must be complemented by policies that guarantee the poor continued access to central hospital services. One sure route to follow is that of implementing a Social Health Insurance Scheme. A SHI scheme would at least provide some assurances that services consumed by vulnerable groups at central hospitals will be paid for one way or the other.

With moves towards devolution the national level of the MOHCW has assumed the role of providing leadership, policy development, the setting of norms and standards, national procurement, resource mobilization and allocation, provision of high level technical support and disease surveillance. In terms of support to the delivery of the essential health package the central ministry of health must ensure:

- ♦ Universal access, social protection and equity
- ♦ Responsiveness to peoples' needs and expectations
- ♦ Mobilization of adequate resources for the delivery of the package of services by both the public and private sectors.
- ♦ That the provincial level provides effective support and supervision to DHMTs.
- ♦ Availability of adequate human resources and staff norms to support service delivery.
- ♦ Availability of adequate stocks of essential drugs, supplies and basic medical equipment.
- ♦ Well co-coordinated mechanisms for quality assurance, pre-service and in-service training
- ♦ An effectively regulated health sector
- ♦ A sound monitoring and evaluation framework

Overall, the referral system is compromised by poor communication systems, including poor road net works which are a major characteristic of rural areas in developing countries. In some cases programs have been developed to link health centers to district or mission hospitals through radio and other methods of telecommunications so that they can request for transport to refer patients to these institutions. Other challenges facing the referral system in Zimbabwe include fuel shortages and an inadequate ambulance fleet to evacuate emergency and other cases that need referral. The shortage of ambulances and poor access to Essential Obstetric Care (EOC) are major contributing factors to increased maternal mortality rates in the country.

Implications of implementing an essential health package

To ensure that the essential health package of services is accessible to the poor the government adopted a policy which stipulated that the package of services would be delivered free of charge at the point of access at all public sector Rural Health Centers and clinics. For patients who are eligible to receive free health services, the package is also available at no cost at the other levels of the health delivery system, provided that the patient follows the established referral system. Patients who do not follow the established referral system are required to pay penalty fees. Furthermore, in terms of the Medical Services Act, this package forms a compulsory minimum benefit package of services to be covered by all health insurance schemes in Zimbabwe. This is likely to be the package covered under the proposed SHI.

Implementation of this package presents an opportunity for the government to target resources to the poor through its chosen strategies for social safety nets which include free access to the package at public health institutions and exemption mechanisms which are tied to accessing the package. The essential health package forms the basis on which central hospitals and urban local authorities claim reimbursement from the Social Dimension Fund (SDF) for services they have provided free of charge to the poor.

The adoption and implementation of the essential health package means that human resource requirements must be planned so as to meet the demands of delivering a comprehensive package at the various levels of the system. The skills base for health staff must be such that staff is competent enough to deliver all the interventions that constitute the package. Whilst the skills mix must respond to the technical requirements of the package, staffing levels are determined based on a combination of workload and staff full time equivalents required to complete the various tasks within the interventions. The total staff requirements to deliver the package form the basis for planning current and future human resources for health. The existing linkages across the interventions within the package require a holistic and integrated approach to in-service training covering all the intervention areas of the package. Training curricula for pre-service training require review and aligning primarily to cover topics in the package.

As indicated earlier, the design of the health center in Zimbabwe is geared towards delivering comprehensive primary health care services. In terms of the essential health package, the health center infrastructure must be able to deliver all the interventions in the package. In this context it is necessary to assess all the stock of health infrastructure to determine the extent to which communities have the potential to access the full package of interventions at existing facilities. Follow up actions on such an assessment may require the upgrading and rehabilitation of some health facilities and, in some cases, the construction of new facilities to improve geographical access. The choice of basic medical equipment must ensure that the necessary technology to deliver the package is available at all levels of the health system. This implies the development of a standard list of equipment for each level of service delivery to enable the delivery of the package.

To ensure the delivery of a quality essential package there must be a compliance framework in terms of service delivery norms for infrastructure requirements, staffing levels, equipment requirements and treatment guidelines for each intervention area within the package. A quality assurance (QA) policy and strategy must address performance monitoring through integrated support and supervision activities as well as addressing other dimensions of quality which include addressing technical competence through monitoring the use of guidelines, standards, norms and clinical audit. Monitoring effectiveness by determining the extent to which the use of guidelines produces the desired improvement in the quality of care. Authorities must develop strategies to monitor interpersonal relations, staff motivation and morale which are significant determinants of the quality of provider client relations. There must be a functional referral system to ensure continuity of care. The system must guarantee safety for both patients and staff through the development and implementation of appropriate infection control practices, the provision of adequate amenities in the form of infrastructure and equipment.

A major constraint in delivering services has been that of weak health systems some of whose elements have been addressed earlier on. It is of course necessary to mobilize and ensure that there are adequate resources to support delivery of the package. In terms of increasing the availability of essential drugs some countries have developed drug lists specific to an essential package, basically prioritizing within priorities. This has involved the development of a list of essential drugs and supplies that are necessary to cover the requirements of the package. To ensure the efficient utilization of these resources, systems for drug and supplies quantification, clearance, stock control, storage, distribution and rational prescription are strengthened.

It is important to recognize that an essential health package is an integral part of the overall health delivery system and must be considered as such. The continuum of care, including cross referrals between hospitals, health centers and the community is crucial, requiring collaboration between health center staff, hospital staff and care givers at community level.

Implementing an essential health package requires a well-financed, well equipped and well staffed health delivery system. Unfortunately the level of available financial resources and the state of human resources for health in most developing countries are major constraints. Furthermore, because boundaries between services and interventions are often difficult to define, there is a need for a clearly defined policy on the type and skills of health professionals required to deliver a package of services. It thus becomes necessary for decisions to be made as to the extent to which health workers must be multi-skilled in order to provide the full package at each level of the health system.

Tensions must be reduced between different service programs delivered within the same facility using the same resources. For example, if a vertically funded STI program has adequate amounts of STI treatment kits in stock, it should be possible for these drugs to be made available to treat other patients who require them irrespective of whether they suffer from STIs or not. It becomes necessary therefore to identify and integrate vertical programs into the essential health service package framework. It is however necessary to determine the possibility and extent to which the integration of some of these programs is feasible without disrupting their efficient delivery. A skills audit must be undertaken, staff retrained, some job descriptions and staffing levels reviewed in order to develop an appropriate skills mix to deliver all the other interventions at the various levels of the health system.

The referral system must be strengthened in order to guarantee its efficiency and effectiveness in supporting the delivery of the package of services at the lower levels. This can be achieved in several ways including ensuring that trained and well motivated staffs are in place and equitably deployed. The design and quality of physical facilities must guarantee an adequate and appropriate environment for the delivery of the interventions, and facilitate the effective management and delivery of outpatient and inpatient services, including speedy handling of emergencies. Well functioning equipment, efficient transport and communications feedback systems and adequate supplies of essential drugs are *"sine quibus non"* for an efficient referral system.

The role of other players in delivering the package

Partnerships are an essential ingredient for effective delivery of essential health services to communities. There are several ways in which the public sector can effectively collaborate with relevant stakeholders in the provision of essential services. The range of potential partners includes public sector health providers such as local authorities and other government departments; not-for-profit organizations such as local and international NGOs, civil society and faith based organizations (ZACH); private-for-profit entities such as private practitioners, commercial companies, nursing homes, pharmacies, private hospitals and clinics.

There must however be effective regulatory mechanisms and a policy framework that guides the operations of the actors in the health sector. In the case of Zimbabwe, the potential of the Medical Services Act, the Public Health Act and the Health Professions Act must be fully exploited. It is necessary for the public sector to consolidate existing partnerships, at the various levels of its organization by entering into contractual arrangements with RDCs, urban local authorities, faith based organizations (missions) and insurance schemes to continue providing the essential package of services on its behalf. These arrangements must be further strengthened by the development of transparent mechanisms for payment or subsidization of contracted services. Standards, norms and a quality assurance program must become an integral part of the contracting arrangements so as to provide a framework within which the performance of contracted parties can be monitored. Existing accreditation systems for health professionals and minimum requirements that govern the establishment of health facilities can be strengthened in order to complement any QA program that is established. Above all, the public sector as the purchaser must ensure that it has the capacity to design, negotiate, manage and monitor the implementation of service contracts.

Development partners collaborate with the public sector mainly at the higher and policy level by providing technical assistance in capacity building, providing financial assistance, involvement in priority setting, policy analyses and joint monitoring and evaluation. Development partners also provide support to service delivery through their support to local and international NGOs. The essential package forms an effective rallying point for the involvement of communities and civil society groups in health service planning, implementation, monitoring and evaluation. The potential for such participation has long been available through existing local governance structures such as local development committees, village health committees which have however proved to be ineffective.

Monitoring the delivery of an essential health package

The main objective of implementing an essential health package is to ensure that the poor and other vulnerable groups have universal coverage and equitable access to basic health services. To this end an appropriate monitoring and evaluation plan must be developed to monitor progress towards the achievement of this objective. The following are some of the areas proposed for monitoring within such a performance framework:

Geographical accessibility
The sector must be able to guarantee that the poor have physical access to the agreed package of services. In order to achieve the above the starting point is to establish a health facilities inventory and map which shows the current distribution of essential health services broken down by the location of fixed facilities, outreach points, mobile clinics and NGO facilities, major roads and natural barriers. The following indicators can be collected to facilitate the analysis:

- Number of clinics, hospitals (per 1000 population) offering the full package of services, broken down by poor and less-poor districts, rural-urban.
- Catchment population living within a given distance of a particular type of facility (e.g. 8-10 km) - broken down by income level, poverty mapping.
- The time taken by a client to reach a facility or service delivery point (e.g. less than an hour).

Availability of essential inputs

The health sector has the responsibility to ensure that there is continuous availability of essential inputs at all levels of the health system. This means that apart from being physically accessible the health facility must have the full complement of essential resources such as staff, drugs and equipment available at all times. Availability surveys can be conducted at health facilities to collect more detailed and reliable information.

Social accountability

The health delivery system must be responsive to the poor and also ensure that the poor are able to exert meaningful influence over health providers. This is in light of the fact that staff in government facilities is often considered to be unresponsive to the plight of the poor. The following areas can be assessed in order to determine aspects of social accountability:

♦ Mobilization of communities for health promotion activities
♦ The engagement of communities in monitoring the performance of facilities or providers through:
   ♦ Measuring the percentage of facilities with functioning community representation in advisory or similar committees.
   ♦ Monitoring how regularly these committees meet.
   ♦ Assessing the presence of an effective complaints system.
   ♦ Assessing the availability and adherence to a Patients' Charter.

Organizational quality and consumer responsiveness

The health sector as a whole, public, private, and/or NGO services, must be responsive to consumer concerns and deliver services in a way that encourages the utilization of these services. The following are some of the several factors that influence the user friendliness of health services:

♦ Attitudes of staff
♦ Hours of operation
♦ Space, cleanliness and comfort of the wards
♦ Waiting time and in certain cultures the gender of service providers
♦ User fees

The above factors affect the manner in which consumers perceive the quality of services and have a significant influence on whether the services are used or not. Measuring indicators for organizational quality relies on both qualitative and quantitative tools such as:

♦ Qualitative surveys.

♦ Focus group discussions: separately for men and women.
♦ Exit interviews with patients: client/provider interactions.
♦ On-site assessment of various aspects of service organization

Utilization of health services
The proportion of specific segments of society, especially the poor, making use of health services in a given year is crucial to monitoring the extent to which basic services are being successfully targeted to vulnerable groups. This is also a key indicator of the extent to which clients come into contact with the health system; public, private and NGO.

♦ The health information system collects data on the use of services: outpatient visits, in patients, vaccinations etc. This information can be analyzed to provide a useful trend analysis.

♦ Household surveys can provide better information on the percentage of a target population making use of a particular service and possibly reasons for non-use.

♦ The quality of services produced in a specific area could be linked through a poverty map to income level.

Timing and continuity
It is important for clients or patients to receive the correct number of contacts for services that require repeated interventions and to ensure that time-sensitive services are delivered and consumed in a timely manner. Such services include ANC visits, vaccinations or essential obstetric care where timing is critical. The following indicators can be used to monitor this category of services:

♦ Drop-out rates.
♦ Vaccine coverage
♦ Children with a full course of immunization
♦ Number and timing of antenatal visits (% beginning in first trimester etc)
♦ Compliance with TB treatment

Technical quality
This is the likelihood that the service, if used, will lead to improved health outcomes. Some aspects of quality depend on effective provider training and supervision, the existence of appropriate treatment protocols, the adequacy of the necessary inputs as well as factors such as provider workload. Technical quality may be poor even when consumers express

satisfaction with the services. Assessing this type of quality requires direct observation of the behavior of providers and a comparison of existing practices against standard protocols. The following indicators are useful:

◆ Perinatal mortality rates
◆ Malaria case-fatality rates
◆ TB cure rates.
◆ Maternal mortality rates
◆ Proportion of health workers adhering to treatment protocols

Allocative efficiency

In the context of a country's Poverty Reduction Strategy scrutiny on whether public health activities aimed at benefiting the poor are adequately funded by the government is essential. It is necessary to ensure that the essential health service package is given priority compared to those interventions that are high cost and low impact. This includes the scrutiny of resources in the private sector as to whether they are being channeled towards cost-effective interventions or not. Public expenditure reviews are a good source of information to compare the amount of resources spent on priority public health activities to those spent on interventions considered to be less essential.

Equity of expenditures

Because of their influence and the information they possess, the rich usually benefit by sidestepping exemption mechanisms at the expense of the poor. It is therefore important to know whether public health and other health interventions actually benefit the poorest groups as intended. As a result, beneficiaries of expenditures on health must be traced and classified by socio-economic groups. Household budget surveys can be used to identify access to different types of facilities by households of different income groups.

Affordability

Out of pocket payments in most developing countries in Sub Saharan Africa contribute at least 10-20% to total health financing in these countries. It is therefore important to know the extent to which households are pushed further into poverty as a result of such out-of-pocket payments. This can be achieved through undertaking assessments that compare current prices of services with the capacity of households to pay and the pattern of utilization at a given price. Such an exercise requires that data on utilization of services and a comparison of household expenditures with services price data must be available (Knippenberg (1986) and Miller (1989).

Conclusions and the way forward

The core health service package similar to that adopted by the MO-HCW in Zimbabwe was estimated to cost least US$22 per capita per annum to deliver. Estimates by the CMH put the annual per capita cost of delivering an essential package in a developing country at between US$34 and US$40.

Current thinking is that the gap between available resources and the means to provide the package is not one of political will but, in most cases, a deep rooted inability of some countries to mobilize adequate internal resources to support the health sector. In the absence of additional resources materializing, it may be necessary for the government of Zimbabwe to reprioritize the contents of its rather comprehensive core health service package to one which it can afford. Other alternatives include improving efficiencies in the utilization of existing resources, mobilizing additional resources from international development partners and entering into partnership with the local private sector to take responsibilities of delivering the essential package.

A new National Health Strategy must be developed to accommodate any new strategic choices that may be adopted. Policy makers must consult relevant stakeholders and apply their better judgment to determine new sector priorities, taking into consideration cost effectiveness, affordability and the political implications of such options. The formal inclusion of HIV/AIDS related interventions like Counseling and Testing, PMTCT and ARV therapy in the package should be a mere formality.

The concept of an essential health service package brings to the fore inconsistencies between its interventions and the existing budgeting framework of the ministry of health. The package is defined on the basis of specific interventions whilst the health sector budget lines focus more on inputs such as drugs, salaries of staff, vertical programs, etc. It is thus a challenge for the ministry to translate the package to match ministry budget lines in order to facilitate its financing. Considering that patients do not choose their illnesses, the delivery of a "selective package" provides a moral dilemma for frontline health workers, especially for patients with conditions outside the package. Experience has shown that selective health packages do not necessarily address issues of equity despite the fact that the interventions may be targeted to benefit the poor (Pearson, M, 2000). In adopting an essential health package caution is advised as to some the package may mean a sort of discrimination, namely, "low cost and/or low quality services" for the poor. Having introduced and adopted an essential package of services, it is important for the government not to commit all its resources to the implementation of such a health service package. Previous commitments and political imperatives call for a more guarded approach. There should be enough room left for maneuver to enable the government to continue to allocate some resources to interventions that are not included in the package. Resources must be set aside and made available to support central hospital services and the referral system to ensure continuity of care. An essential health package should not only refer to health service interventions but must consider health support systems as an integral part of the package.

Review questions

1. There are several ways in which countries can set their health priorities; using DALYS, selective PHC approaches, vertical programming, etc. Describe a transparent and accountable method of priority setting that is well suited to your country.

2. Justify the introduction and adoption of a core health service package (Essential Health Care Package) in the health delivery system of a country you are familiar with.

3. Specify any disadvantages that are likely to be experienced by the health sector of a country which has adopted an essential health care package.

4. The core package of health services is best delivered in an integrated manner. Describe the concept of "integrated service delivery" and how integration can be achieved in a health system characterized by vertical programs.

5. You are a consultant assigned to a developing country to assist the Ministry of Health with the costing of its package of essential health services. Present your detailed end of mission report to the head of the ministry.

8

THE SECTOR WIDE APPROACH (SWAp)

Introduction

'The domestic political and commercial environment ensures that an agency's aid program conforms to the country's foreign policy and is responsive to domestic commercial interests, most notably through tied aid (Nancy G, 1986).

Whilst the above statement was true at the time, the question is whether it is still true today. It is also true that governments in African countries also have political considerations which are similar to those of their developed country counterparts, one of which is to stay in power. They have to, and must be seen to pay attention to their power base and fulfill some of the promises they make to their electorates.

Reference to the above statements has been given as one of the reasons for the failure of development assistance to African countries. The argument being that aid often follows political rather than development objectives; that there is a lack of "ownership" of development projects and programs by countries receiving assistance. It has also been noted that the lack of co-ordination among development partners also compounds the above situation (Kanbur R. et al, 1999).

International co-operation in health remains poorly understood and difficult to implement effectively. In some cases, foreign assistance does not benefit the intended beneficiaries as much as it does the various intermediaries, both inside and outside the recipient country. There is the added dimension where technical assistance is always tied to development aid, usually as a condition upon which aid is released. In other cases donor countries have terminated the benefits of assistance or development aid without any reference to the recipient country.

Some African countries have analyzed the role and impact of foreign aid in health development and demonstrated the evolution of the country's dependence on external resources to maintain their health services. This has resulted in most of these countries gradually losing control over their own doctrines and policies. Policy makers in African countries and the rest of the developing world have complained, from a position of weakness, that they spend more time trying to fulfill donor requirements and co-ordinating donor actions rather than discussing with their own people the soundness of home grown development strategies. African countries need the freedom to be able to assess their own needs and to design their own development strategies and systems necessary to effectively coordinate development partners.

While accepting the right of donors to impose stringent criteria in the disbursement of development aid, the question is whether it is right for them to force governments to adopt policies and strategies that they do not believe in. This is much more unnerving when different donors impose totally different conditions to the same government. The current view is that donors should give up some of their rigid control over development assistance to the governments of developing countries and move more towards partnerships (Kanbur R, et al, 1999).

Traditionally development assistance was delivered either as being project specific or sector specific. The flow of development assistance funds into the country can either be through government institutions, the private for profit sector or NGOs. In some cases aid can come in the form of technical assistance, in the form of human resources or the sharing of knowledge. Development assistance can also come with explicit or implicit conditionalities.

Donors have provided project support for a long time and continue to do so. Because projects are usually separate from government management systems they have high transaction costs to both the donor and the recipient country. Such costs arise from the need to manage, monitor and evaluate projects separately from each other and from the systems used by the government. There are separate missions conducted by project sponsors which require ministry of health staff to write equally separate reports. Whilst the popular view may be that project financing is on the decline this is probably the best approach to supporting fragile states.

General budget support on the other hand, channels development assistance to recipient countries through the national treasury by supporting the country's general budget process. This implies that development assistance supports government priorities across the whole spectrum of the government's development program. However because of the fungible nature of government finances, it is possible that where governments do not consider health as a priority, resources meant for the health sector may be diverted to other government programs.

The other method of delivering development assistance is the Sector Wide Approach (SWAp) which became the preferred method of delivering aid in the mid 1990s.

Defining the Sector Wide Approach (SWAp)

The SWAp is a *"method of working between governments and donors, where significant funding for the sector supports a single sector policy and expenditure program. The government is in the lead and together with the other parties adopts common approaches across the sector. On their part donors are expected to adhere to national priorities"* (Cassels, 1997).

There are several key words and phrases that are associated with the Sector Wide Approach, namely: 'a coherent policy framework, local stakeholders in the driving seat, all donors sign in, common implementation arrangements, and minimal long-term technical assistance' (Forster M, 1999). What is crucial is that '*the partner government and development agencies agree on the policies and plans for the development of the sector, including the allocation of resources*' (Peters D and Chao S, 1998).

Why some countries have embarked on the SWAp

There are several reasons why some countries adopted the SWAp:

- ♦ Incoherent sector policies and budget frameworks resulting from project aid
- ♦ Increased administrative and recurrent (transaction) costs associated with projects as a result of the establishment of project units and disjointed technical assistance.
- ♦ Rigid administrative procedures and decision-making processes associated with projects.
- ♦ Islands of excellence created by projects which prevent the achievement of equitable distribution of resources.
- ♦ Various conditionalities on project aid associated with each of the development partners.
- ♦ The need to harmonize donor missions and reporting requirements
- ♦ The SWAp as part of aid conditionality

The SWAp arrangement confers some perceived advantages to either or both partners in the SWAp, Box 8.1. Donors assume more influence on the development of sector policies and develop a closer working relationship with all stakeholders within the sector than before. With closer working relationships and a common development framework it becomes unnecessary for the development partners to deploy many of their staff to field offices. This has the potential to reduce administrative costs and improve efficiency in the allocation of resources from development assistance.

When a government assumes real control of the situation, there is a possibility that home grown policies will be implemented as opposed to those "imposed" by development partners. In a SWAp framework resources are deployed over a wider area and contribute towards equity as opposed to the concentration of resources in projects that are located in isolated geographical areas. It is envisaged that with a single strategic framework and plan that is spearheaded by the government there is greater flexibility and targeting of available resources. Experience to date has shown that in the context of a SWAp the justification and mobilization of additional resources from the donor community becomes much easier.

The concept of ownership

"Government ownership is at its strongest when the political leadership and its advisers, with broad support among agencies of the state and civil society, decide of their own volition that policy changes are desirable and choose what these changes should be and when they should be introduced" (Killich, et al 1998).

Other views on ownership deal not only with where the policy emanates from but with whether there is commitment or the government accepts the policy (Morrissey, O, 2002). Ownership has been defined as a combination of commitment, technical and administrative capacity to conceive, negotiate and implement reforms. Aid conditionality on the other hand is considered an obstacle to country ownership. The two are considered to be incompatible. Situations however arise when development partners want to induce partner countries to adopt policies or programs that they would otherwise not adopt on their own.

Box 8.1 Perceived advantages of the Sector Wide Approach

Advantages to Development Agencies	Advantages to the Governments
• Opportunities for donors to influence sector policies. • Improved partnership in program implementation with the government and closer links with NGOs. • Reduction in management costs. • Perceived improvement in resource utilization, disbursement and accountability by recipient government.	• Government takes the driving seat and is in charge and determines its own priorities and policies. • Increased flexibility in the use of funds (pooled funds) rather than having earmarked funds. • It is easier for the government to influence and control the flow of external funding and to justify it. • Plans from a single strategic framework are easier to develop and evaluate. • Less pluralism on policies and priorities.

According to Johnson and Wasty (1993), "ownership" consists of several dimensions which include the *locus of initiative* which gives a clue as to whether a policy is *government centered or not*. The level of intellectual conviction among policy makers is referred to as the *technocratic dimension* of ownership. In true ownership the top leadership is seen to be acting and speaking in support of the initiatives (reforms), an aspect referred to as *the political dimension* of ownership. There must also be visible efforts towards consensus building among various constituencies in order to demonstrate how widely the support is spread beyond government.

Building partnerships

It must be stressed that the principles of partnership require a right mixture of political commitment, ethical precepts and technical expertise. Partnerships in development co-operation are based on strategies that are owned by the government, communities, development partners and civil society. The key words that must guide such collaboration are; ownership, country leadership, broad based participation and accountability. Objectives to achieve the above can be accomplished through multiple partnerships among agencies, between agencies and governments, between different governments, between sectors and between governments and the people.

Partnerships require an approach that integrates development assistance into the local health development process in a collaborative manner and on an equal basis. The attitudes of parties involved in a partnership must reflect mutual respect. In this context, African countries must be supported and given the opportunity to develop their own homegrown strategies and plans in consultation with their own people and constituencies. All stakeholders to a partnership must be prepared to share risks, trust each other and develop appropriate mechanisms to deal with any problems that arise. Externally imposed conditionality is not effective, sustainable or conducive to country ownership or lasting partnerships.

According to Cassels A, (1997) there are different kinds of partnership arrangements that are essential for a successful SWAp; a joint statement of intent to proceed with a SWAp, a collaborative program of work with annual agreements on performance objectives, a formal Memorandum of Understanding amongst the partners and an agreed Code of Conduct to assist in dealing with disagreements within the partnership, especially with respect to activities that may not be consistent with sector programs.

Framework for developing the Sector Wide Approach (SWAp)

Defining the health sector

A health sector is defined as a coherent set of activities which can be relevantly distinguished in terms of policies, institutions and finances, and which need to be looked at together to make a meaningful assessment, that is, the entire network of public, private and voluntary institutions financed, managed or regulated by the ministry of health. Such a definition however excludes some important health promoting and sustaining activities that do not fall directly within the realm of the ministry of health, e.g. nutrition, water, sanitation and some aspects of population interventions.

The SWAp planning process

It must be recognized that the role of the public sector in health is only part of what happens in the health sector and that public expenditures need to be supplemented by those from the private sector. The institutional mechanisms for the SWAp must be decided in the context of other national policies and reforms such as decentralization and the delegation of powers to local government structures.

The sequence of events in the planning process must result in:

♦ A Strategic plan or framework which defines, within the policy direction, priorities, the financial framework and resource allocation indications

♦ A short to medium term plan and the activities to be undertaken

♦ Annual plans developed through a bottom-up process, aggregated at the regional and national levels and forming the basis for an annual budget.

♦ A joint evaluation strategy for the sector

The work plans must be detailed enough to be able to identify major activities within the sector and indicate funding by source and must require donors and governments to be explicit about what each intends to fund. The adoption of a broad based program approach in the sector means that all resource inputs contribute to a single strategic joint program of work for the whole sector. All donors must agree to contribute collectively to a coherent program of health services delivery and phase out individual projects which require separate financial management and accounting procedures. Resource projections must include those available from public, private and donor sources.

Managing the SWAp process

It is important that the management process of a health SWAp is; to the extent possible, based on existing government structures and systems. The SWAp must thus become part and parcel of the core business of the ministry of health. SWAp governance structures should include a high level committee of policy makers from different departments of government supported by a body that coordinates the SWAp implementation process consisting of all stakeholders in the sector, including donors. Several technical working groups are usually established to support the work of this implementation body. Harmonized joint review procedures, reporting, monitoring, evaluation and audit mechanisms are usually developed and must satisfy the requirements of all partners to the SWAp process. Monitoring is usually based on the follow up of agreed indicators at the sector level, including milestones in the reform process itself. The development of parallel structures has been found to be disruptive and frustrating to efforts aimed at achieving local ownership.

Planning, budgeting and monitoring processes

Since the SWAp process is coterminous with the business of the organization it must follow the planning and budgeting cycle of the government within the Medium Term Expenditure Framework (MTEF). The program of work developed through the SWAp process must also fit into the strategic expenditure framework of the government. The review of the performance of the SWAp is based on joint annual performance reviews intended to replace individual review missions undertaken by different development partners at different times of the year. In a pure SWAp it is not possible to separate results and attribute them to inputs by a particular donor. This is particularly true where pool funding arrangements have been adopted within a SWAp arrangement. Where a common fund has been established, it is expected that participating partners will be satisfied with the targets and impact achieved through the use of pooled funds, ideas, influence, technical assistance, advocacy and action.

Table 8.1 Major steps in preparing a SWAp

Steps	Key Issues
1. Government and development agencies (DAs) agree to work towards a SWAp.	How to ensure all relevant parties understand the approach and what is required? Who in government will lead policy development and strategies? How will DA's input to this and agree on it? What will be the mechanism for coordination between DAs and the government?
2. Agree on policy framework, identify main strategies based on resources available and show how resources will be allocated.	*Policy issues to be tackled:* Content of affordable essential package at each level. How to improve the quality of services. Role of the private sector and NGOs. Decentralization and changing the role of the ministry of health. How much are DAs likely to provide? Details of the required budget allocation over 5 years.
3. Review management and organizational implications of the change to a SWAp.	What are the implications of the SWAp and decentralization plans on the role and structure of the ministry of health? How will vertical programs be affected?

4. Develop first year work plan with milestones.	With sufficient detail to identify major activities and easy to monitor. Involve those responsible for implementation in preparing the work-plans, keeping realistic budget ceilings. Work plans must show funding by source. DAs to be explicit about what they will fund. Include plans for institutional development, capacity building and further policy development.
5. Agree on funding mechanisms and terms.	Decision on whether to have pooled funds and what these can be used for. Are proposed conditions for releasing funds achievable and do they leave scope for flexibility?
6. Agree procedures for approving expenditure, disbursement and procurement.	Are work plans with budgets sufficient for approving expenditures? How will procurement rules be agreed?
7. Agree on monitoring & reporting arrangements including financial reporting and audit.	How to get agreement on a limited, shared list of indicators? How will government monitor activities as well as expenditures during the year? How will value for money be assessed/verified, frequency of financial audit?
8. Establish a Memorandum of Understanding and working arrangements.	How to allow for changes in the sector program based on experience. How to deal with disagreements during implementation.
9. Identify transition steps required, including development of capacity and systems.	*Preparatory steps may include:* Preparing for the end of program funding. Communications to staff and the public on policy and SWAp related changes. Development of information and finance systems plus supporting training. Collection of baseline data for use in subsequent evaluation.

Under such an arrangement it becomes necessary to convince the donors that the information available from joint annual reviews is adequate and accurate enough to give them the assurances that they require. This effectively means that the review process must include independent assessments, be thorough enough to provide confidence and be relied upon. Independent assessments are necessary because routinely collected data is neither adequate nor sufficient to assess the overall performance of a health sector. An independent team is usually engaged to undertake the review process based on Terms of Reference agreeable to all stakeholders. Monitoring of the SWAp process requires a consensus amongst the government, NGOs, civil society and development partners on the indicators to be used, targets to be achieved and systems to monitor performance. Consensus must be reached even before the start of the joint program of work. The SWAp monitoring process focuses on higher-level indicators and aims to achieve results that may be considered not tangible, such as institutional development and local ownership which are difficult to measure quantitatively and objectively.

As the ultimate objective of a SWAp is to improve the health status of the population in an equitable manner, indicators that only monitor the impact of the reform process are not adequate. It is necessary to select additional performance indicators which reflect equity, access, efficiency, effectiveness and sustainability. The indicators should be selected such that they are appropriate to the goals and stakeholder interests in a particular country. Hotton, G (2000) has proposed a set of indicators to consider in monitoring SWAps, see Table 8.2.

Common procedures in financial management

The main objectives of the SWAp in this area are to ensure that sectoral plans become the basis upon which all funding to the sector is prioritized, that government financial management systems are strengthened as opposed to developing parallel systems and to reduce the number of accounts managed by ministry of health staff.

Evidence shows that 80% of SWAps being implemented in 2004 used project disbursing and accounting procedures. This was mainly a result of the fact that most of the donors are not yet prepared to take risks and use government financial management systems which they consider to lack transparency and accountability. In other cases donors are not allowed by their principals to co-mingle their funds. Hybrid SWAps currently being implemented have been adopted as a compromise not to exclude those donors with difficulties in using common procedures.

Table 8.2 Selected indicators for monitoring a health SWAp

Access	Equity	Quality	Effectiveness	Efficiency	Sustainability
Proximity to services	**Economic incentives**	**Health infrastructure**	**Mortality**	**Technical efficiency**	**Financing source**
Time and Distance	Government subsidies	Changes in staffing patterns	Maternal mortality ratio	Outpatient visits per staff	% spending from tax
Full essential package	Gini coefficient	Minimum standards met	Infant mortality rate	Inpatient days per staff	% spending from user fees
Facility with a doctor	Means testing availability	Personnel	Under five mortality rate	Hospital bed occupancy	% spending from donors
Pharmacy	Free exemptions granted	Equipment	AIDS mortality rate	Salaries payments on time	Financing schemes set up
District hospital	**Risk pooling availability**	Essential drugs	Disease specific mortality rates	Performance incentives	**Size of the health sector**
24 hr ambulance service.	Population with access	Treatment guidelines used	**Prevalence**	Levels of wastage, theft, etc.	Health spending versus total spending
Staff population ratio	**Voluntary services**	**Quality assurance**	AIDS prevalence	**Economic efficiency**	Health spending versus GDP
Cost of:	Availability of NGO services	Minimum standards	Malaria	Nurses per doctor	**Spending**
Outpatient illness episode	Use of NGO services	Normal consultations	TB notification rate	Nurses per hospital bed	% government spending on EHP
Inpatient hospital stay	**Health spending**	Emergency referrals	Diarrhea prevalence	Doctors per hospital bed	% government spending to preventive services
Health care utilization	Consumption per head	Non-emergency referrals	Pneumonia	Cost per outpatient bed	**Institutional**
Outpatient consultations	Per capita expenditures	Client understanding	Post partum hemorrhage	Cost per hospital bed day	Foreign doctors
			Malnutrition	% personnel expenditure	Annual staff outputs (training)
		Adverse outcome due to poor quality care	Low birth weight	% expenditure on drugs	Donor research and training
Inpatient admissions	Spending on the EHP		**Treatment options**	**Allocative efficiency**	
Hospital delivery	Use of resource allocation formula	**Patient satisfaction**	Tuberculosis	% spent on public services	
Immunization coverage	**Access**	Respect for persons	Malaria	% spent on the EHP	
Bed net coverage	Poverty and housing	Client orientation	**Demographic indicators**	% spent at district level.	
Clinic hours	Food supply		Life expectancy	Referral system functions	
			Total fertility rate	Average length of stay	
			Crude birth rate		
			Crude death rate.		

Source: Hotton, G (2000)

Policy implications of the SWAp in the African context

The SWAp process provides an opportunity for the government, development partners, NGOs and civil society to actively participate in the policy formulation process as "equal" partners. A far cry from the era of purely project based support. The SWAp provides structures for effective participation by all stakeholders in the prioritization process, resource allocation, strategic and operational planning, technical discussions and program reviews.

The SWAp provides a framework for a policy development process which is explicit about resource allocation priorities, is in line with the Medium Term Expenditure Framework and ensures that both government and donor expenditures are tracked against the national budget. For example, if a country has a policy to implement an essential health package, the allocation and expenditures on these services are monitored with respect to the extent to which the package has been implemented.

It has long been argued that health policies in African countries are decided externally by financial institutions such as the World Bank, the World Health Organization, UNICEF etc. Over the years the influence of the World Bank and the IMF in health development has become considerable, especially through the conditionality of Structural Adjustment Programs (ESAPs) imposed on poor countries. In the majority of cases ESAPs resulted in reduced spending on social services, including the health sector. Where ESAPs have been implemented the World Bank and the IMF have been accused of influencing other development partners to follow suit and put pressure on African countries to adopt World Bank inspired policies and conditionality.

From the time the World Bank became a major player in health sector investment in developing countries it has pursued several health policy themes that developing countries have had to implement over the years. The Bank has supported Primary Health Care initiatives, inflexible infrastructure development projects, cost effective health packages, HIV/AIDS programs and health reforms which have emphasized cost recovery and the diminished role of the state in the provision of health services. The Bank is currently encouraging countries to adopt the SWAp which it links to the development and implementation of Poverty Reduction Strategy Papers. The World Bank continues to encourage increased reliance on the market to finance and deliver health services without taking due regard to the potential for market failures. Market reforms have obvious implications on policies that African countries have adopted with respect to universal coverage, free access to primary health care services and access to pro-poor health interventions which these governments have promised to their electorate.

As the World Bank consolidates its position as the major investor in health in developing countries and increasingly assumes a co-coordinating role among other agencies, it is likely to impose its policies on countries that rely heavily on development assistance in financing their health services. This has huge implications on the future of the SWAp in many countries, most of which are heavily indebted. This is however not to say that World Bank polices are wholesale retrogressive but that they certainly need to be considered with caution, especially the manner in which they are imposed on poor, helpless and hapless countries. The main problem is that of advocating policies on the basis of the principle that, "one size fits all".

There is a known and proven link between governance and development. Governments that do not acknowledge that they have an obligation to be accountable to their own people are not likely to pursue development policies and strategies that lead to poverty reduction and social progress. They are likely to pursue policies that favor minority elite groups, such as particular social, ethnic or economic classes. In this context, there are those who argue that the SWAp should be supported only in those countries where there is "legitimacy of government structures" in the form of accountability of public institutions, (Gould et al, 1998). It is heartening to note that the World Bank's 2007 Health, Nutrition and Population Strategy adopts a more holistic approach and focuses on health systems strengthening, including human resources for health issues.

It is also a fact that development partners have their own agenda when it comes to the content and orientation of sectoral policies and that they have an edge over recipient or African countries. However the reality of the matter is that, if policy must culminate in a joint agreement between donors and the government, the leadership role of government in its own development programs must at least be acknowledged even if it is not allowed to manifest itself.

Experiences in the implementation of the SWAp

By 2006 there were several countries in Africa who were either planning or implementing the SWAp and these included: Burkina Faso, Egypt, Ethiopia, Ghana, Kenya, Malawi, Mali, Mozambique, Rwanda, Senegal, Sierra Leone, Tanzania, Uganda and Zambia. Gill Walt et al

(1994) observe that some countries in the Sub-Saharan region have had varied experiences in implementing health reforms. "Zambia" for example, "embraced reforms wholeheartedly and enjoyed positive relations with donors, at least until 1998". "Other countries became cautious reformers as they achieved stability or peace after years of disruptions, as is the case in Mozambique." "Malawi was extremely slow to take up reforms (Mvula and Munthali, 1997) and "Tanzania has been likened to a driver implementing reforms with one foot on the accelerator and one foot on the brake" (Pavignani, 1999).

The SWAps currently being implemented in some countries are characteristically hybrid arrangements where some resources continue to flow in the form of program support and others as project aid. In all these countries there are still project accounts for individual donors though in certain cases these are gradually being phased out. A survey of 16 SWAp like sector programming by the Strategic Partnership with Africa (SPA) revealed that 80% were still relying on project disbursement and accounting procedures (Forster and Fozzard, 2000). From some of these country experiences it is clear that, after all, the ideas that make a SWAp are not new but constitute what should have been happening all along in reinforcing national leadership in the health development agenda.

According to Peters and Chao (1998) Zambia and Mozambique are countries that made firm commitment to support and implement the SWAp. By 2000 Tanzania had what could be described as a fully-fledged SWAp and the government of Zambia was implementing a hybrid SWAp arrangement. The government of Malawi completed its SWAp mission report in November 2002 and proceeded to develop a SWAp joint program of work which was completed and agreed to by the partnership early in 2004. In 2000 there were no signs that the governments of South Africa, Swaziland and Zimbabwe had any intentions of implementing SWAp arrangements in their health sectors.

In most of the African countries that are implementing the SWAp, budget processes have received priority attention. Expenditure programs have been prepared mainly in a context of Economic Structural Adjustment Programs (ESAP). Uganda, Zambia and Tanzania have translated such frameworks into Medium Term Financing Plans rolled into 3 year and short-term annual budgets. Gill Walter et al indicate that in Zambia and Tanzania the SWAp has translated into an increase in resource inflows into the health sector. The problem however has been the lack of adequate capacity to implement the SWAp in both countries.

Zambia was the pioneer in the establishment of pool fund arrangements as far back as in 1997. At the time only five donor agencies supported the pooling of funds which did not cover all the areas within the SWAp program of work. The pooling arrangements mainly supported Primary Health Care activities and excluded the payment of salaries for health workers.

The review of experiences with the SWAp shows that all the countries that have implemented joint funding arrangements have placed particular emphasis on approval mechanisms for district plans. They also spelt out the conditions under which districts are considered eligible to receive allocations from pooled funds. For its SWAp program the government of Tanzania adopted a comprehensive financial management system that is based on systems developed as part of the changing overall government financial management systems. In some of the countries where pooled funds support a comprehensive health program, experience shows that there are delays in the release of funds which often frustrate staff efforts to implement programs.

According to Ortendahl, C (October 2007), the SWAp in Uganda which was considered to be a model in its early days later declined in its performance. Several factors have been cited as contributing to this phenomenon. These include a decline in government health expenditures, weakening government leadership, poor governance in the health sector and changes in aid modalities.

In their study which explored the contributions of the SWAp to resource allocation in Zambia, Collins, C et al., (2008) indicated that after more than 10 years of implementing the SWAp, transaction costs of aid management remained high; budget execution did not improve though funding levels at district level increased, at the expense of hospital funding. The study reveals that development partners continued to support the health sector through multiple projects. The disbursement from basket funds was however more predictable and timely than government funding.

The major highlight in the SWAp experience in Mozambique has been the operation of the Global Fund through the SWAp common fund, "PRO-SAUDE". According to Martinez, J (2007), this decision was facilitated by the existence of a firmly established "set of common principles, objectives and working arrangements that functioned relatively well". However, despite this achievement, operationally things did not work as planned as there were long delays in the disbursement of GFATM funds into the common fund. These delays resulted in a financial gap that adversely affected the implementation of the 2007 operational plan. The delays were a result of triggers which continued to be required for the release of GFATM funds. To avoid similar problems, by mutual agreement, in 2008 the minister of health directed that funds from the GFATM, though still complementary to PROSAUDE, be managed outside the PROSAUDE framework. The GTAFM however remains signatory to the SWAp process.

In the case of Zimbabwe, the closest the MOHCW came to adopting a SWAp type arrangement was when it entered into a Health Sector Program Support (HSPS) with the Danish Development Agency (DANIDA). The MOHCW developed a National Health Strategy (NHS) covering the period 1997-2007. The NHS clearly defined the policy framework and values that would guide national investment in the health sector during the plan period. The guiding principle of the HSPS was to support the development of partnerships through a national framework and sector program to be implemented on the basis of annual rolling plans.

Central to the HSPS was the introduction of innovative organizational and administrative procedures, systems and capacity building at all levels of the health delivery system. This collaborative arrangement focused on increased accountability and transparency within the health sector, the principles of which are central to a SWAp or sector wide thinking. The HSPS reinforced the need for the coherence of institutions, budgets and policies within the health sector as a whole.

In order to institutionalize these arrangements the MOHCW created a Policy Development and Planning Department which housed the Strategic Development Unit (SDU). This move was aimed at strengthening the capacity of the MOHCW in planning, policy development and analysis. The SDU was responsible for:

♦ Coordinating the implementation of the reform process.
♦ Coordinating the planning process within the MOHCW.
♦ Providing management support and advice to the provinces, districts, central and provincial hospitals.
♦ Coordinating the development of health information systems to support the reform process.
♦ Advocacy on health reforms through the production and distribution of a quarterly MOHCW newsletter, *"Lifelines"*.
♦ Coordinating DANIDA and EU Technical Assistance within the MOHCW.

The Health Services Fund (HSF), established within the framework of the HSPS, proved to be a crucial component which facilitated the pooling of funds from donors, the government and revenue from user fees and their smooth flow to the district as well as within the district. The HSF became a key mechanism for direct financial support to the operational level of the ministry of health. The horizon of the HSPS collaboration had been envisaged to cover a period of between 10 to 15 years. Unfortunately this was not to be as DANIDA prematurely terminated its development aid commitments to the government of Zimbabwe in 2001 because of political differences between the two governments.

The SWAp Memorandum of Understanding (MoU)

Facts on the ground show that despite genuine commitments to partnership, power relationships between development partners and governments that are implementing the SWAp remain asymmetrical. Developed countries continue to unilaterally terminate bilateral aid agreements for reasons not directly related to health sector support. Examples of such unilateral breaches of cooperation agreements include those by DANIDA in Malawi and Zimbabwe in the turn of the millennium.

The SWAp process includes the development of "rules of the game" that govern and bring sanity in the area of development cooperation. Countries that have implemented the SWAp have developed and signed Memoranda of Understanding and Codes of Conduct meant to regulate the conduct of partners within the SWAp process. Such documents are however more of 'gentlemen's agreements' based more on trust than being legally binding documents. Experience shows that during the drafting of such documents there has been a general tendency for development partners to gain the upper hand by including conditional phrases which are biased against recipient countries. The documents lean towards demanding recipient governments to "act in certain ways" and for development partners "to consider undertaking certain commitments" as opposed to 'agreeing to act" in a certain way.

A general review of these agreements reveals the following similarities in content:

+ Obligations or undertakings by the government.
+ Obligations or undertakings by the development partners.
+ Obligations of both the government and development partners.

+ Modalities for fund pooling, financial management and procurement procedures to be adopted.
+ Specification of the areas of cooperation within the partnership.
+ Regular joint monitoring and review procedures and processes.
+ Conditions, under which the MoU can commence, be amended or terminated.
+ Conditions for co-opting additional partners.
+ Steps to be followed in resolving differences and misunderstandings that may arise during the course of the SWAp implementation process.

The Memorandum of Understanding (MoU) is usually supported by annexes in the form of Terms of Reference (TORs) for committees, guidelines, code of conduct and other relevant documentation. The guiding principle of a Memorandum of Understanding (MoU) is TRUST which some have likened to a glass which once broken can never be the same again, (Collins, T, June 2000).

Conclusions and the way forward

External resources have become the norm in health development in almost all African countries. However, to be effective these resources must be provided in a timely and predictable manner, support agreed country priorities, guarantee sustainability and be utilized in a transparent and responsible manner. Cooperation agreements involving development assistance must conform to the principles of joint control and ownership.

External assistance works best when co-operation is based on respect, a common purpose and actions and when both sides contribute at least some resources to the common goal. Transformation from assistance to co-operation requires better co-ordination in the objectives and activities of both bilateral and multilateral organizations. Such a transformation demands that there be a change in the vocabulary from 'donors and recipients' to 'partners'.

The SWAp has the potential to achieve expected results as long as there is consensus on some form of agreed policy framework between the government and its partners. The government must truly be in the lead with development partners adhering to national priorities and being seen to give up some of their control to the government. Experience in implementing the SWAp shows that power relationships between development partners and governments in recipient countries remain in favor of development partners. Unfortunately, indications are that this situation is unlikely to change in the near future, especially with the aid architecture becoming increasingly dominated by vertical funding. As a result African governments will continue to be faced with the dilemma of being unable to hold development partners accountable for their commitments. It remains to be seen the extent to which this situation will change as a result of implementation of the Paris Declaration on aid effectiveness and the International Health Partnership (IHP).

Skepticism about the SWAp will always be present, reinforced by the amount of pressure and implicit conditionality that development partners exert on poor countries. The credibility of the SWAp will continue to be undermined as long as some of the development partners are either not willing to or are unable to participate in pooling their resources together with other partners. This is usually compounded by a lack of visionary leadership in the health sector in most of these countries. The increase in vertical or disease specific funding in the early 2000s from organizations such as the Global Fund, GAVI, PEPFAR and charitable organizations are an emerging and serious threat to the SWAp process. A positive spin to this threat has been a renewed willingness by these institutions to support the strengthening of health systems which enable these disease programs to be effectively implemented.

Burnside and Dollar (1996) state that in countries where there are poor policies, development aid did not result in the desired impact. Furthermore, relationships which are based on conditionality often undermine the basis of achieving reciprocity between development partners and the recipient government, largely due to asymmetrical power relations. The current view is that conditionality has failed as a means of promoting sustainable policy reform in African countries. This is because under conditionality there is no ownership of any proposals for reform and development partners often do not have the determination to take action to enforce the prescribed policy conditions.

Some development partner organizations have proposed that African countries should be assessed to determine the extent to which they are committed to undertaking health sector reforms and the extent to which they are prepared to lead and assume ownership of this process. The following predictors have been proposed for such an assessment:

♦ The extent to which the government is willing to take a leadership role in the SWAp process and secure the support of development partners.
♦ The extent of national involvement in policy debate.
♦ The resolve with which the government has faced up to difficult policy choices in the past.
♦ The level of endorsement or frustration of sector policies at the levels of cabinet, parliament and other stakeholders.
♦ The level of knowledge and understanding of the sector program at the operational and policy levels.

It should be accepted that there are situations where the SWAp will simply not work. If the government is either unable or is unwilling to take a leadership role within the health sector, a SWAp may not materialize. Furthermore, the SWAp is not a panacea to all the problems affecting the health sector in low-income countries; it only provides the means by which some problems can be dealt with in a more coherent manner. Countries that have embraced the SWAp tend to be those that have inadequate institutional and management capacity to plan, co-ordinate and/or implement programs. From this perspective one may be justified to say that a SWAp is doomed even before it takes off the ground under conditions of poverty, lack of political will and a sheer lack of capacity.

Predetermined policy conditions are not an effective approach to accountability between the government and its development partners, they are counter-productive. Any government can easily sign a formal document in which it undertakes to be accountable to development partners by implementing health reforms. No amount of cohesive pressure can take the place of government commitment and ownership of policy reforms.

Development partners have had their share of concerns about the SWAp, especially those that are traditionally associated with vertical programs. One major concern is the potential loss of attribution of funds to a specific development partner or program. In a SWAp pooled fund arrangement development partners are in a dilemma as to how they will justify to their principals how they have used their resources. Such concerns result from a lack of confidence in government financial management systems by development partners and the absence of guarantees that the funds will not be abused. Those developed countries who have invested in vertical programs mourn the potential loss of the gains achieved in specialized training, procurement and management systems built over the life of such programs.

The issue of attribution within pooled funding can be resolved through the development of detailed implementation plans which include activity costs by source of funding. Where a country has opted to provide a package of services, funds for special programs can be ring-fenced, at least in the initial stages of the SWAp.

Because the SWAp is based on trust, development partners must at some point accept that governments are unlikely to change quickly in order to meet the reporting requirements of external partners who must also be prepared to adapt their own systems.

After all, how far true is it that in countries where the SWAp is being implemented policy reform is largely driven by domestic influences and not by external aid agencies? *"The SWAp approach aims to achieve progress which will ensure that all significant funding for the sector supports a single sector policy and expenditure program, under government leadership, adopting common approaches across the sector, and progressing towards relying on government procedures to disburse and account for all funds".* At the same time it has been said that such a state of affairs can only be tenable in highly aid dependent countries (Forster M. 1999) – the same countries that do not have the capacity to hold development partners accountable for the commitments they have pledged.

Review questions

1. Some have said that, "The Sector Wide Approach (SWAp) is what should have been happening all along" – i.e. leadership by the government, commitment to shared goals, a collaborative program of work and comprehensive plans. Elaborate on this statement.

2. How feasible is it for a highly aid dependent country to hold development partners accountable to fulfilling their financial commitments to a joint program of work? How useful is the Memorandum of Understanding in ensuring that development partners fulfill their end of the bargain?

3. In the context of a SWAp what do you understand by the terms "ownership of the policy process and ownership of the Program of Work"? What factors would you consider to be helpful in putting this concept into practice?

4. The SWAp is relevant only to highly aid dependent countries. Discuss this statement.

5. You have been given an assignment to provide technical assistance to the ministry of health to develop a Sector Wide Approach. Describe the stages in the development of the SWAp that you would outline for the ministry of health.

9

REGULATION, COMMERCIALIZATION AND SUBCONTRACTING

Introduction

This chapter deals with the implementation of market-oriented health reforms in African countries. These are mainly a result of challenges concerning the role of the state in the provision of health services, the poor performance of government run institutions and in some cases pressure from multinationals and the World Bank who apply an economic approach to health and exercise their dominance over country specific approaches. These moves are also a response to the globalization of public health policies. Although governments retain the primary responsibility for health, health determinants and means to address them transcend health ministries and national governments. It is becoming the norm rather than the exception that in order to develop and adopt national policy objectives governments find themselves having to increasingly turn to international development partners. Under this model of reforms the government's role is confined to policy formulation, monitoring, coordination and regulation.

Traditionally African countries have implemented the integrated model to health provision which combines public financing with public ownership of hospitals and the employment of salaried health professionals. It is through this model that some governments have been able to develop and successfully implement policies that have ensured universal coverage and equitable access to health care in the absence of viable third party payers. However, like any other policy strategy this model has had its share of criticisms which include those of being entrenched bureaucracies, inefficient and non responsive to public demands.

The introduction of market mechanisms in the health systems of African countries has meant that some services previously provided by the public health sector are now delivered by private companies under contract with the public sector. The public contracting model provides services to patients through negotiated contracts between governments and independent providers of care and in some cases with local authorities. The strategy is to use government funds to purchase clinical or non-clinical services from private providers in order to improve the productivity of public resources by purchasing the gains in efficiency perceived to be characteristic of the private sector.

The establishment of semi-autonomous hospitals and the commercialization of some government departments are meant to improve the efficiencies and effectiveness of public sector organizations and to ensure that they become financially viable. This has meant that governments have had to adopt and develop performance management systems and appoint professional managers to run these hospitals on short term performance related contracts meant to provide them with incentives to perform effectively. The tradeoff between the achievement of efficient resource allocation and utilization means that the principles of equity are sacrificed in some instances. There is also a need for an increased capacity to monitor the various actors in the delivery of contracted services.

The Government of Zimbabwe (GOZ) follows the Beveridge model of financing the health sector which is based on the collection of taxes and the provision of services organized through publicly owned and managed institutions. The state defines the overall framework of the country's health sector through legislation and the regulation of the actions of the various providers, including autonomous actors in health provision. Current theories on the management of social services call for the state to move away from the direct provision of health services. Such a policy move requires effective laws and an efficient regulatory environment.

The Ministry of Health and Child Welfare has over the years implemented policies on decentralization, commercialization of some departments and subcontracted some of its non-core functions. Some of these reforms meant that the MOHCW entered into service agreements with non state providers of health services in order to distance itself from the direct provision of health services. Such reforms were meant to improve efficiency and effectiveness in the management of health services, ultimately improving the quality of services and increasing equity in access to health care.

The MOHCW operates in an environment in which it administers a number of health and health related legislation which include:

♦ Anatomical Donations and Post Mortem Examinations Act, 1976(No. 34 of 1976).
♦ Atmospheric Pollution Prevention Act (Chapter 318).
♦ Dangerous Drugs Control Act (Chapter 319).
♦ Drugs and Allied Substances Control Act (Chapter 320).
♦ Food and Food Standards Act (Chapter 321).
♦ Hazardous Substances and Articles Act (Chapter 322).
♦ Mental Health Act, 1976 (No 23 of 1976).
♦ The Public Health Act (Chapter 328).
♦ Termination of Pregnancy Act, 1977 (No 29 of 1977).
♦ Traditional Medical Practitioners Act, 1981 (Chapter 224).
♦ Zimbabwe National Family Planning Council Act, 1985 (No 1 of 1985).
♦ Health Professions Act (Chapter 27:19 of 2000)
♦ Concealment of Births Act (Chapter 57).
♦ Government Medical Stores Commercialization Act (2000).
♦ Medical Services Act (1999)
♦ National AIDS Council of Zimbabwe Act (Chapter 15:14) of 1999.

The bodies responsible for putting into effect some of these legal instruments include the MOHCW itself, regulatory bodies such as the Health Professions Authority (HPA), the Medicines Control Authority of Zimbabwe (MCAZ) and local authorities through enforcing relevant by laws. A study carried out by Hongoro (1997) revealed that the regulatory framework which is based on the existing legislation in Zimbabwe was very weak and that the Acts as they stood did not adequately address the needs of a dynamic health environment.

The expansion of the private medical sector over the past decade has made it increasingly necessary for the government to put in place a more effective regulatory framework for the sector as a whole. One of the objectives has been to prevent the proliferation of substandard health facilities, to monitor malpractice by both registered and unregistered professionals and to prevent professional negligence by unscrupulous practitioners. Additional concerns include those that relate to equity, quality and the escalation of health care costs as a result of an unregulated private medical sector.

A challenge faced by regulatory authorities in the health sector concerns "self regulation" in which groups of pears are vested with some authority to license and sanction colleagues. Though this mode of regulation is a lot less expensive there are general concerns about its transparency.

Regulation of the health sector

According to Allsop and Murray (1996), regulation in the health sector has several roles which include "controlling market entry, competitive practices, market organization, remuneration, standards, quality and ensuring safety". Changes in the roles, responsibilities and ownership within the health sector in developing countries and the rapid growth of the private medical sector has in some instances come with general misuse of privileges, medical malpractice and medical negligence and inequalities. Regulations are also necessary to ensure that quality standards are met and that other abuses are prevented.

The structure and function of the HPC as it was known then had over the years been a subject of public interest, debate and scrutiny. The HPC had been accused of being secretive and protective of the medical fraternity at the expense of the general public. It was alleged that even in cases where unscrupulous practitioners had harmed patients the council often failed to act in a proper and fair manner, opting instead to protect the interests of practitioners. Other professional groups within the HPC had complained that the medical profession was marginalizing them and that they were unfairly represented in council structures.

Reform of the Health Professions Council (HPC)

After an extensive consultative process a new Act of Parliament was enacted in 2000 to regulate professional practice and conduct within the health profession. This Act, the Health Professions Act, established the Health Professions Authority (HPA) of Zimbabwe as the organization which succeeded the Health Professions Council. The major change brought about by the Act was the establishment of 8 independent professional councils:

1. Allied Health Practitioners' Council of Zimbabwe.
2. Medical and Dental Practitioners Council of Zimbabwe.
3. Natural Therapists Council of Zimbabwe.
4. Nurses Council of Zimbabwe.

5. Pharmacists Council of Zimbabwe.
6. Medical Laboratory and Clinical Scientists Council of Zimbabwe.
7. Environmental Health Practitioners Council of Zimbabwe.
8. Medical Rehabilitation Council of Zimbabwe.

These independent councils each have the following responsibilities:
+ The Registration of persons in that particular health profession and the issuing of practicing certificates to registered persons.
+ The exercise of disciplinary powers in relation to registered persons.
+ Disabilities of and offences by unregistered persons who perform acts specifically pertaining to health professions in respect of which a register is kept and who present themselves to be practitioners in any such health profession.
+ The Registration and control of health institutions and the regulation of services provided therein or there from.
+ The development and approval of curricula pertaining to their professional groups.
+ In some cases to set and grade professional examinations.

Each of the councils is required to establish committees of council which include; an Executive Committee, a Practice Control Committee, a Disciplinary Committee and an Education Committee. In addition to the above the councils are required to appoint a registrar and keep a register of practitioners and issue practicing certificates to its members who qualify.

The Act also repealed the following Acts:
+ The Chiropractors Act (Chapter 27:04).
+ The Medical, Dental and Allied Professions Act (Chapter 27:08).
+ The Natural Therapists Act (Chapter 27:09).
+ The Psychological Practices Act (Chapter 27:01).

The Health Professions Authority consists of 15 Members, 8 chairpersons of each of the councils, 6 ordinary citizens who are not associated with the practice of the health profession and the Secretary for Health. These 6 ordinary citizens are appointed by the Minister of Health and Child Welfare from submissions by a variety of civil society groups which are specified in the Act.

The number of members proposed to be appointed by the Minister became a controversial issue during the consultation process. The initial Bill proposed that the Minister of Health would appoint the majority of members constituting the Health Professions Authority. This was however rejected by professional and civil society groups on the grounds that such an "Authority" would not be independent and that it could be manipulated and subjected to undue political influence by the Minister.

The other area of contention was on the powers the Bill conferred on the Minister of Health to intervene directly in the day to day operations and decisions of the HPA. This clause was also considered to be a threat to the independence of the HPA. The agreed position was that the Minister, as was the case in all other similar Acts, had powers to give *"directions of a general nature"* as appear to him/her to be in the national interest.

As soon as the HPA became operational in 2001 all the councils increased registration and membership fees. This was to ensure that as independent entities, the councils would be financially viable under the new legislation. In cases where councils experience viability problems in the future, the Act provides for the merger of some of these councils. The Act also provides for the establishment of new councils if it were to be found necessary to do so in the future.

The Health Professions Authority is empowered to raise revenue to cover operating expenses through levying an agreed fee on the revenue raised by the different councils from their membership. The HPA has to date also relied on a meager annual grant from the MOHCW for its running expenses. According to the MOHCW resources from this grant cannot be used by the HPA to subsidize the running expenses of independent councils. It is important that the HPA maintains its financial and operational independence from government so as to guarantee its independence. Due to the increased number of Zimbabwean medical practitioners practicing outside Zimbabwe (in the Diaspora), in 2008 the Medical and Dental Council of Zimbabwe introduced a special register for these practitioners. Their registration and retention fees are denominated in foreign currency.

Accreditation of health professionals

As was the case with the previous Act, all health professionals and paramedics must be registered with the HPA and be in possession of current practicing certificates if they are to legally practice their profession in Zimbabwe. Whilst in the past practicing certificates were automatically renewed on the payment of an annual fee, some councils now require members to accrue continuing educational credit points for their practicing certificates to be renewed. For example, in 2003 the Medical and Dental Practitioners Council adopted a resolution requiring its members to participate in compulsory continuing education. The achievement of stipulated continuing education points is one of the conditions necessary for the renewal of annual professional practicing certificates. It was also proposed that medical professionals obtain mandatory malpractice insurance coverage.

Under the new Act, as was the case with the previous one, independent councils of the HPA have the power to impose additional conditions on professional practice. They can restrict the scope of practice of any practicing health professional. Such conditions can restrict a professional to practice only at government or other designated institutions. The councils can restrict a practitioner from undertaking private practice. In case of professional negligence the HPA and its councils have the authority to take appropriate disciplinary action which may result in the removal of the practitioner from the register of health professionals. It is illegal for the MOHCW or any health institution or organization in Zimbabwe to employ health practitioners who are not registered with the HPA.

Accreditation of health institutions

In 1995 the Health Professions Council made a decision that all health institutions, both public and private, were required by law to be registered with the HPC before they could be allowed to operate. Registration is preceded by an inspection to determine if the facility meets the specified minimum standards. However, because the HPC's inspectorate did not have the required capacity to undertake such work, it entered into an informal arrangement with urban local authorities to undertake some of these inspections within the areas of their jurisdiction.

The criteria used in these inspections have generally been limited to the design, physical structure, type of health staff employed and their registration status. The inspections do not adequately review the technical quality of health care provided at both public and private institutions. In cases of malpractice and professional negligence the HPA relies on reports and complaints from patients, the general public or whistle blowing from professional colleagues. The medical school, the HPA and the MOHCW conduct inspections and assessments of teaching hospitals, though it has been very difficult for them to follow through any of the adverse reports that have so far been made on some of these institutions.

Regulation of the pharmaceutical industry

Experience shows that many developing countries have serious problems with the registration of pharmaceuticals, prescription practices and quality control. Where regulatory intervention is inadequate there is extensive illegal sales of counterfeit drugs and a large black market in medicines. The Medicines Control Authority of Zimbabwe (MCAZ) keeps a register of all outlets that prescribe, manufacture and dispense drugs and medicines. The authority also requires all private general practitioners who wish to dispense medicines at their private surgeries as part of patient management to take a professional examination on the management of pharmaceuticals and dispensing procedures. According to the law private surgeries are ordinarily not allowed to dispense drugs or prescription medicines if they are located within a stipulated distance from an established pharmacy or drug store. The MCAZ, together with law enforcement agents, conducts regular and sporadic raids on street vendors and outlets that illegally trade in pharmaceuticals.

The Medical Services Act (1998)

Regulation of the health market is also aimed at achieving social goals of improving equity and distributive justice and the protection of individuals from discrimination and exploitation. This has traditionally included restrictions, controls and incentives.

This Act was enacted in April 1998 and seeks amongst other things to:

♦ Register and license private hospital development.
♦ Classify public hospitals as being open or closed depending on whether private practitioners are allowed to admit private patients or not.
♦ Regulate the operations of Healthcare Funders (Medical Aid Societies) - voluntary health insurance schemes.
♦ Provide for the Minister of Health and Child Welfare from time to time to fix fees and charges for government and state aided institutions.
♦ Delegate the administration of the regulations to rural and urban authorities and any other appropriate agency.
♦ Provide for the registration of Health care Funders by specifying the conditions under which a medical aid society can be registered, including the requirement to provide a specified minimum benefit package of services.

The Medical Services Act of 1979 which was considered to be discriminatory on race was repealed by the Minister of Health in February 1981. The Act promoted the existence of a dual hospital system based on racial grounds.

Regulation of public and private hospitals

There are several factors that prompted the government to pursue hospital reforms. These include the challenges faced by the authorities to monitor the performance of both public and private hospitals. The unreliable flow of funds from government resulted in substandard care at government institutions and in some cases vulnerable groups were denied access to specialist services by both sectors.

The objectives of hospital reforms were to ensure that those patients who were able to pay for services outside the basic package did so, to improve the quality of care, management practices and to encourage efficient utilization of public resources. It was also expected that if the private medical sector were to absorb a sizeable portion of the patient workload government resources could then be used to provide public health interventions targeted at the poor. Public health goods being those services that require public financing if they are to be provided at all and whose benefits accrue to the public at large as opposed to benefiting individuals. The policy shift was also to establish semi-autonomous institutions managed by independent boards.

To facilitate the implementation of the above objectives the Medical Services Act provides for:

♦ The Minister of Health and Child Welfare to approve the establishment of private hospitals.
♦ The prevention of discrimination in the exercise of the right to admit patients.
♦ The Minister of Health and Child Welfare to approve the fees charged at private hospitals.

Under the Medical Services Act it is possible for the MOHCW to enter into contractual agreements with private hospitals to purchase health care services on behalf of the public sector. Normally private hospitals require patients to pay up front or provide evidence that they are covered by health insurance before they treat them. This Act allows private hospitals to stabilize emergency cases for up to 24 hours and transfer them to the nearest government hospital. In such cases the government will pay the private hospital for the treatment of those patients who would normally be eligible for free treatment at public health facilities.

To ensure that the public or communities participate in the governance of public hospitals the Medical Services Act provides for the establishment of Community Health Councils at government hospitals. These councils facilitate the exercise of citizen's rights, ensure patient welfare and are expected to enhance hospital responsiveness to community needs. The terms of reference of these councils are detailed in Statutory Instrument 208 of 2001 and ensure that:

♦ Catering standards are maintained and that patients receive a nutritious diet.
♦ Visiting hours are convenient to the public.
♦ Hospital equipment is properly maintained.
♦ Wards and departments are hygienically maintained.
♦ Hospitals are adequately staffed and effectively managed.
♦ Complaints related to the management of the hospital are investigated.
♦ The hospital adheres to the provisions of the Patient's Charter.

Experience shows that the learning curve of these councils is very slow and characterized by a decline in interest, mainly because they cannot exert any meaningful influence or authority over health workers. At the core is the political context, patronizing attitudes of civil servants and government regulations, procedures and legal instruments that empower and determine the accountability channels of civil servants. Very few members of these councils have a great sense of altruism and are thus not ready to sacrifice benefits to themselves for the greater good and benefit of society.

Regulation of Health Insurance Schemes

Health fees charged for services offered by the private sector have over the years been determined through negotiations between the Zimbabwe Medical Association (ZIMA) and the Association of Health Funders (formerly National Association of Medical Aid Societies (NAMAS)). In case of any disagreements or dispute between the two parties in the determination of these fee levels there was no legal provision for any arbitration process. Neither the MOHCW nor the Minister of Health and Child Welfare had any legal powers to arbitrate in such disputes. In 1997 the impasse between the two parties became so serious and took so long to resolve that patients on medical aid could not access health care from private providers unless they paid cash up front. This situation led to a lot of suffering especially among pensioners who had no sources of ready cash to pay private providers cash up front. Medical aid societies refused to pay or reimburse patients the level of fees demanded by private providers of health care. Private providers of care, especially the medical doctors, refused to accept the fees that the medical aid societies were prepared to pay.

A similar situation arose in 2003-2004 where because of the very high rate of inflation of over 600% doctors in private practice demanded an increase in medical fees to match the prevailing rate of inflation. The medical aid societies refused to accept the proposed fee hike on the basis that the fee levels demanded by the private doctors were not based on any rational consideration. Compared to the prevailing monthly minimum wage of Z$13 000 general practitioners charged consultation fees of up to Z$ 90 000 for a single consultation, paid in cash up front. This time around the situation was also compounded by the fact that the country was experiencing a severe shortage of cash. This meant that even patients who would have normally been able to pay cash were not able to do so. The situation was eventually resolved after more than four months of an impasse. By August 2008 the rate of inflation had reached an unprecedented 11000 000%.

The Medical Services Act gives the Minister of Health the authority to arbitrate in case of a dispute between third party payers and private providers of health. Regulations to the Act also provide for the establishment of a Tariffs Committee which includes, amongst other members, persons nominated by the Association of Health Funders of Zimbabwe, the Private Hospitals Association of Zimbabwe, the Zimbabwe Nurses Association (ZINA) and the Zimbabwe Medical Association (ZIMA).

The main objective of the Tariffs Committee is to devise a tariff of fees for services provided by general practitioners, state aided and non-state aided private health institutions, and local authority health facilities. In determining the fees the committee takes into account the social obligations of state aided institutions in providing services to those patients who cannot afford treatment on the same terms and conditions as those admitted to private hospitals.

Since their establishment in Zimbabwe, health insurance schemes (formerly called Medical Aid Societies), had never been regulated through any legal instrument. They were merely required to be registered with the Ministry of Finance for tax purposes. As a result some of them had developed wayward and discriminatory tendencies against patients considered to be high risk; the elderly, the poor and those with chronic conditions such as HIV/AIDS.

Some health insurance schemes have established pharmacies, laboratories and diagnostic services and denied their membership the choice to receive similar services from institutions established by other providers. It could however be argued that the establishment of such facilities is a conflict of interest. Health insurance schemes are now regulated under the Medical Services (Medical Aid Societies) regulations of 2000 and are required to support the MOHCW core health package as their minimum benefit package for their members.

The Commercialization of MOHCW departments

The Government Medical Stores

The Treasury established the Government Medical Stores (GMS) in 1958 as a Trading Account of the Ministry of Health responsible for procuring and distributing drugs and medical supplies within the public sector. The GMS had a long history of operational problems and an inability to satisfy the requirements of the public health sector. This was mainly attributed to inadequate capitalization of the trading account, poor and inefficient management and corruption.

Efforts to improve the operations of the GMS include financial and technical assistance provided by DANIDA in the early 1990s to recapitalize, reorganize the GMS and strengthen its management capacity. The GMS infrastructure was rehabilitated and expanded to improve storage capacity, stock holding and management. New information and data processing systems were developed and staff trained in supplies management.

The benefits from technical assistance were however, compromised by a continued decline in government expenditures on health and a decline in the capitalization of the GMS, which led to wide spread shortages of essential drugs in the public sector. Persistent poor management and massive drug leakages further discredited the operations of the GMS to an extent that more drastic solutions were sought to improve the drugs supply situation in the country.

This resulted in the enactment of the GMS (Commercialization) Act in 2000 which established a publicly owned drugs and medical supplies procurement company, the National Pharmaceutical Company (Natpharm) which is managed by a Chief Executive Officer who is responsible to a Board of Directors. The Board reports to the Minister of Health and

Child Welfare. The Secretary for Health represents the interests of the MOHCW at the board meetings. The board has powers to hire, fire and set the conditions of service for its employees, outside those of the civil service. At its inception the company started on a clean slate, acquiring all the assets previously owned by the GMS with the exception of the debt (liabilities) which remained with the government (MOHCW). The company's mandate is to *"purchase, sell, deal in and store medicines, medical equipment and other goods and articles for use in hospitals, clinics, pharmacies and other medical establishments".*

The company relates to MOHCW institutions purely on business terms, though the management board requires ministerial approval on decisions relating to setting or reviewing "mark-up" on drug sales. Being a publicly owned and not-for-profit entity the company has a social obligation to ensure that the public sector can afford to purchase medicines so as to guarantee affordable health care to vulnerable groups. In a truly business sense MOHCW institutions are required to pay for goods purchased strictly within a 30-day period and failure to do results in the company withholding further sales to defaulting institutions. This is unlike in the past when public health institutions defaulted from paying the GMS for up to as long as twelve months in extreme cases.

The Medicines Control Authority of Zimbabwe (MCAZ)

The Medicines Control Authority of Zimbabwe, established through an amendment to the Medicines and Allied Substances Control Act (Chapter 15:03) of 1996, succeeded the Drugs Control Council (DCC). The MCAZ which is responsible for regulating the pharmaceutical industry in Zimbabwe is empowered to inspect and license all pharmacies. Responsibilities of the MCAZ include:

+ The Registration of medicines on the basis of quality, safety and efficacy, cancellation and variation of the conditions of registration of medicines.
+ To monitor Adverse Drug Reactions (ADR).
+ The declaration of specified medicines.
+ Control of advertisements of medicines.
+ To exercise powers of search, forfeiture and safe custody of prohibited drugs and their distribution.
+ Post marketing surveillance.
+ Licensing and control of pharmaceutical premises and persons.
+ To inspect pharmaceutical premises.

- The management of the Zimbabwe Regional Medicines Control Laboratory which is a WHO collaborating center.
- To control and monitor clinical trials.
- Keeping the Medicines Register.
- The provision for certain prohibitions, controls and restrictions relating to medicines and other substances.

The MCAZ is managed by a board which has powers to determine the conditions of service for its staff that are not part of the civil service. The MCAZ is expected to raise its operational costs from the revenue raised from providing services to the public. Despite good corporate management practices, the poor macroeconomic environment prevailing in Zimbabwe in the early 2000s proved to be a major challenge to the organization's financial viability.

Proposals to establish semi-autonomous hospitals

Semiautonomous central and provincial hospitals were effectively established in terms of the Medical Services Act (1998). Statutory Instrument 208 of 2001 of the Medical Services Act [Chapter 15:13] established Hospital Management Boards (HMB) at central and provincial hospitals by providing for the composition, the powers and functions of such boards. Because the Act does not empower Hospital Management Boards to hire and fire staff, the implication is that these boards do not have complete jurisdiction over the staff they manage. Semi-autonomous hospitals remain government owned and an integral part of the public health delivery system. This fact is underscored in Part II, Section 4 (2) of S.I. 208 of 2001 which states that the board shall, in managing these institutions, have due regard to the social obligations of the hospital as a government institution and provide for the needs of the public. As a result when these institutions develop their management policies they must ensure that the principles of equity in access to health care are upheld at all times. Government's overriding objective in establishing semi-autonomous hospitals is to improve institutional management, resource utilization, and the work environment for health professionals and the quality of health care provided. Additional anticipated benefits from this reform objective include:

- Ability to generate and draw upon local goodwill, especially through Community Health Councils, response to local expectations.

♦ Freedom to develop their own human resources strategies, to set their own pay levels and remuneration packages thus enabling them to attract and retain qualified and experienced staff.

♦ Freedom to treat private patients and generate income, subject to fulfillment of the hospitals' social obligations.

♦ Achieving efficiency in the mobilization and utilization of financial resources.

In operating both as public health institutions and semi autonomous institutions these hospitals are likely to face challenges from several fronts. As public health oriented institutions they are required to ensure that all individuals who require health care receive it irrespective of their ability to pay. As institutions that have to be financially viable they will need to develop admissions and financing policies that reflect the fact that they do not depend on the government for their operational costs. Some government policies on user fees are likely to restrict the hospitals from fully relying on user fees as a main source of revenue, unless there is a fully operational Social Health Insurance Scheme.

The shortage of resources in terms of skilled manpower and finances has the potential to limit the extent to which quality service delivery can be achieved. The massive loss of experienced managers from the public sector is likely to influence the capacity of these institutions to adopt a corporate management culture. The semi autonomy of different institutions within a government policy framework may result in fragmented policy interpretation and implementation by different management boards, especially with respect to levels of user fees and exemption criteria for vulnerable groups.

Too much emphasis on cost recovery has the potential to adversely affect government efforts to achieve equity in access to specialist services by the poor. With respect to provincial hospitals, not all of them have the infrastructure to provide the necessary package of specialist services.

Powers, responsibilities and freedoms of semi-autonomous hospitals

In terms of the Second Schedule, Section 4 (3) of S.I. 208 of 2001 and the amended Parirenyatwa Hospitals Act:-

♦ Semi-autonomous institutions are operationally independent and not subject to centralized bureaucratic procedures and processes or pressure from the MOHCW.

♦ Semi-autonomous institutions will be able to develop their own staffing levels and structures and set their own terms and conditions of employment, subject to the general guidelines of the Health Service Board.

The Minister of Health and Child Welfare is responsible for appointing members to these Management Boards who are responsible for:
+ Determining the overall policy of the hospital.
+ Monitoring the execution of agreed policies.
+ Ensuring the financial viability of the hospital.
+ Appointing the Chief Executive Officer of the hospital.

The remuneration of the board members is subject to approval by the Minister of Health and Child Welfare. The hospital management board is expected to adhere to a minimum code of conduct:
+ Retain full and effective control over the hospital and monitor executive management.
+ Ensure a clear division of responsibilities to ensure a balance of power and authority, so that no one individual has absolute powers of decision.
+ Ensure that the direction and control of the institution is firmly under its control.
+ Agree on procedures for board members to undertake their responsibilities.
+ That all members of the board follow board procedures.
+ That applicable rules and regulations are complied with.
+ Board members are free from any business or other relationships which could materially interfere with the exercise of their independent judgment.

In terms of S. I. 208 of 2001 the Hospital Management Boards are accountable to the Minister of Health and Child Welfare through the following and other tools:
+ An annual (business) plan: on services, financial projections and capital development plans.
+ An annual report of the previous years' performance.
+ Annual accounts.
+ Regular financial monitoring information.
+ Submission of core statistical data necessary to support the Minister's public accountability.
+ Submissions of major capital schemes that require Treasury approval.

The Chief Executive Officer is responsible to the HMB, gives effect to its policies and performs the day-to-day management of the hospital. He or she is expected to have extensive management experience, preferably in the health sector, and a relevant qualification in organizational management. A qualification or experience in a health related field is an advantage but not a requirement. The Chief Executive Officer is the accounting officer for the hospital and will answer any questions relating to hospital accounts on behalf of the Hospital Management Board. The CEO's tenure is based on a 3-year performance contract which can be renewed by the board in consultation with the Minister of Health and Child Welfare, subject to satisfactory performance. The performance of the Chief Executive Officer is judged according to agreed criteria which may include those listed below, though not necessarily exhaustive:

+ The development of an acceptable business plan for the hospital.
+ The timely production of audited annual accounts.
+ Production of accurate, up-to-date, regular and acceptable financial monitoring reports.
+ The establishment and implementation of a viable quality assurance or clinical audit program and the maintenance of acceptable clinical and nursing standards.
+ The development and enforcement of a financially viable and equitable admissions policy for the hospital.
+ Achievement of acceptable staffing levels for the institution.
+ An acceptable report on the performance of the previous year.
+ The maintenance of a financially viable institution with effective budgetary control systems.
+ Any other performance criteria that the HMB may deem necessary for its purposes.

The work of semi-autonomous hospitals should be underpinned by the following values:

+ Accountability: everything done by those who work for these institutions must be able to stand public scrutiny and judgment on propriety and professional codes of conduct.
+ Probity: there should be an absolute standard of honesty in dealing with the assets of the hospital, integrity should be central to all personal conduct in decisions affecting patients, staff and suppliers and in the use of information acquired in the course of their duties.

♦ Openness: there should be sufficient transparency about hospital activities to promote confidence between the hospital and its staff, patients and the public.

As part of the public health delivery system semi-autonomous hospitals are bound by the same mechanisms of accountability as all other publicly owned health facilities. The following provisions, laws and statutes, amongst others, apply:

1. The Patient's Charter and the hospitals' complaints procedures.
2. The Medical Services Act.
3. The Health Professions Act [Chapter 27:19].
4. The Public Health Act.
5. The Audit and Exchequer Act [Chapter 22:03].
6. The Mental Health Act [Chapter 15:06].
7. The Dangerous Drugs Act [Chapter 15:03].
8. Hazardous Substances Act [Chapter 15:05].
9. Medicines and Allied Substances Act [Chapter 15:04].
10. Termination of Pregnancy Act [Chapter 15:10].
11. Constitution of the Health Services Fund.
12. Lotteries and Gaming Act [Chapter 10:26].

Financing and financial management issues

In the foreseeable future, the bulk of the finances for these institutions will continue to come from government as a grant appropriated by an Act of Parliament and largely based on the hospital's business plan. Other sources of finance include:

♦ Revenue from fees or charges for services and facilities provided.
♦ Donations or grants from well-wishers which are permitted by the Minister of Health and Child Welfare.
♦ Income derived from investment.
♦ External borrowing.
♦ Disposal of assets.
♦ Lotteries and gaming.

The hospital's financial resources are expected to be managed through the Health Services Fund as constituted in terms of Section 30 of the Audit and Exchequer Act [Chapter 22:03]. The institutions are expected to keep proper accounting records and draw up accounts each year as laid down by the Comptroller and Auditor General. The accounts must show a "true and fair view" and in general drawn up using acceptable accounting standards. In case of borrowing, the HMB must demonstrate that they are getting value for money, the best terms available. It is not acceptable for the hospital to borrow at low rates from government and deposit it in an account at higher interest rates in order to generate income.

Choice of services and arrangements for patient referral

The package of services to be offered by provincial and central hospitals must be based on:

+ The need for such services (geographical, burden of disease, etc).
+ The institution's role in the teaching of health professionals.
+ Available financial, material and human resources.
+ The need to avoid duplication of services in a particular geographical area.

The Ministry of Health and Child Welfare will continue to provide general guidance on the core services expected to be delivered by central and provincial hospitals, respectively, to ensure that the health system maintains an effective and efficient referral system throughout the country. Semi-autonomous hospitals are encouraged to enter into collaborative arrangements with each other in order to avoid duplication of services in a particular geographical locality.

The referral of patients is guided by clinical rather than financial reasons and ensures patient access to essential referral services. The following arrangements for the referral of patients are proposed:

1. Referred patients who are not entitled to 'free' health care pay for their own referral services at semi autonomous institutions.

2. In terms of patients who are entitled to 'free' health services, to consider the following options:

   + Individual central or provincial hospitals enter into contractual arrangements with district or other institutions for a fixed amount of money to cover referrals, irrespective of their number – based on a simple block contract.

   + A central or provincial hospital charges a referring institution based on the cost of each case referred - cost per case basis.

   + For patients who are eligible for "free" health care in terms of prevailing government policies, the provincial or central hospital attends to the referrals at no cost at the point of service delivery and claims for a refund from the Social Dimensions Fund (SDF) or a Social Health Insurance (SHI) scheme.

Staffing and the management of human resources

During the transition period, it is envisaged that Hospital Management Boards will be responsible for identifying staff to be transferred to their (semi-autonomous) hospitals. The HMB is expected to develop its own human resources strategy to motivate staff to higher levels of performance and to offer employment packages which are sufficiently attractive. It is further envisaged that management boards will have the freedom to set the terms and conditions of service for the staff they employ. In doing so, the boards are expected to be guided by the Health Service Board and its regulations. In terms of the relevant legislation, the conditions of service for the Chief Executive Officer are subject to ministerial approval.

Should staff be transferred from the Health Service Board to the HMB they are expected to continue contributing to the same pension scheme in terms of the Public Service (Pensions) Regulations, 1992 (S.I. 124 of 1992). Alternatively, HMB can opt for staff to join other pension schemes, provided the employees consent to such arrangements.

Staff opting for voluntary or early retirement from the Health Service Board as opposed to being transferred to semi-autonomous hospitals will be free to do so, provided that the Health Service Board agrees. Those employees, whom the HMB is not able to employ and the Health Service Board is not able to re-deploy within the service, shall be retired on abolition of office. This is provided that in terms of Section 32B of the Public Service Act as amended, the HMBs will not employ staff that have been granted retirement on abolition of office before the lapse of a period of 10 years from the date on which they would have left the Public Service. Exceptions can only be granted by the Health Service Board.

The Hospital Management Boards are expected to adhere to government policies and strategies on health manpower training and development. They are also required to employ recognized training grades such as Junior Resident Medical Officers (JRMO), Senior Resident Medical Officers (SMRO), Registrars, trainee nurses etc. Central hospitals are expected to ensure that they make the necessary effort to remain as designated institutions under the Health Professions Act for the purposes of training medical doctors and other health professionals.

Responsibility for the costs of pre-registration attachment and basic training of health professionals that take place at semi-autonomous hospitals must be appropriately assigned. In the interim, the MOHCW is expected to sponsor such training posts. The MOHCW has the responsibility to plan for and allocate the number of training posts in line with national training requirements and in consultation with Hospital Management Boards, the private sector and other training institutions. Central and provincial hospitals will continue to provide clinical placement for trainees in the health profession.

Due to the critical shortage of professional health staff in the country, HMBs are encouraged to consider other options of managing human resources such as:

+ Time-based arrangements to match staffing to work-load (use of different shift patterns, working hours).
+ Contract based arrangements for organizational flexibility e.g. temporary staff and fixed term contract staff.
+ Contracting out some hospital services.

Roles and responsibilities of consultants and specialists

In 1995 the MOHCW put to paper job descriptions for all categories of medical doctors employed in the public sector. The major amongst many reasons was to ensure accountability within this group of health professionals. Consultants and specialists where thus required to develop job plans in agreement with their institutional heads. Draft contract documents were also developed to guide the transition towards the employment of consultants and specialists on performance contracts. Contracts were to come into effect concurrently with the establishment of semi-autonomous hospitals. The contracts would be signed between the doctor and the board to ensure that:

1. Together with colleagues the specialist provides a service to the hospital(s) with the responsibility for the prevention, diagnosis and treatment of illness.

2. The specialist undertakes out of hours responsibilities in the form of rota commitment.

3. The specialist is on call for emergencies on a rota which ensures that at all times a consultant is available for the management of emergencies. It is the responsibility of the consultant to ensure that the hospital is able to contact him or her in case of emergency for his or her patients.

4. The specialist fulfills any requirements agreed to for the provision of cover for consultant colleagues who may be on leave.

5. The specialist provides professional supervision and management of junior staff.

6. The consultant fulfills his or her responsibilities to teach junior staff the principles and practice of his or her specialty during ward rounds and formally through tutorials, lectures etc. and to devote time to this activity on a regular basis.

7. The consultant fulfills responsibilities to carry out teaching, examination and accreditation duties as required and contributes to post-graduate and continuing education activities. Each consultant or specialist is encouraged to seek honorary lectureship with the local medical school. The consultant is also required to participate in medical audit and relate it to continuing education within his or her specialty.

8. Where the hospital has other obligations such as providing services to other agencies, e.g. district or provincial hospitals, prison services etc., to ensure that the consultant provides such services.

9. The consultant conducts all scheduled ward rounds on all in-patients under his or her care and at all times to be responsible for management decisions on his or her patients.

10. The consultant undertakes regular outpatient clinics and attends to all patients referred for specialist opinion. Surgeons were required to undertake all regular theater duties.

The proposal is for Hospital Management Boards to employ consultants and specialists under the following general contractual terms and conditions:

- Three (3) year contracts with an option for renewal.
- Consultants or specialists required to develop work programs to include a weekly timetable of commitments in consultation with their peers and the head of institution.
- The work programs to include fixed and flexible commitments indicating the hospital(s) where the commitments would be undertaken.
- Fixed commitments which clearly state the following types of work programs, which are not exhaustive:
  - Outpatient clinics.
  - Theater lists and/or lists for special procedures.
  - Ward rounds.
  - Medical audit.
  - Teaching commitments.
  - Call duties.

The flexible commitments include administrative duties such as compilation of medico-legal reports, evaluation of junior doctors, writing departmental reports and attending meetings etc. Two types of contracts would be considered for the employment of consultants and specialists:

(i) *FULL TIME CONTRACT*
In which a consultant is required to work a total of 4.5 days a week, perform a minimum of two (2) calls per week.

(ii) *PART-TIME CONTRACT: SESSIONAL CONSULTANT*
In which a consultant is contracted for a mutually agreed number of hours of work and is paid on a pro-rata basis, based on the basic salary of a full time consultant. In addition, the consultant is allowed privileges to admit and treat his or her own private patients in the hospital, see Box 8.

Maintaining quality of care

In order to ensure that the hospitals maintain the desired quality and standards of care semi-autonomous hospitals are expected to pay particular attention to:

1. Patient rights and ethical issues: -
   a. Adherence to the Patients' Charter and complaints procedures.
   b. Develop and implement guidelines in the following areas:
   + The conduct of research involving patients and the need for supervision by an ethics committee.
   + Guidelines for the involvement of patients in teaching.
   + Procedures for consent to treatment (informed consent).
   + Procedures for the retention and access to patient records.
   + Confidentiality of patient records and information.
2. Public Health issues:
   + Notification of adverse drug reactions.
   + Compliance with some codes of practice e.g. disposal of clinical waste, notification of specific diseases, post exposure and injury on duty policies (occupational safety issues), infection control practices and guidelines for the use of blood and blood products.
   + Inspections in relation to the control of dangerous drugs.
   + Discharge of patients from hospitals.

       ◆ Development and implementation of guidance on the discharge of patients from hospitals.

4. Clinical Audit:
   ◆ The hospitals are expected to make arrangements for implementing an effective system of clinical audit.

5. Information provision:
   ◆ The hospitals to provide certain statistical and financial information to the Minister of Health and Child Welfare, e.g. annual financial activity report, 3 year forward plan, regular financial data for central financial monitoring, manpower and patient related activity data and other epidemiological data.

6. Disaster preparedness.
   ◆ The hospitals are expected to participate in emergency and contingency planning arrangements.

7. Procurement procedures.
   ◆ The hospitals are required to follow government procurement policies and procedures with respect to tendering for commercial contracts and supplies.

Box 9.1 Specimen contract for the employment of the Chief Executive Officer

SPECIMEN PERFORMANCE CONTRACT OF EMPLOYMENT
ENTERED INTO BY AND BETWEEN
...Mpilo...HOSPITAL MANAGEMENT BOARD
ESTABLISHED IN TERMS OF THE MEDICAL SERVICES ACT,
Statutory Instrument 208 of 2001.
AND Dumisani Nyathi (HEREIN AFTER REFERRED TO
AS THE CHIEF EXECUTIVE OFFICER
NOW THEREFORE IT IS AGREED THAT:

Mpilo Hospital Management Board (hereinafter referred to as the Board) in consultation with the Minister of Health and Child Welfare employs the Chief Executive Officer who hereby accepts the appointment on the following conditions.

1. PERIOD OF EMPLOYMENT.

This appointment shall be subject to a probation period of 1 year from the date of commencement of duty. The Chief Executive Officer shall work full time for...Mpilo .Hospital in the capacity of Chief Executive Officer for a period of 3 years commencing on 7th July 2004 or the date of assumption of duty, whichever is the sooner.

The Board may renew the contract thereafter after consulting with the Minister provided that if the Minister/Board does not intend to renew the contract, they shall give the Chief Executive Officer a period of notice of six (6) months before the date of expiry of the contract.

If the Chief Executive does not wish to renew the contract he/she shall give the Board a period of notice of six (6) months before the date of expiry of the contract.

2 DUTIES

Key responsibility Areas.

The Chief Executive Officer shall be accountable to the Mpilo Hospital Management Board. The Hospital Management Board shall allow the Chief Executive Officer to exercise initiative in the performance of his/her duties and which duties can be varied by the Hospital Management Board from time to time provided that the powers of the Board to prescribe, vary or alter the Chief Executive's duties shall not entitle the Board to reduce or diminish the Chief Executive Officer's status.

3. JOB SUMMARY

+ To provide leadership and strategic vision which enable the hospital to provide effective management which ensures that the clinical, financial, legal and contractual obligations are met.
+ The Chief Executive Officer is the Accounting Officer of the institution.

4. CORPORATE RESPONSIBILITIES

+ To lead the executive team in corporate management and strategic planning.
+ To actively promote the hospital's health care and management objectives.
+ To implement the policies of the Management Board.
+ As a Member of the Board, to contribute to decision-making and participate in effective discharge of the Board's functions.
+ To promote a positive image of the institution with external agencies and the media.
+ To ensure the institution and its activities continue to meet the challenges of the health reforms and policies.

5. LEADERSHIP AND VISION
The Chief Executive Officer shall: -
  a. Ensure the active and positive participation of clinicians and other health professionals in the management and leadership of the Hospital.
  b. Develop a clear management style and culture for the institution and provide leadership to senior managers, and other staff in the achievement of the institution's objectives.
  c. Manage and monitor the hospital management team's achievement of responsibilities delegated to them.

6. SERVICE PLANNING AND DEVELOPMENT.
  * Ensure the preparation of strategic and business (operational) plans.
  * Promote service development and ensure financial viability of the institution through maximization of income and control of costs.
  * Provide leadership in an environment which encourages initiative, enterprise, research and delivery of clinical and supporting services.

7. MANAGEMENT OF RESOURCES
  * Review the use of resources and value for money.
  * Ensure proper systems are in place to support the standing orders and financial instructions, the production of business plans, regular financial reports, annual reports and timely statements of accounts.
  * Development of the institution's budget.

8. PERSONNEL.
  * Ensure management and organizational structures are continually reviewed to meet the changing needs of the institution.
  * Ensure effective arrangements for recruitment, training, development and management of staff.
  * Ensure the development of a human resources strategy and policy for the institution.
  * Ensure there is a code of conduct for staff employed by the Board.
  * Ensure that the institution fulfils its training obligations with respect to the training and secondment of medical doctors, nursing staff, and other allied health professions as may be required by the Health Professions Authority.

9. QUALITY ASSURANCE
  * Ensure specific standards of service delivery are set, understood and monitored.
  * That clinical audit responsibilities are undertaken and that there is continuous development of strategies for quality.

10. ACCOUNTABILITY.
The Chief Executive Officer shall be accountable to the Chairman of the Hospital Management Board who shall delegate duties to him/her from time to time.

11. HOURS OF BUSINESS
The normal hours of business as practiced in the Civil Service shall apply, as well as any other duties required from time to time, and no overtime shall be paid.

12. REMUNERATION
Subject to an annual review, the Hospital Management Board shall pay the Chief Executive Officer, a gross annual salary of Z$ .... per annum payable monthly in arrears less any deductions required to and made by the laws of Zimbabwe.

The Chief Executive Officer's salary shall be subject to (annual) review by the Hospital Management Board in consultation with the Minister of Health and Child Welfare. In discharging this exercise the Hospital Management Board shall take into account the Chief Executive Officers' performance in the discharge of his/her duties in terms of this contract.
+ Performance Award. [Up to .... of Annual Salary.]
+ Housing Allowance.
+ Telephone Allowance.
+ Entertainment allowance.
+ Domestic Worker Allowance.
+ Education allowance. [Equivalent to fees paid at government schools for up to three (3) dependents].

13. OTHER BENEFITS.
+ Pension Contribution 50%.
+ Personal Use Vehicle
+ Medical Aid- Contributory.
+ Vacation Leave as per Health Service Board (General Leave) Regulations as amended.
+ Annual leave.
+ Sick Leave- as per HMB Regulations.
+ Notice period- ...... months.
+ Insurance Cover- Group Accident Cover.

14. CONFIDENTIALITY.
The Chief Executive Officer shall not, either before or after the termination of this agreement (excerpt in so far as shall be necessary in the ordinary course of his/her duties) disclose to any person any information as to the practice, business dealings and/or affairs of the Hospital Management Board or any other matters which may come to his/her knowledge by reason of his/her employment as aforesaid.

15. TERMINATION OF CONTRACT
The Hospital Management Board in consultation with the Minister of Health and Child Welfare may terminate this contract forthwith at any time on grounds recognized by law and Code of Conduct as contained in Statutory Instrument 65 of 1992 Public Service (disciplinary) Regulations 1992.

The contractual approach to service delivery

The Medical Services Act (1998) provides for contractual relationships to be entered into between the MOHCW and other providers of health services in Zimbabwe. It is thus necessary to clarify and agree on the roles and responsibilities of the government, local authorities, the private-for-profit-sector and the private-not-for-profit sector consisting of faith based organizations and other NGOs in the provision of health services in Zimbabwe.

The proposed contractual arrangement is based on service contracts between the Provincial Medical Directors (on behalf of the MOHCW) and local authorities, faith based institutions, or private (for profit) health providers to provide curative and /or public health services. The contracts should specify the cost and volume of services to be provided so as to make it easy for faith based organizations and local authorities to know in advance the amount of money they expect from the government for the delivery of services. A similar arrangement is expected to govern the relationships between the MOHCW and semi-autonomous institutions as recipients of a health grant from the government.

This type of arrangement requires a quality assurance framework to enable contracting parties to monitor the performance of the contracts. Faith based organizations have over the years been required to declare all health related donations they receive from other sources in addition to those they receive from the government. This was meant to ensure that the government allocated grant money to faith based organizations in a rational manner.

The contractual agreement is to be guided first and foremost by the trust that exists between the parties to the agreement and based on the premise that a contract is a voluntary alliance between independent partners who mutually expect to derive benefits from the agreement. The expected benefits in this case include cost savings, effectiveness, responsiveness, improved quality, accountability and equity in service delivery. In order to achieve these objectives the contracts are meant to combine service targets and performance measurements and derive legal sanction from the shared need to conduct business together rather than being based on classical contractual models. The contracting parties have several contractual models at their disposal, namely:

Intra-governmental performance contracts and partnership contracts are linked to the devolution of programs or funding from the national to local governments. The national level provides funding to local government in exchange for the provision of specified levels of services. Such service contracts are common in the education, health care and labor markets where the national government may still retain final responsibility and accountability for the provision of service but finds that local authorities more effectively implement the programs. This is the preferred model for a devolved health delivery system.

Organizational performance agreements are agreements between the Minister and the Permanent Secretary (PS) or between the PS and senior managers. These agreements breakdown overall strategic goals into program elements, set specific and detailed operational, process and output oriented and targeted resource allocations. Such contracts include the budget in exchange for increased operational autonomy in achieving the agreed targets.

Purchaser-provider agreements focus on separating the role of the purchaser from that of the provider of services. Such arrangements ideally should specify the outputs required in terms of timing, volume, cost and quality.

Customer service agreements detail service standards and specify the quality and quantity of services to be provided as well as the avenues for redress and compensation where services fail to meet the standards. Such services are usually developed through consultations with customers (Claude, B, 1999).

MOHCW's experience with contracting clinical services

The contracts piloted by the MOHCW required the following information to be made available to enable performance monitoring:

+ Basis of agreement with the parties to the agreement.
+ The duration of the agreement.
+ Arrangements for variation including specifying those able to sign for each party.
+ Arrangements for arbitration.
+ The type of services to be covered.
+ Quality standards.
+ Service contract price.
+ Payment schedules.
+ Monitoring and performance evaluation features.
+ Protection of consumers.

Some of the experiences that the MOHCW in Zimbabwe has had with contracting health service delivery include entering into a contract with Hwange Colliery Hospital (a private for profit institution) in 1994 to provide referral clinical services to patients who would otherwise be eligible for free health services at government institutions. Hwange Colliery Hospital was established as a mine hospital offering health services to mine employees, mine pensioners and their dependents. The contract covered patients referred from hospitals within Matabeleland North province where the government did not have specialist referral hospitals. The nearest government hospital capable of providing referral services is more than 300 kilometers away.

According to the contract the mine hospital submitted monthly statistics on patients attended as well as financial information. For each case treated, the hospital was required to provide evidence that the patient had been assessed as eligible to be treated under the contract, the authority given by the District Medical Officer, the date of treatment and details of the treatment given. The hospital would then be paid on a cost per case basis within 30 days of submitting the bill. The MOHCW established a government almoner's office at the hospital's outpatient department which was responsible for screening patients for their eligibility to receive "free" treatment at the Hwange Colliery hospital under the contract. The fees charged were based on the Relative Value Schedule (RVS) current at the time the treatment was provided. Prescriptions were to be generic and in line with the Zimbabwe Essential Drugs Action Program (ZEDAP) and the Zimbabwe Essential Drugs List (EDLIZ).

The MOHCW estimated that the total payments made to Hwange hospital on an annual basis were enough to pay for the running costs of a typical district hospital. As a result the ministry found it difficult to continue to justify the amounts of money the government was paying to this hospital. On these and other grounds both parties agreed to terminate the contract in 1999. Subsequent to the termination of this contract the government made a political decision to construct a new district hospital within 10 kilometers of the Hwange Colliery hospital. In the meantime the Catholic Church had completed building a district type hospital within the same radius, purportedly to fill the gap created by the termination of the Hwange contract by the government.

The more rational course of action would have been for the MOHCW to renegotiate a more acceptable contract and let the private hospital continue providing local referral health services. What has since transpired is that Hwange district has an oversupply of hospital beds with five hospitals serving a population of about 300 000. The district is thus served by the Colliery hospital, Lukosi rural government hospital, St Patrick's mission hospital, the Victoria Falls (government) hospital and the Hwange Government District Hospital. All these institutions are understaffed and compete for scarce financial and human resources.

Contracts between the MOHCW and local authorities

The Ministry of Health conducted trial runs on contracting the delivery of health services to Rural District Councils. Contracts were entered into between some Provincial Medical Directors and Rural District Councils, requiring RDCs to provide the core health service package to communities living in their areas of jurisdiction. The contracts which operated during the 1999-2000 plan period were supervised by the DHMTs and the PMD's office and paid for from the HSF. Lessons learned from this rather limited experience are likely to inform the contracting process when the decentralization agenda is revived in the future.

Collaboration with faith based health institutions (ZACH)

The MOHCW and religious missions have had an informal collaborative arrangement in the provision of health services in rural areas dating back to 1969. The interests of faith based organizations, also called missions, are represented by their umbrella organization, the Zimbabwe Association of Church Related Hospitals (ZACH). Mission facilities were historically located in very remote rural areas where the colonial government did not provide adequate health facilities to the local population. When the government of Zimbabwe embarked on its infrastructure development program in the rural areas it took cognizance of the existence of these mission facilities as an integral part of the national health delivery system.

Because there was no regulatory framework governing the establishment of these institutions, the result has been a diversity of structures of differing types which are difficult to classify within the district based health system. Some of the mission institutions have over the years been upgraded to district type facilities, resulting in 13 of them being designated by the MOHCW as district hospitals. In addition to providing health care services mission institutions train nurses on behalf of government. To facilitate this process, the MOHCW has over the years allocated faith based hospitals nurse-training posts and paid the allowances and salaries for the trainees and their tutors.

The treasury allocates health grants to missions, Rural District Councils and urban local authorities through the MOHCW. Over the years these grants have constituted about 7% of MOHCW expenditures. The following criteria have been applied over the years in the allocation of grants to mission facilities:

+ 100% salary grant for approved staff.
+ 80% for other recurrent expenditures.

♦ 100% grant for drugs purchased from the National Pharmaceutical Company (Natpharm).
♦ 100% grant for approved capital development projects.
♦ 100% support for approved nurse training posts.

However, despite being considered an integral part of the health delivery system mission facilities have over the years suffered from serious under funding especially considering that they are the major source of health care in rural areas. It is estimated that mission hospitals have half the required staff establishment and receive two to five times less recurrent budget support from government compared to what government institutions of a similar size receive. One of the problems cited by the MOHCW has been that these institutions do not disclose the amount of resources they receive from other sources, especially in the form of overseas donations. Without this information it is difficult for the Ministry of Health to accurately estimate the exact requirements of these institutions without prejudicing allocations to district hospitals that are wholly financed by the government.

A point of contention has been the fact that mission institutions charged user fees for the services they provide despite a government policy to the contrary. Because they receive a government grant faith based institutions are bound by the policy not to charge user fees for primary health care. Information from the National Health Inquiry of 1946 indicates that mission facilities have been at loggerheads with the government on user fees since that time. The Inquiry proposed an increase in grant support to those missions who agreed to abolish charging fees to "Africans". More than 60 years later the same problem is yet to be resolved as mission facilities continue to defy similar government policy directives not to charge "user-fees".

A proposed way forward to resolve this issue is for the government and missions to enter into a contractual relationship based on the delivery of the core health service package at a well defined cost. This would ensure that missions are paid the economic cost of the services that they actually provide as opposed to grant support whose calculation is not based on objective parameters.

Subcontracting non-core services

The implementation of government civil service reforms saw the MOHCW commercializing some of its institutions and entering into contracts with different private companies to provide selected non-core services. Services so far subcontracted include hospital laundry, hospital cleaning, hospital security, grounds maintenance and the provision of staff meals. The cleaning of specialized departments such as theaters and intensive care units have proved to be a challenge as they require professional expertise and very close supervision. It has also been impossible to get a sufficient pool of private providers to compete to provide these services in rural areas where most district hospitals are located. As a result subcontracting has generally been limited to facilities in urban areas where there is sufficient competition amongst potential providers.

Available evidence has indicated varying degrees of satisfaction with the performance of the contracts entered into by the different hospitals. There have been concerns about the quality of services provided by some contracted firms who demonstrated a lack of preparedness to take on these tasks. It has also been evident that the MOHCW did not have the capacity to monitor the implementation of these contracts, both at the central and operational levels of the system.

In some cases the contractors are not paid their contract sums at the agreed times partly due to inadequate budgetary allocations for this item as well as poor management capacity within the ministry. This has often led to the contracted services being provided on an ad hoc basis. In other cases the contracted parties do not have the necessary equipment nor adequately trained manpower to provide the services. Some contractors expected the hospitals to provide them with the detergents and cleaning materials for them to use in carrying out their work. This rather confused state of affairs invariably resulted in poor or no services being provided to the institutions, at least at the initial stages of the contracting process.

Where the MOHCW was not satisfied with the performance of the contractor it was very difficult to take any corrective action or terminate the poorly performing contracts. The Ministry of the Public Service, Labor and Social Welfare, which was responsible for overseeing this process, often interfered on the basis that all the ministries were bound by the government policy of affirmative action which required retrenched civil servants to be given preference and guarantees in the awarding of such contracts. The government did not wish to see companies formed by retrenched civil servants having their contracts terminated, even if they were not performing satisfactorily. Such double standards made it impossible for the ministries to benefit from the potential efficiencies often attributed to the operations of the private sector.

The Patients' Charter

According to the Medical Services Act both public and private providers are required to develop institutional Patients' Charters. It has become a norm that most hospitals display copies of their Patients' Charter for the public to view. These "charters" specify, amongst other things, the following rights of patients:

- That every individual has the right of access to competent health care and treatment without discrimination.
- That the patient has a right to be treated with dignity.
- That every patient shall have the right to have details of their condition, treatment, including such records relating to patient care to be treated as confidential unless:
  - Authorized in writing by the patient that confidentiality should be broken.
  - It is desirable on medical grounds to seek a patient's consent but it is in the patient's own interest that confidentiality should be broken.
  - Information is required by due legal process.
- That the patient's consent must be obtained for inclusion in any research or teaching program.

The Patients' Charter is expected to be complemented by a complaint's procedure which requires that:

- Hospital authorities attend to every complaint within a reasonable and specified period of time.
- The complainant is made aware of his or her rights to complain to the Health Professions Authority and the Secretary for Health and Child Welfare.

In Zimbabwe the Patients' Charter forms part of the quality assurance and public relations agenda of the MOHCW.

Conclusions and the way forward

Devolution comes with a need for the MOHCW to develop a capacity to monitor the performance of RDCs so as to ensure that they effectively fulfill their new roles and responsibilities in delivering quality health services. Furthermore, the MOHCW has to ensure that institutions that train health workers and professional practice are well monitored and regulated. This responsibility is much more crucial in an environment in which the private medical sector is growing rapidly.

Semi-autonomous hospitals must operate on the basis of business plans which clearly state the services they intend to provide, the actual cost of the services, the institutions' comparative advantages and fulfillment of prescribed social obligations.

Staffing levels at semi-autonomous and other health facilities are expected to be determined based on workload analyses than on traditional methods that determine fixed establishments. The Health Service Board is not expected to interfere with the responsibilities conferred on Hospital Management Boards to determine the remuneration of the CEO and senior hospital managers. It may however be necessary to amend the Medical Services Act in order to empower Hospital Management Boards to have some autonomy in setting the conditions of service for all staff employed at their institutions, hiring, disciplining and firing staff. The role of the Health Service Board should be that of providing general guidelines on human resource issues within the sector as a whole. According to the laws of the country, the arbitration process for health workers is based on the prevailing labor laws that govern all workers in Zimbabwe, irrespective of industry or profession.

Provincial hospitals are unlikely to be able to sustain their operations from user fees, in the near future. The MOHCW will thus have an obligation to provide "block grants" for the operation of these institutions, probably on a contractual basis. It is highly likely that resources required to support the operations of semi-autonomous hospitals will be a permanent feature of the ministry's budget allocation. What is needed is the strengthening of mechanisms for accountability for these resources. User fees are however expected to contribute some revenue through voluntary private insurance schemes and any compulsory health insurance scheme that may be established in the future. These hospitals need to strengthen their billing and accounting systems so as to prevent corruption and leakage of revenue from the system. Decisions on the need to review the level of user fees and exemption mechanisms must be handled promptly to avoid unnecessary delays which may compromise the predictability and steady flow of revenue to these institutions.

It is crucial that the establishment of semi-autonomous institutions does not interfere with the efficient function of the country's referral system. Referrals from the district and provincial hospitals must have continued and guaranteed access to specialist services at central hospitals, irrespective of the patient's socioeconomic status and other characteristics. The MOHCW must seriously consider allocating financial resources to district, probably provincial hospitals as well, for the specific purpose of paying for the referral of those patients who are eligible for "free" health services. Whatever arrangements are agreed to, they must ensure that every patient who requires specialist referral services is able to access them.

Whilst competition for patients amongst these institutions may be desirable, at least initially, it may not be the best way to conduct business. Geographical location rather than market forces currently determines the patronage of both provincial and central hospitals. An element of deliberate zoning currently plays a significant role in determining where referrals to each of the central hospitals come from. Central hospitals located in the same geographical area will, in the future, need to rationalize the services they provide so as to concentrate on those services in which they have a comparative advantage. It is necessary to avoid duplication in services delivery, especially in an environment of scarce financial and human resources. The range of services provided by individual central hospitals need to be clearly defined and publicized so that patients know exactly where to go for what services. Apart from making it easier for patients the definition of services will also make it easier for the hospitals to accurately cost their business plans. Due to the shortage of specialists it will probably take some time for most provincial hospitals to provide meaningful specialist services.

Experience from elsewhere shows that even after commercialization establishments continue to experience bureaucratic interference from parent ministries and politicians. Clauses that impose social obligations on these quasi government institutions usually deprive them of the freedom to conduct their business on a commercial basis. Price and other controls imposed, for example, on drug procurement companies by parent ministries tend to exacerbate their viability problems. In this case it will be imperative for the minister of health to act with utmost restraint in exercising his or her powers over Natpharm's policy on drug prices and the fee structure of semi-autonomous hospitals.

Hospital reforms aim to improve the quality of clinical services through improvements in management practices, efficient resource allocation and effective utilization. With the establishment of semi-autonomous hospitals, some improvements have been realized in areas of resource mobilization through the retention of revenue from user fees, improved accountability and human resources management. In the majority of these cases the gains have not been sustained for long periods. Admissions and financing policies are often skewed towards raising revenue and in the process making it difficult for the poor to access specialist services. The future lies in putting in place strategies that will not undermine equity or lead to the deterioration of public health services and throw the baby with the bath water.

Review questions

1. Some of the objectives for establishing semi-autonomous hospitals include the need to achieve management efficiency, improved quality of care and public accountability. Describe how such an initiative can achieve these objectives.

2. A combination of subcontracting, service agreements and the implementation of a core health service package has the potential to either improve or adversely affect equity. Discuss the logic and implications of this statement.

3. One of the major concerns in the establishment of semi-autonomous institutions is their financial viability. Suggest how best this can be achieved in an African country of your choice.

4. Briefly describe the issues that need special attention in the regulation of:
   + General practitioners.
   + Private hospitals.
   + Public hospitals.

10

COMMISSION OF REVIEW INTO THE HEALTH SECTOR IN ZIMBABWE

Introduction

The Chief Secretary to the President and Cabinet proposed that a Commission of Inquiry into the health sector in Zimbabwe be constituted. In the MOHCW's view there was no need for a commission of inquiry but a Review Commission on the health sector. The agreed objectives of the review were the examination of the operations of the health sector in Zimbabwe, its organization, staffing, staff remuneration and the constraints the sector faced in discharging its mandate.

In 1946 a National Health Services Inquiry had proposed, amongst other things, the establishment of a national health service based on the creation of 4 Regional Health Authorities to be headed by Regional Medical Officers of Health. In the scheme of things Regional Health Authorities would be responsible for all state curative and preventive health services.

The Inquiry had further recommended the establishment of a voluntary user fee scheme in which those patients who were not willing to accept the services of salaried hospital consultant staff would be required to pay the full economic rates at the hospital, in addition to their private doctor's fee. This decision was aimed at preventing the government from inadvertently subsidizing private doctors.

This was the first time the government had allowed Government Medical Officers at district level to undertake private practice. However, the fees paid by the patients did not accrue to the doctor but were credited to a hospital fund. The medical officer was paid an allowance in lieu of private practice. Private practitioners were not allowed to use the hospital outpatient departments as consultation rooms for their private patients, except in cases of emergencies.

Faith based institutions or mission institutions would continue to receive grants from the government provided they stopped charging fees to rural "African" populations and agreed to inspections by the government. The commission also recommended the following rates of Government grants to mission institutions:

+ Subject to approval of building plans, 50% of the cost of new buildings.
+ 50% of the cost of approved equipment.
+ 75% of the cost of approved drugs.
+ Two-thirds of the mission doctors' salaries,
+ Two-thirds of the salaries of nurses, nursing orderlies corresponding to grades in government employment.
+ Two-thirds of the cost of maintaining hospital beds.
+ 50% of the cost of maintaining midwives, nurses, orderlies and nurse assistants in training.

Proposals were made for mine hospitals to be paid similar grants to provide health services to patients from surrounding areas free at the point of delivery, the cost being borne by the government.

State of the public health sector at the time of the Review Commission on Health

For a decade post independence the Zimbabwe health delivery system made impressive and consistent progress in the areas of health, population and nutrition. Between 1980 and 1988 government expenditures on health rose by 48% in real per capita terms and from 2.2% of GDP to 3.1% by 1990/91. During this period Zimbabwe pioneered many of the cost-effective primary and community based health interventions considered to be examples of best practice.

During the same period the government achieved health care coverage whereby 85% of the population lived within 8 kilometers of a health facility. There was also considerable increase in the supply of drugs to these facilities. Life expectancy at birth increased from 56 years in 1980 to 61 in 1990, the Infant Mortality Rate (IMR) declined from nearly 100 deaths per 1000 live births to about 50, weight for age malnutrition in children less than three years of age fell from 22% to 16% and universal childhood immunization was achieved in 1990 from a baseline coverage of 25% at independence. At that time the average Infant Mortality Rate for the Sub-Saharan Region was estimated to be 93 per 1000 live births. In Zimbabwe the mortality rate in children under the age of five years was reduced to 77 per 1000 live births compared to a regional rate of 170 per 1000 live births. The goal for eliminating neonatal tetanus, that is less than 1 case per 1000 live births per district, had been achieved at the time the Review Commission conducted its work.

Whilst the major policy thrust at independence had been to correct the imbalances inherited from the pre-independence era the health status of the rural population has remained worse than that of their urban counterparts. Rural children are twice as likely to suffer from Acute Respiratory Infections (ARI), to be malnourished, stunted, etc. The worst health indicators are found in resettlement and farm households located in large scale commercial farms. For example 38% of births in rural areas occur at home compared to only 9% in urban areas.

The HIV/AIDS epidemic has since 1988 become a crisis of major proportions in Zimbabwe. In 1989 more than 30% of women attending antenatal clinics (ANC) in Harare were found to be HIV positive compared to 22% in the rural areas. Since then the situation has deteriorated further to more than 35% of women attending ANC being HIV positive (2000). AIDS has become the single leading cause of death in children between the age of one and four years and in adults between 15 and 49 years of age. The impact of HIV/AIDS on TB is such that annually reported tuberculosis cases rose from 13 000 in 1989 to more than 53 000 in 2000. Child health indicators have since the epidemic deteriorated. The Zimbabwe Demographic Health Survey (DHS, 1999) indicated that the Infant Mortality Rate had increased from 53 in 1994 to 65 per 1000 live births in 1999 and child mortality from 75 per 1000 live births in 1988 to 102 per 1000 live births in 1999.

Health Sector Reforms

At the time the Review Commission on Health commenced its work the MOHCW was in the midst of implementing its health reforms. The health reform process combined elements of redesigning the ministry's organizational structure, redefining roles and relationships, the development of innovative ways to mobilize additional resources and improvement of managerial processes within the health sector. The reforms resulted in a shift in the role of the central ministry of health from that of direct service provision to policy formulation, monitoring, coordination and regulation of the health sector.

A Strategic Development Unit was established and given the responsibility for coordinating planning, policy analysis, review and formulation within the ministry as part of strengthening its planning capacity. The unit was also responsible for monitoring progress in the implementation of the ministry's plans and the reform agenda and the development and implementation of a capacity building program meant to prepare health workers for their role in a decentralized health system. At the time the MOHCW had completed its National Health Strategy (1997-2007) as a framework to guide the health sector beyond the year 2000.

Financing the health sector

Records indicate that between 1990/91 and 1995/96 financial years public sector spending on health as a proportion of total government spending declined by more than 30%, from 6.4 % in 1990/91 to 4.3% in 1995/96. Expenditures on health declined from 3.1% of GDP to 2.1% of GDP over the same period, (World Bank, 1996). The 1995/96 budget allocation for health represented a 40% decline in real per capita spending from its peak in 1990/91. This level of public spending on health was the lowest since the country attained its independence in 1980, (World Bank, 1996).

The share of public resources spent on preventive care declined from 39% in 1992/93 to 36% of total Ministry of Health and Child Welfare outlays in 2000. Public spending on Primary Health Care (PHC) was US$6 per person as opposed to US$9 per person considered to be necessary to provide a basic package of health care in Zimbabwe. This shortage of financial resources resulted in drug shortages throughout the public health system. The public were increasingly concerned about the deteriorating quality of services at a time the government had reviewed hospital fees upwards. Central hospitals were no longer able to function as referral hospitals because an increasing number of patients by-passed lower level facilities which were experiencing chronic shortages of drugs and other essential supplies. There was thus an increasing lack of confidence in the public health system by both the consumers of services and health workers.

Grants from central government to local authorities continued to decline, resulting in local authorities resorting to levying user fees in defiance of the prevailing government policy. Overseas donations to faith based hospitals, even combined with the meager grant from government, were no longer adequate to support the operations of these institutions which resorted to charging user fees, also in defiance of government policy.

In order to adopt more rational and objective means of preparing its budget, in 1995 the MOHCW developed a package of core health services. The annual cost of delivering this package of services was estimated to be US$22 per capita. This per capita expenditure formed the basis upon which the MOHCW arrived at its annual estimates of expenditure.

In a milestone decision in 1997 the government of Zimbabwe approved that revenue from user fees collected at health facilities be retained and used locally. This move meant that the revenue would supplement the government budget allocation to MOHCW institutions for purposes of improving the quality of services. It was further emphasized that this revenue was in addition to and not a substitute of the amount the government allocated to the health sector. A Health Services Fund was thus established through an Act of Parliament to facilitate financial management and accountability for these resources. In order to improve their rate of debt recovery, health institutions were authorized to engage private debt collectors.

Human resources

The implementation of the Economic Structural Adjustment Program (ESAP) resulted in a public sector freeze on employment and establishment of new posts in government. This move affected the Ministry of Health and Child Welfare which, at some point, was not able to employ all the nurses that it trained. This situation resulted in nurses either roaming the streets unemployed, some seeking employment in neighboring countries and others changing careers to work in other sectors of the economy. Despite the fact that the ministry did not have enough Environmental Health Technicians (EHT), about 100 of these professionally trained health workers remained unemployed. This was indeed ESAP without a human face!

Table 10.1 Annual government expenditures on health between 1980/81 and1995/96

Year	Total real health expenditure		Total real health expenditure per capita	Health expenditures as % of GDP.	Health expenditures as % of total govt. exp.
	Z$ (millions)	US$ (Millions)			
1980/81	256, 24	376.0	35.62	2.0	5.3
1981/82	306,60	344.5	41.44	2.2	5.6
1982/83	300,10	312.6	39.44	2.1	4.8
1983/84	289,61	301.7	36.74	2.2	4.8
1984/85	291,97	304.1	35.92	2.3	4.9
1985/86	331,00	344.8	39.48	2.5	5.3
1986/87	355,64	114.7	41.14	2.8	5.1
1987/88	384.10	120.8	43.08	2.8	5.5
1988/89	412.18	129.6	44.82	2.6	5.4
1989/90	478.88	150.6	50.50	2.8	5.9
1990/91	564.49	100.8	57.72	3.0	6.2
1991/92	511.97	75.1	50.76	2.5	5.1
1992/93	458.18	67.2	44.00	2.4	5.3
1993/94	412.88	60.5	38.45	2.2	5.1
1994/95	424.33	51.4	38.31	2.2	4.5
1995/96	409.71	44.9	35.86	2.2	4.2

Based on information from the Government of Zimbabwe (various years) and Report of the Comptroller and Auditor General, Harare

The period during which Zimbabwe was implementing the ESAP saw the salaries of civil servants being eroded by as much as 40%. This resulted in a marked increase in the attrition rate of health professionals to the local private sector, neighboring and overseas countries. It is estimated that the public health sector in Zimbabwe lost close to 450 medical doctors to the Republic of South Africa alone. At one time more than 70% of doctors working in rural areas were expatriates as the few local doctors remaining shunned working in rural areas. They preferred working in urban areas where they could easily supplement their salaries by moonlighting in the private sector.

Poor conditions of service for civil servants, the absence of credible collective bargaining mechanisms and the slow decision making processes in the Public Service Commission led to increasingly agitated demands for improved conditions of services, salaries and allowances by different categories of professional civil servants such as nurses, doctors, teachers and legal practitioners. Between 1991 and 2004 Zimbabwe experienced more than 14 episodes of industrial action by health professionals.

It became evident that over the years the Ministry of Health had not invested adequately to develop its capacity to set policies, establish national priorities, develop strategic plans, and monitor performance and the capacity to enforce policies. The ability of the MOHCW to carry out these functions largely depended on the good will and commitment of the few health workers who remained in the MOHCW. Experienced professionals required to organize and manage the strategic functions of the sector left the country for "greener pastures". The shelf-life of a Permanent Secretary in the Ministry of Health and Child Welfare was the shortest in the whole of Government, resulting in poor leadership and a lack of institutional memory.

In its fragmented approach to human resources development the government approved a policy that allowed civil servants to undertake private practice related to their professions. This privilege included private practice by health professionals. However poor management of the policy resulted in some medical doctors neglecting their government duties and spending more time at their private surgeries.

In an attempt to manage the situation the MOHCW published job descriptions for medical doctors employed in the public sector. The guidelines were meant to assist hospital managers, especially Medical Superintendents, to monitor the work of health professionals at their institutions. The guidelines required consultants and specialists to develop job plans. Unfortunately there was a lack of commitment from both the consultants and the Medical Superintendents to adhere to and monitor these job plans, respectively. In some cases the Medical Superintendents were found wanting as they abused the privileges of private practice.

Amongst other incentives, the government made a decision to provide onsite accommodation for junior doctors. Where it was not possible to provide accommodation, the government reimbursed the junior doctors a reasonable proportion of the rent they paid. Junior doctors were also afforded a car loan purchase scheme payable over 7 years and guaranteed by the government. It was agreed that all on-call and other allowances for health workers would be reviewed regularly in line with salary adjustments and inflationary pressures.

The policy of the Ministry of Health and Child Welfare was always to deploy junior doctors to rural areas when they completed their second year of internship. The doctors serve rural communities for at least a year before they are considered eligible for post graduate training.

The other policy decision made by government was to decentralize general nurse training to provincial and general hospitals. This decision was made in 1997 when the Ministry of Health and the Health Professions Council approved the training of Registered General Nurses at these institutions throughout the country. This move increased the total annual output of nurses from government and mission training institutions in Zimbabwe from about 400 to at least 1 200 by the end of the year 2000.

The Review Commission on Health

In the eyes of the MOHCW the Review Commission on Health merely confirmed and led credence to the problems that every stakeholder in the health sector had echoed over the previous 10 years or so. According to the MOHCW it was a simple matter in which; government expenditures on health had been declining, a poor macroeconomic environment and poor conditions of service for staff which had resulted in an increase in the attrition of health professionals and a shortage of essential supplies that had led to the deterioration in the quality of services delivered at public health institutions. It was the Ministry of Health's position that the whole of government needed to commit itself to increasing health sector financing and improving the conditions of service for health staff. In the health sector there was no substitute for well motivated and well trained health workers in achieving the objectives of improving the health of the nation. The renowned achievements of the country's health system had been the result of the high levels of staff commitment, despite working under very poor conditions. Health professionals were of the view that the government did not appreciate the sacrifice and commitment they continued to make on behalf of the nation.

Terms of Reference of the Commission

The Commission of Review into the health sector looked into the following issues:

- ◆ The role of Government in the provision of health services.
- ◆ The provision of an organized, cost-effective and efficient health care delivery system that is both affordable and accessible to the

most vulnerable in society and yet addressing the nation's health priorities within the context of the government policy of planning for equity in health.

♦ An appropriate organizational framework and managerial processes for the public health delivery system with particular attention to administrative, financial and legislative provisions necessary to provide such a health delivery system.

The review was to address more specifically the following issues:

♦ Organizational capacity and accountability.

♦ Organizational structure, responsibilities and roles within the public health delivery system with particular reference to the policy of decentralization.

♦ Elimination of structural barriers to achievement, in terms of delegated powers from the center to the district, the formal relationship between the technical, administrative and political actors in the system and the budget structure.

♦ The relations between the Ministry of Health and Child Welfare, missions, local authorities and the private medical sector, including the financing arrangements.

♦ Health, disease problems and priorities:
  ♦ The major health and disease problems of the nation, priorities needing special attention and action and how these could be addressed.

♦ Service quality:
  ♦ The quality of health infrastructure and its maintenance, availability of essential drugs at public health facilities and the protection of preventive and promotive services through primary health care.
  ♦ The role of the Health Professions Council (Authority) of Zimbabwe in setting professional standards and maintaining discipline amongst the professionals.

♦ Financing the health sector:
  ♦ In the light of a drastic decrease in public health expenditures by government, the mobilization of adequate resources to deal with priority health problems of the nation.
  ♦ Government policy on cost recovery, safety nets for the poor, flexibility in the non-salary budget, financial management and accountability.
  ♦ Planning and resource allocation systems, decentralization and the capacity of local authorities.

- Human resources management systems:
  - Addressing shortages and high attrition, poor attitudes and low morale among professional staff, achieving quality and productivity gains. Strategies for the retention of professional staff.
  - Private practice by health workers employed by the state.
  - Salaries, recruitment and conditions of service for health workers in light of the recommendations that may be made on the privilege to do private practice.
- Managerial and control posts:
  - Secretary for Health as the Chief Medical Officer and Chief Health Officer.
  - The Principal Medical Director.
  - Provincial Medical Directors and Medical Superintendents.
  - Conditions of appointment for consultant staff and specialists.
  - Doctors deployed in rural areas, the special role of the District Medical Officer.
  - Nursing staff.
  - Local decision making in relation to personnel management in a decentralized health delivery system.
  - The role of the Public Service Commission in the recruitment, appointment, promotion and determination of conditions of service for the public health system.
- Any other matters as the Commission may deem necessary to pursue in the spirit of addressing and uplifting health services in Zimbabwe.

Composition of the Commission

The Commission consisted of the following members appointed and sworn in by the state President, see table 10.2.

Table 10.2 Membership of the Review Commission on Health

Member's name	Organization
Chairman	
Dr. E. Tarimo	Former Director of the Division of Analysis, Research and Assessment; WHO, Geneva.
Members	
Dr. F.B. Chikara	Consultant Psychiatrist, UZ/MOHCW.
Dr. C.P.E Kostermans	Senior Public Health Specialist, World Bank.
Prof. L.F. Levy	Neurosurgery Department, University of Zimbabwe
Mrs. C.S. Nondo	State Registered Nurse, Chairperson and Lecturer, Department of Adult Education, University of Zimbabwe and President of the Zimbabwe Nurses Association,
Rev. Dr. C.C.G Mazobere	Minister of Religion.
Prof. G.I Muguti	Associate Professor of Surgery, University of Zimbabwe.
Dr. B.B. Nyathi	Public Health Specialist, former Director of Health Services, City of Bulawayo.
Mr. R.D. Nyenya	Executive Secretary, Zimbabwe Association of Church Related Hospitals (ZACH).
Mrs. M.P. Torongo	Pharmacist in the Private Sector.

Summary of the report of the Review Commission on Health

The Report of the Review Commission on Health was presented to government and approved by Cabinet in 1999. The MOHCW held the sarcastic view that the substance of the recommendations of the Commission consisted in the main of issues already on its implementation agenda. However, despite Ministry of Health's rather unenthusiastic view of the report, it must be appreciated that when problems are presented by a high profile body like the Presidential Commission they tend to be more visible and attract renewed interest. One major weakness of the report was the absence of cost estimates for implementing the recommendations. Details of the Commission's recommendations can be found in the commission's main report.

The Commission's recommendations are categorized into four (4) main areas:

- Delivery of health services:
  - The need to intensify the fight against HIV/AIDS, TB and Malaria.
  - Declaring HIV/AIDS a national disaster.
  - Giving particular attention to improving the quality of MCH services.
  - The re-introduction of the Village Health Worker Program.
- Human Resources:
  - Improved personnel information systems.
  - Putting in place a Human Resources Development Plan.
  - The establishment of a second Medical School in Bulawayo.
  - The implementation of a realistic package of conditions of service to retain health staff.
- Organizational issues:
  - The formation of a Health Service Commission to carry out, amongst other functions, those of the PSC.
  - The establishment of Hospital Management Boards.
  - The gradual decentralization of district health services to RDCs.
  - The review of the role of the provincial office and ministry of health headquarters.
- Health Financing:
  - To increase the per capita allocation or expenditure on health to at least US$23.6.
  - The establishment of a Social Health Insurance Scheme.

Implementation of the recommendations of the Review Commission on Health

The following tables present a synopsis of progress made by the end of 2008 in the implementation of the more strategic recommendations of the Review Commission on Health.

Table 10.3   Recommendations on public sector health services

Public Sector Health Services	
Recommendations	**Progress**
Re-introduction of the Village Health Workers.	The VHW Program was re-established in the MOHCW in 2000.
Establishment of the National AIDS Council.	The National AIDS Council (NAC) was established in 1999 and the board constituted in same year.
Sustainable strategies to mobilize resources for HIV/AIDS pursued.	In 1999 the government introduced an AIDS levy and established an AIDS TRUST FUND financed through an ear marked tax regime. Zimbabwe's first application to the Global Fund on HIV/AIDS was approved in 2002.
Declaring AIDS a national disaster.	Zimbabwe declared HIV/AIDS a national disaster in 2002.
Comparative costs of universal use of anti retroviral treatment against medical, economic and social costs to be worked out.	The socio-economic and demographic impact of HIV/AIDS in Zimbabwe undertaken in July 1998. Nevirapine introduced in the prevention of mother-to-child-transmission (PMTCT) of HIV. Zimbabwe introduced ARV therapy in public health facilities in 2004. A local pharmaceutical company started manufacturing ARVs in Zimbabwe in 2004.

Table 10.4   Recommendations on clinical services and the private health
sector

Clinical Services	
Recommendations	**Progress**
The grant for recurrent expenditures and staffing levels for Mission Hospitals should be at the same level as for comparable government institutions.	Not achieved (2009). Policy of MOHCW since 1993 was that mission facilities should be financed at the same level as government institutions. However the allocation from treasury continued to be inadequate to meet these requirements.
There should be formal contracts between the MOHCW and missions clearly defining the relationship between the two parties.	Not achieved (2009) Under the reform program the MOHCW proposes entering into contractual relationships with RDCs and missions to provide the core health service package.
District hospitals to be built in Harare and Bulawayo to reduce congestion at central hospitals.	Not achieved - 2009 Proposals on the PSIP since 1995.
The establishment of a provincial hospital in Matabeleland North Province.	Included in PSIP budget since 2003, not achieved by 2009.
All central hospitals should have management boards.	Achieved by 2003 as provided for in the Medical Services Act, Statutory Instrument 208 of 2001.
There should be a clear equipment policy in the MOHCW covering essential elements such as procurement, maintenance, upgrading, replacement and inventory and disposal.	No meaningful progress recorded
Improved procurement, supply and distribution of drugs.	The Government Medical Stores (GMS) commercialized into a Section 26 company, "NatPharm" managed by a Board of Directors.
All drugs and raw materials for the manufacture of drugs in the EDLIZ to be exempted from customs duty.	Achieved.
Nurses in private homes should only prescribe and dispense drugs that they are legally allowed to do so.	Not achieved – 2009.
The Private Health Sector	
That a public-private sector Committee be established to draw up mechanisms for coordination of these sectors.	Not achieved- 2009.
Traditional Medicine: the monitoring of Traditional Medicine practice to be strengthened through ZINATHA and other related organizations.	Achieved. The Traditional Health Practitioner's Act reviewed to include other organizations of Traditional healers in addition to ZINATHA. MOHCW established a unit responsible for coordinating Traditional medicine - 2008
That alternative medical practitioners set up institutions and facilities, separate from those of existing conventional practice.	The Health Professions Authority Act and the Traditional Health Practitioners' Act provide for this separation.

Table 10.5 Recommendations on human resources

Human Resources	
Recommendations	**Progress**
The ratio of nurse aides to nurses to be increased to 3:1 and the introduction of a new grade of health worker who is multi skilled.	2002 - The Primary Care Nurse introduced. Output of Primary Care Nurses pegged at 600 per year.
The MOHCW should increase the intake Registered General Nurses (RGN).	Achieved – 1999. 2001 - National annual training output of nurses increased from 400 to 1 200 per year. Provincial and general hospitals now train RGNs.
To increase the supply of doctors by having effective recruitment policies and enhancing the capacity of the present medical school and establishing a second medical school in Bulawayo.	Intake of the Harare Medical School increased over the years from 80 to about 120 per year. A second medical school established at the National University of Science and Technology, NUST.
All health workers forming a core group should be employed on a performance contract.	Draft contracts developed for employment of junior doctors approved by the PSC in July 2001 & Junior doctors employed on contract. 2001 - Student nurses engaged on a contract basis. 2001 - Chief Executive Officer for Parirenyatwa Central Hospital, Clinical Director, Director of Operations and the Director of Finance employed on contract.
Full time employees of the MOHCW to undertake private practice only with the permission of the Hospital Management Board (HMB) and to undertake this privilege only outside official working hours.	2009 - No new policy development
A well-laid out policy to be developed for injury or infection on duty.	Infection control policy operational in MOHCW. Guidelines on Post Exposure Prophylaxis (PEP) for HIV/Hepatitis in place.

Table 10.6 Recommendations on organizational capacity

Organizational capacity and accountability	
Recommendations	**Progress**
A Health Service Commission to be established.	2004 - Health Service Board constituted.
The Commission recommends a gradual process of decentralization to districts beginning with deconcentration to the District Health Executive.	Government adopted 13 Principles to guide the decentralization process. The decentralization of health service delivery stalled in 2001.
To revive the Community Health Movement by strengthening the role of VHWs and involving communities in planning and management of health activities.	2000 - Village Health Worker Program re-established in the MOHCW.
A reasonable portion of the Health Services Fund (HSF) should support the community health movement.	The MOHCW proposed that 40% of the HSF be allocated to the RHC and community levels.
The government needs to regulate the growth of the private health sector.	The Medical Services Act, Statutory Instrument 208 of 2001 enacted for this purpose.
The MOHCW to establish a national program on Quality Assurance as soon as possible.	2000 – unit responsible for QA established in the MOHCW
The Medical, Dental and Allied Professions Act 1971 should be reviewed to provide legal recognition to medical interventions carried out by Clinical Officers and other health workers.	The Health Professions Act enacted to establish the Health Professions Authority of Zimbabwe. 2009 - role of the Clinical Officer yet to be reviewed.
The fixing of medical fees should involve the MOHCW and all partners.	The Medical Services Act provides for an all inclusive tariff committee and an arbitration process in case of tariff disputes between GPs and third party payers in health.
The MOHCW and Medical Research Council of Zimbabwe should develop an overall Health Research Strategy.	An Essential National Health Research agenda was developed, the MOHCW allocates a budget for research – to the National Health Research Institute and within the MOHCW to the Provincial Medical Directors. In 2002 US$600 000 was allocated for research activities as part of the MOHCW budget.
That a task force be formed to rethink the fundamental structure of the MOHCW as outlined in figure 4.1 of the main Report of the Commission.	No task force formed. Reorganization of MOHCW structure approved by PSC in 2001 and another by the Health Service Board in 2008

Table 10.7 Recommendations on health financing

Health Financing	
Recommendations	**Progress**
That in the short term the government increases its contribution to the health sector to at least the level of the per capita expenditure US$23.6.	Since 2000 the annual per capita expenditures on health have declined to less than US$ 13. Zimbabwe is in the category of countries that require spending at least US$ 34 to US$ 40 per capita per year on health services
Consideration is made to introduce earmarked taxes, tax exemptions.	In 1999 the government introduced the AIDS Levy to support HIV/AIDS prevention and control efforts. Essential drugs and their raw materials enjoy tax and duty exemptions.
That the Social Health Insurance (SHI) be considered.	Not achieved -2009 Feasibility study on SHI was conducted in 1997. 2006 - SHI legislation enacted
That the government demonstrates more interest in and encourages good management and efficiency in Medical Aid Societies.	The Medical Services Act of 2001 regulates the establishment and conduct of (Medical Aid Societies) Health Funders of Zimbabwe 2002 - All health insurance schemes to be registered and regulated by the MOHCW.
That user fees be instituted for hospitals, RHCs and Clinics. No fees are levied for children under the age of five years, preventive programs such as MCH and the treatment of some infectious diseases.	According to the MOHCW fee policy no fees are levied at RHCs and Clinics, no fees are levied for the treatment of children under the age of 5 years, MCH services and some infectious disease conditions. In January 2009 the government introduced an option for public health institutions to levy user fees in foreign currency (US$ and South African Rand) for those patients who are willing and able to pay in foreign currency. Private practitioners started charging consultation fees in foreign currency in 2008
Empower appropriate committees at village level to grant exemptions, collect and manage funds at RHCs and Clinics.	Elected representatives (councilors) issue exemption letters for patients attending district hospitals where fees are levied. No funds are collected at RHCs and Clinics
The department of Social Welfare and the MOHCW should work out appropriate exemption guidelines and mechanisms to recognize those not able to afford to pay for health services.	The Department of Social Welfare developed guidelines for reimbursement of central hospitals and urban councils for exempting patients from paying. Local councilors also issue exemption letters in rural areas.
Fees should be fully retained at the facility level.	1997 - Act of Parliament established a Health Services Fund (HSF) which facilitated the retention of user fee revenue at health facility level.
The MOHCW should encourage more donor support through the Sector Wide Approach (SWAps) or Budget Support.	2009 - No SWAp implemented in Zimbabwe SWAp expected when donors decide to resume Overseas Development Assistance to Zimbabwe
Government and the MOHCW should improve its financial information system in line with National Health Accounts.	2004 - Integrated Financial Management System (IFMIS) rolled out to MOHCW. 2001 - First round of National Health Accounts completed. 2004 - Second round of NHAs started and still not completed by 2009.

The commission recommends the introduction of a mathematical formula for the allocation of government finances.	1997 - Resource allocation formula within the MOHCW developed in 1997 and continues to be reviewed.
The MOHCW should move gradually with contracting out, assessing and evaluating services that are suitable for contracting out – central and provincial hospitals.	1999 – Contracting out introduced for Laundry. Security. Cleaning and Grounds maintenance.

The unfinished business

The Reform Agenda:

♦ Decentralization of health services
  ♦ A review of existing legislation to provide for the establishment of appropriate RDC structures to facilitate effective management of the delivery of a decentralized health service.
♦ Employment of staff in the MOHCW on performance contracts.
  ♦ Not all institutions employ consultants and specialists on performance contracts.
♦ Other outstanding issues on the recommendations of the Review Commission on Health
  ♦ Establishment of contracts or service agreements with mission hospitals and local authorities.
  ♦ The construction of district hospitals in Harare and Bulawayo.
  ♦ The introduction of a Social Health Insurance Scheme.

Conclusions and the way forward

The establishment of the Review Commission on Health provided an opportunity for the general public, politicians, professional groups, development partners and civil society groups to contribute to the MOHCW's reform process, which had hitherto been likened to a closely guarded secret of the top management within the MOHCW. The Commission was also a demonstration of the government's recognition of the problems faced by the health sector and an opportunity for it to redeem itself in the eyes of the general public.

As a direct result of the Commission's work the government has demonstrated some interest in improving the conditions of service for health workers. It is now incumbent upon the MOHCW and the rest of government to follow through, in a coherent manner, the recommendations of the Commission and to seize this opportunity to improve the management and function of the health system in Zimbabwe. In the same vein the government must, more than ever, commit adequate resources for this to be achieved.

In the final analysis it is reasonable to argue that the work of the Review Commission on Health is yet another endorsement of the MOHCW's reform agenda by the cabinet, the legislature, and the public and civil society groups who participated and contributed to the work of this Commission.

Review questions

1. The report and recommendations of the Review Commission on Health in Zimbabwe reiterated the problems and solutions that the MOHCW had always known and articulated over the years. Comment on the validity of this statement.

2. What powers should the Health Service Commission or Board have if they are to make any difference in the conditions of service of health workers?

3. In your opinion, what is the most significant contribution of the Review Commission on Health to the health sector in Zimbabwe?

11 .

HEALTH REFORMS AND EQUITY

Introduction

Soon after independence the government of Zimbabwe adopted Primary Health Care (PHC) as a strategy to achieve its policy objective, "Planning for Equity in Health". The main objective was to reverse the inequities of the past and achieve distributive justice and an acceptable health status for the country's population.

In the foreword to the document, "Zimbabwe Health for All Action Plan" the Minister of Health states that *"Having been deprived of social justice for so long, our main preoccupation following our struggle for independence was the establishment of social justice in health for the betterment of the life of our previously oppressed people. Our first major task in the health sector was to correct the gross inequities in health service provision, to which the masses had been subjected."* The plan period for the "Health for All Action Plan" ended in 2000 and was succeeded by the National Health Strategy (1997-2007) which was dubbed, "Working for Quality and Equity in Health".

Society is concerned about disadvantaged groups that have poorer survival chances and die younger than more favored groups in society. Such groups not only suffer a heavier burden of illness than others but also experience chronic illness and disability at a younger age. Human rights also advocate for the provision of essential health services to all, of course within the limits of available resources. In virtually all communities there are inequities of one kind or the other. Social privilege is evident in the differences in socio-economic status, geographical location, gender, racial or ethnic differences and age, including other dimensions of time. Such inequities are evident in the differences in morbidity and mortality rates between occupational classes, gender and in different age groups. In the United Kingdom men and women in Class V were observed to have double the probability of dying before retirement age compared to those in

Class I. Several factors were found to be associated with these variations in health; ethnic, geographical, socio-economic and gender (Black et al, 1980).

The divided society in the history of Zimbabwe meant that there was great variation in the distribution of health problems and health services. *"The most marked characteristics were the inequitable geographical distribution of services,"* (MOH-Health for All Action Plan, 1986). At the time the new government took over in 1980 only 20 percent of the rural population had access to adequate water and sanitation. Preventive and promotive services were sacrificed at the expense of the provision of selective and high quality curative services accessed only by a privileged few. This discrimination in access to health services was reflected in the burden of ill health which was concentrated more amongst the poor, who were mainly resident in rural areas.

Aday (1980) defines an "equitable distribution" of health-care services as one in which illness (as defined by the patient and his or her family or by health care professionals) is the major determinant of the allocation of resources. Some have defined equity in health as implying that ideally everyone should have a fair opportunity to attain their full health potential and that no one should be disadvantaged from attaining this potential if it can be avoided. Others see equity as being about creating equal opportunities for health.

The major objective of an equity-based health policy is not to eliminate all differences in health but rather to reduce or eliminate mainly those that are possible to do so because they are avoidable and unfair. It is not possible to achieve a state where everyone has the *"same level of health suffers the same type and degree of illness and dies after exactly the same lifespan"* (Whitehead, 1992).

Equity has moral and ethical dimensions to it and refers to disparities that are unnecessary, avoidable and are considered unfair and unjust. A distinction has been made between equity and inequality, equality being a particular interpretation of equity which is concerned only with equal shares. If justice is to prevail in the distribution of health services there must be an assurance of an equitable pattern of its provision irrespective of cost to the rest of society. In order to describe a situation as being inequitable the root cause must be judged to be unfair in the context of what is going on in the rest of society.

The notion of vertical equity requires that differing needs be provided with equally differing inputs or that "un-equals" are treated unequally.

However, is it just (or fair) for those with greater ability to pay, to pay more in proportional terms? Or should one condition enjoy a higher standard of care just because somebody judges it to be more important (Donaldson, C, 1982)? The corollary to vertical equity is "across the board equity", or horizontal equity which advocates for the equal treatment of equals.

The following are some of the operational definitions of equity that have been used in the literature:

Equal access per capita

This means several things to different people; for example, an equal number of doctors or nurses per capita or equal average distance to a health facility per capita. The weakness in this definition is that it does not take into account the differences in need per capita, for example if there are geographic differences in disease distribution.

Equal access for equal needs

This definition refers to equality in opportunities to use versus actual use. It however does not take into consideration that people may tend to use services differently due to social and cultural factors which determine peoples' perceptions of their state of health and the appropriateness of different providers.

Equal expenditure for equal needs or demand

This means that planners must take into account the factors that influence need and demand for health like population distribution, age and sex distribution, morbidity and mortality patterns, etc. In this case resources refer to revenue allocation per capita and other inputs like hospital beds, doctors and nurses per population. This definition does not take into account that inputs in health can differ among populations not only because of variations in need but also due to differences in the cost of providing the services in different communities. In such cases equal expenditure means unequal services.

Equal health status

This is considered to be a very ambitious definition of equity as it requires that the health status must be the same in all regions and social groups. Such an expectation is extremely unrealistic as the determinants of health go beyond the remit of the health sector.

Equal utilization for equal needs

This definition calls for a system whereby the use of health services is allocated pro-rata with need or demand. It is however possible that some people may choose to exercise their right not to utilize health services due to various reasons which may include religious grounds or ethical reasons.

For the purposes of establishing a working definition focus has been placed on accessibility, quality and acceptability of the care offered to all sections of the population (Whitehead, M., 1992). "Using this approach, equity in health care is defined as:

+ Equal access to available care for equal need.
+ Equal utilization for equal need.
+ Equal quality of care for all."

Equal access *"implies equal entitlement to available services for everyone. A fair distribution of health services throughout the country based on health care needs and ease of access in each geographical area, and the removal of other barriers to access"* (Whitehead, 1992). Factors that contribute to unequal access to health care maybe due to people being turned away at health facilities because they are not able to pay, because of race, sex or religion. Clinics may have inconvenient opening hours and thereby exclude workers that finish work late in the evenings. In some cases long waiting times increase the opportunity costs of using health services. Language may also be a barrier to health care in certain minority groups (Daniels, N, 1982).

People exercising their right not to use health services, for religious reasons, may inhibit the utilization of health services by others; other people give less importance to their health status than others even if they have similar needs. In some cases there is excessive utilization of some services merely because of excessive activity in those particular services, e.g. high caesarian sections amongst certain segments in society. At times there is a need to equalize the use of some services such as immunizations by introducing outreach services to make it easier for populations in remote areas to access these services.

Equality of care is important where certain social groups are afforded preferential treatment opportunities over less favored groups on the basis of race or ethnic origin. Equality in quality of care implies that health workers will aim to put the same commitment into the services they provide to all sections of the community so that everyone gets the highest quality of care.

Equity and the reform process

The impact of health financing options

During the first decade of Zimbabwe's independence central and provincial hospitals accounted for 45 percent of public health resources compared to district and rural health centers. This was despite the fact that, combined, district and health centers dealt with a larger disease burden. In 1981 the proportion of expenditures by the four central hospitals was 60 percent of the total ministry of health budget. This led to the implementation of a policy which over the years reduced this proportion to 35 per cent of total public health expenditures.

When countries implement health reforms they must consider their potential consequences on equity in health. For example, the introduction of market mechanisms raises concerns about the ability of the poor to access primary health care services. The rapid increase in poverty levels in Zimbabwe and the poor macroeconomic environment has raised the specter of the majority of the population having no access to health services. Studies in Zimbabwe and elsewhere have indicated that when the poor are required to pay for health services at the point of delivery, there is a significant decline in total utilization levels. Another study conducted in Zimbabwe demonstrated that after the introduction of user fees there was a 30% decline in the demand for services (Zigora, 1997). The increase in fees also led to a decline of 30% in deliveries taking place at public health institutions compared to the same period the previous year. There was also an increase in the number of babies born before arrival at health facilities as pregnant women delayed their arrival at health facilities in order to reduce the length of hospital stay as a cost saving measure.

Due to inadequate capacity attempts to implement exemption mechanisms in many developing countries have been ineffective in protecting the poor. Difficulties have been experienced in the development of clear criteria for eligibility, though disease and health condition specific exemptions such as free TB treatment and free maternal and child health services seem to have been met with some success.

Ideally Health Insurance Schemes should be able to transfer resources from the healthy to the sick and from the wealthy to the poor. Such schemes are usually more effective in achieving equity goals if they are compulsory, income related and the benefits determined on the basis of need. Where contributions are tax-exempt they effectively translate into public subsidies to members subscribing to health insurance schemes. The contention is however that these subsidies are achieved at the expense of public funds that could have been used to provide better services for the poor through the public health sector. This underscores the need for health reforms to be complemented with appropriate safety nets to cushion the poor and mechanism to monitor their impact on equity as an integral part of the reform process.

Contractual arrangements and government subsidies

The adoption of a policy to contract-out health services has the potential to undermine equity in health. It is possible that services which are less profitable as opposed to less efficient can be phased out or completely neglected as providers are likely to shun or avoid disadvantaged communities if serving them is likely to generate losses. The process of "contracting out" also provides opportunities for the private sector to complement public sector efforts and increase the availability of health services. Examples include the government contracting "for- profit" or "not-for-profit" organizations to provide health services in places where the government does not have facilities of its own or the capacity to do so. In doing so the government must ensure that it is not in any way subsidizing the private for profit sector. A study by Mudyarabikwa (2000) showed that there were various ways in which government influenced equity through explicit and implicit subsidies, Table 11.1.

Table 11.1 Impact of subsidies on equity and other consumer benefits

Type of Subsidy	Impact on Equity and consumer Benefits (Strength: +/-)
Subsidies for Financiers	
1. Tax exemptions. 2. Private benefits/tax relief. 3. Co-use of public facilities. 4. Low user fees at public facilities.	Less impact on equity as the subsidies only cover the formal sector. The subsidies also do not directly benefit consumers. They also reduce public sector revenue for reinvestment in health since the public sector remains the largest provider of health for the majority population. (Strength: --/+)
Subsidies: Private for Profit Providers	
1. Tax Credit: land, buildings and tools. 2. Tax relief: associations. 3. Co-use of public facilities. 4. Low user fees at public health facilities. 5. Liberalized private practice. 6. Manpower training and development. 7. Contracting out of services.	Impact on equity is low to moderate for these subsidies. They are inequitable because they are mostly applied to the formal sector, therefore subsidizing the already well to do. They also allow for availability of more providers for those consumers who cannot afford the fees. (Strength: +/--)
Subsidies: Not-for-profit	
1. Running costs grants. 2. Staff salaries. 3. Capital development costs.	These probably have the highest impact on equity and consumer benefits for all subsidies. They enable missions to provide adequate curative and preventive services in rural areas for the majority of poor consumers. (Strength: + + + +)
Subsidies: Private Sector to Public sector.	
1. Service provision. 2. Designation as District Hospital. 3. Nurse Training. 4. Out of pocket user fees exemptions.	High impact on equity and high benefits from majority consumers, especially the poor in rural areas. Missions take the responsibility of what are otherwise public sector duties. (Strength: + + +)
Subsidies for consumers.	
1. Fee exemptions. 2. Free MCH services, TB treatment. 3. Tax credits- medical aid. 4. Tax relief-invalid appliances. 5. Training and manpower development.	These also have high impact on equity and high benefits to consumers. Such public sector subsidy is mostly provided to cushion the poor who are the majority consumers who cannot afford the services and including those provided by the private sector. Similarly, training guarantees availability of skilled, competent and appropriately trained personnel for the benefit of consumers. (Strength: + + + +)

Based on Information from Mudyarabikwa (2000)

Decentralization and equity

Decentralization encourages localized decision making in the development and management of health facilities. This has the potential to increase geographical access which in turn may lead to increased equity. However, because decentralization has a tendency to fragment policy interpretation, policy implementation and lead to a lack of uniformity in decision-making, it can compromise equity. In their newly found autonomy, different local authorities could decide to abolish user fees, introduce or increase existing user fees to generate revenue. At the micro economic level, some districts may be very poor compared to their counterparts and thus not able to provide quality services, or indeed any services at all from revenue generated locally. Disparities in the development of the various districts can also result in some of them being unable to attract health professionals to work in their health facilities.

Challenges in achieving equity in health in Zimbabwe

As stated earlier on, it is not possible to completely eliminate all disparities or inequities in any society. As such the Zimbabwe health system is still characterized by obvious disparities in access to health and health care between different social groups and between different geographical areas. The issue is on the extent to which efforts are being made to reduce avoidable and unjust inequalities. At independence Zimbabwe's health services and resources were concentrated in urban areas with most of the health resources directed at the private sector, which mainly benefited the minority elite. Health care expenditures per person were 100 times more for whites than for blacks.

Income levels

With the continuing decline in the economy the real incomes of rural peasant farmers has been much more adversely affected compared to those of their urban counterparts. The poor quality of agricultural land in communal areas has been cited as a major factor limiting access to a viable resource base for peasants in Zimbabwe. This and other factors have led to a depression in household consumption though it is not possible to tell the extent to which this depression has affected household expenditures on health, (Lowenson, R, 1991).

In 1980 the average income for the white population was 39 times more than that of their black counterparts. As a result the rural population suffered predominantly from preventable diseases and conditions associated with poverty and poor socio-economic conditions. A state of affairs that has hardly changed and is probably considerably worse in some cases, especially considering the increasing levels of poverty in the country. The vicious cycle between income and health means that poor health leads to poverty and poverty leads to poor health. Socio-economic inequalities lead to inequality in health in as much as increases in absolute living standards are expected to lead to improvements in health. Wilkinson (1992) has suggested that once a certain level of affluence has been achieved, it is the degree in inequality in the distribution of income that is the major determinant of population health rather than the average level of income. An income growth for the poor leads directly to better health. Unemployment has adverse effects on health as it increases inequality in income distribution. In this context it is worth noting that in 2003 unemployment levels in Zimbabwe had reached an estimated 70%.

Literacy levels

Improved literacy has a direct and positive impact on the health status of a population. In 1980 the government of Zimbabwe made concerted efforts to increase access to education by removing school fees and introducing free primary education. By 1989 primary school enrolment had increased from 900 000 to almost 3 000 000. However, with the introduction of ESAP the government was forced to impose school levies on households in both urban and rural areas. This resulted in an increase in school dropouts, mainly affecting children in rural areas, from poor households and the girl child.

Education level is a proxy for socio-economic status and offers potential access to a wide range of opportunities and resources that include knowledge, better incomes, food, safe water and sanitation. Female education is also a major determinant for improved health status, especially in women, children and the whole family. Education leads to improved knowledge about health and disease and facilitates the adoption of health improving behavior. The census of 1992 showed that the proportion of women aged 15-49 years without education was up to 42 percent in some of the worst affected provinces.

Indicators of coverage, access and health status

Morbidity indicators show that rural areas are still worse off compared to urban areas. Assessments of the nutrition status of children under the age of 5 years show that as poverty levels increased the levels of malnutrition followed suit. The average proportion of stunted children in the provinces (rural) peaked between 8 and 9 percent for the worst affected areas. During the same period the proportion of stunted children in urban areas ranged between 4.8 and 6.4 per cent. Children whose mothers had primary or secondary education were more likely to be better nourished than those of mothers without, (DHS, 1999).

In 1980 the infant mortality rate (IMR) for the black population was between 100 and 150 per 1000 live births and that for the white population was 14 per 1000 live births. There were also disparities in IMR between those blacks living in the rural areas (140 per 1000 live births) and those in urban areas, (40 per 1000 live births). The mortality experience of infants in Zimbabwe improved over the years until the early 1990s when it began to stagnate at about 66 per 1000 live births. By the turn of the millennium (2001) the IMR had reached 76 per 1000 live births.

Studies conducted in the early 1990s indicated a pattern of persistent and significant differences in life expectancy at birth amongst the country's administrative provinces. In 1992 life expectancy ranged from as low as 57 years in Manicaland to 66 years in Matabeleland South (CSO, 1992). A similar pattern emerged when analyzing Infant Mortality Rates (IMR) with Manicaland showing the highest IMR of 85 per 1000 live births and Matabeleland South the lowest.

Manicaland province happens to have very low rates of adult literacy compared to the rest of the country's provinces. The province also has a very high population of a religious group that discourages the utilization of formal health services, especially the immunization of children. It is reasonable to infer that these factors may be contributing to the poor health indicators recorded in the province. In 1992 the child mortality rate in urban areas was 20 per 1000 live births compared to 30 per 1000 live births in rural areas. Again Manicaland province had the highest rate of child mortality compared to the other provinces. In terms of the crude death rate (CDR) three provinces emerged as having the worst mortality experiences; Masvingo, Manicaland and Mashonaland East. Data from the 1992 census indicated that the maternal mortality rate (MMR) for Zimbabwe was below 400 per 100 000 live births, with provincial rates ranging between 200 and just over 500 per 100 000 live births.

Zimbabwe has over the years had one of the highest contraceptive prevalence rates in Sub-Sahara Africa with up to 54% of eligible women using modern contraceptives, (DHS, 1999). Urban areas have higher contraceptive prevalence rates (55 %) than rural areas (36 %). The highest prevalence rate at provincial level was 40 percent with the lowest being 30 percent. The Total Fertility Rate (TFR) for urban women is 3.1 children per woman while that for rural women is 4.1 children per woman. Women with no education at all had a TFR of 5.2 whilst their counterparts who had attained primary education had a TFR of 4.7. Those who had reached secondary level education had a TFR of 3.3.

The immunization coverage and attendance at clinics for antenatal care increased significantly over the years throughout the country. Urban areas have continued to have a better coverage of above 90 per cent with rural areas achieving universal coverage of at least 80% in 1990.

In 1999, 69 percent of the women in rural areas delivered at health facilities compared to over 90 percent in urban areas. Only 46 percent of those women with no education delivered at health facilities compared to 70 percent of those with primary education. There are wide variations between provinces in the proportion of women delivered by health workers. The three worst affected provinces have less than 50 percent of women being delivered by trained health workers. This is a result of poor access to health facilities, religious beliefs and probably a low ratio of maternity beds to population.

The health worker-population ratio is very high in rural compared to urban areas. In 1999 the doctor-population ratio was one doctor per 80,000 persons in rural areas compared to one doctor to 5 to 8,000 persons in urban areas. There is a private to public sector mal-distribution of health manpower which translates into an urban-rural bias in both access and quality of care. Inequalities in the utilization of health services occur in rural areas because these areas have an undersupply of health staffs, people have to travel longer distances and traverse several natural barriers to access health facilities compared to people living in urban areas. The distribution and availability of health facilities as calculated by the number of hospital beds per population show a national average of 2 beds per 1000 population (1999). This indicator does not take into account the distances traveled in order to access health facilities in rural areas or the population density in the various parts of the country.

Data on the utilization of health services which is derived from routine health information is difficult to interpret. Such information is usually based on outpatient attendances as a proportion of the population below or over the age of five years. Children under the age of five years utilized health facilities more than individuals over the age of five years throughout all the provinces. Utilization of public health facilities by the older age group was low in urban areas compared to rural areas (National Health Profile, 1996). Regions with low population densities had low rates of utilization of health services most probably due to long distances traveled by patients. Opportunity costs in terms of travel time are higher in rural compared to urban areas as a result of natural barriers and an under developed road infrastructure.

Poverty Reduction Strategy Papers (PRSP)

In 1999 the World Bank and the International Monetary Fund (IMF) developed the concept of Poverty Reduction Strategy Papers (PRSP). This development was within the Comprehensive Development Framework of the World Bank which is based on country ownership, partnerships and long term and holistic perspectives. PRSPs are part of the conditions developing countries must fulfill in order to be eligible to receive debt relief through the Highly Indebted Poor Countries Initiative (HIPC). The general expectation is that such strategies will be country driven and based on a poverty country situation analysis of the determinants of poverty and with the involvement of all stakeholders such as the government, civil society, communities and development partners. Central to this process are decisions on how best to channel resources from non-priority activities to PRSP priorities on a sustainable basis. A sound Public Expenditure Management (PEM) framework is also essential in order to assess and define overall resource constraints likely to impede the implementation of the PRSP. The PEM also ensures that government expenditures are closely linked to policy goals and outcomes.

The PRSP process is expected to be open and participatory with all stakeholders included; the private sector, civil society, trade unions, women's groups, direct representation of poor people and development partners. The process provides an opportunity for the country to analyze the poverty and social impact of economic and social policies, including intended policy actions. It is essential that the PRSP is integrated into the existing processes of government so as to ensure clarity of its context and relationships to government planning and strategic actions.

From a health perspective the PRSP builds on the human capital development principle by ensuring that the poor attain a health status and education level that can lift them out of poverty. It also provides safety nets for those unable to benefit from economic empowerment strategies. Some countries have developed essential health packages as health interventions targeted at the poor in a context of the PRSP.

Poverty and health

Tables 11.2, 11.3 and 11.4 demonstrate the relationships between poverty and equity in access to health as well as its impact on other health indicators in Zimbabwe. The stack reality of a poor person is the lack of access to effective curative health care and other determinants of social well being. There is a clear pattern of disparities that emerges between the poor and the well off members of each of the communities in both rural and urban areas. Urban dwellers in their own right have better health indicators.

Table 11.2 Health, Nutrition and Population (HNP) and Poverty by Gender (1994) in Zimbabwe

Indicator	Male		Female	
	Poorest	**Richest**	**Poorest**	**Richest**
IMR	56.7	56.4	46.9	26.1
U5MR	84.4	72.4	84.7	39.6
Children Stunted (%)	25.7	12.4	21.6	12.3
Under weight (moderate)	22.0	9.6	15.2	8.7
Severe	3.7	2.3	1.8	0.6
Service Indicators				
Immunization coverage, all (%)	72.3	90.5	71.2	81.6
Treatment of Diarrhea: Prevalence	29.0	19.0	28.8	15.8
Oral Re-hydration Therapy use:	79.7	92.3	83.4	Sample small
Acute Respiratory Infection Prevalence:	34.8	15.3	35.0	16.7

Based on Gwatkin, D et al (2000)

Table 11.3 National: HNP and Poverty (1994)

Status	Total Population		
Indicator	**Quintiles**		
	Poorest	**Middle**	**Richest**	**Population Avg.**
IMR	52.0	47.4	41.6	51.2
U5MR	84.5	62.4	56.3	75.9
Stunted children (%)	23.7	22.9	12.3	21.4
Moderate Malnutrition (%)	18.6	13.7	9.1	15.5
Severe malnutrition (%)	2.8	4.4	1.5	3.0
TFR	6.2	4.3	2.8	4.3
Service Indicators			
Immunization coverage all (%)	71.8	84.6	85.7	80.1
ARI treatment Prevalence (%)	34.9	25.0	16.0	25.4
Diarrhea prevalence (%)	28.9	25.0	17.0	23.5
ORT use (%)	81.5	84.9	95.6	86.3
ANC > 2 visits (%)	88.0	90.1	92.0	90.5
Delivery attended by trained person (%)	55.1	65.5	92.8	69.4
% of deliveries occurring in public facilities.	53.2	64.5	84.5	66.6
Deliveries at home (%)	45.0	34.3	7.3	30.3

Based on Gwatkin, D et al (2000)

Table 11.4 HNP and Poverty: Urban-Rural Residence

Indicator	Urban		Rural	
	Poorest	**Richest**	**Poorest**	**Richest**
IMR	(Sample not enough)	39.7	52.0	69.4
U5MR		54.7	84.6	90.5
Stunted children (%)		12.0	23.7	18.0
Moderate malnutrition (%)		9.0	18.6	13.6
Severe malnutrition (%)		0.9	2.8	2.8
TFR		2.8	6.2	3.2
Service Indicators				
Immunization (all) (%)		85.6	71.8	81.7
Diarrhea treatment prevalence (%)		16.7	28.9	22.6
ORT use (%)		95.5	81.5	94.3
ARI prevalence (%)		15.5	34.9	24.8
ANC >2 visits (%)		91.9	88.0	93.7
Delivery attendance by trained personnel (%)		93.8	55.0	71.2
Delivery at home (%)		6.3	45.1	28.1
Use of contraceptives (F)		54.9	31.1	68.2

Based on Gwatkin, D et al (2000)

The MOHCW resource allocation formula

In attempting to address the question of "equal access for equal need" the MOHCW developed a resource allocation formula to allocate financial resources within the ministry. The historically based system of allocating resources had tended to perpetuate inequities that had been imbedded in the system for a very long time. This allocation had largely depended on the number of health facilities present in a geographical area irrespective of whether they were being fully utilized or not. It did not take into account whether the district had used all the financial resources allocated to it or not. As a result those provinces or districts with many facilities always attracted and received more resources at the expense of those with fewer health facilities. Those who had historically always received more resources, for whatever reason, continued to do so irrespective of changing circumstances.

The introduction of a resource allocation formula in any situation is always marred by controversy. The major issues that needed to be resolved included how much weighting was to be attributed to each parameter and how much each parameter would contribute to relative need. The formula was developed over a two-year period and adopted by the MOHCW in 1993. At the time it was agreed that the following parameters would initially be included and that the formula would be reviewed on an annual basis and as necessary:

+ Population: male, female and total.
+ Surface area: total area of the administrative province or district, epidemic potential, distances to be covered (road network).
+ Number of health facilities: both mission and government given similar weight, bed capacity and occupancy.
+ Workload or utilization: outpatient attendance, total in-patient days per unit of population.
+ Staff establishment: for salaries and allowances.

Apart from the weighting of the above parameters on the basis of their perceived impact on a particular budget item, the allocation was deliberately split into 35% for central hospitals and 65% for the provinces, (provincial, district, health center and community levels). The parameters used in the formula did not include poverty related indicators even after the poverty assessment data became available from the 1995 Poverty Assessment Survey. It proved inappropriate to apply all the parameters equally to all the vote items in the budget. For example surface area only related to field based activities such as vector control and outreach programs and not to curative services.

The formula was criticized for being biased towards hospital services and not well suited for the allocation of financial resources to public health programs. As a result in 2001 the MOHCW resorted to a demand based resource allocation strategy. This involved the provinces, central hospitals, district hospitals and other units within the MOHCW submitting plan based bids within a specified global MOHCW ceiling from Treasury. This involved the allocation of resources to cost centers on a pro-rata basis depending on the budget estimates submitted. This allocation method is not very different from incremental or historical allocation and does not address equity issues. Since 2003 the MOHCW has been considering the adoption of an equity based allocation formula. This is a follow up on a study initiated by the MOHCW and the Training and Research Support

Center (TARSC) in 2001 to explore and propose variables that can be used in the resource allocation formula, (TARSCO/MOHCW/Equity Gauge Monograph 4/2001). This process is yet to be concluded.

Measuring and monitoring equity

In order to pursue equity in an objective manner it should be possible to measure disparities in terms of health or other appropriate indicators in the different segments of society. Inequities due to health interventions can be measured using changes in incidence, case fatality rates, disability rates and coverage according to population groups. Where specific indicators of inequity are not available, more general data can be used such as maternal mortality, infant mortality and other similar parameters.

Measures of health status can also be used, for example, mortality and morbidity rates like they were used in the Black Report (Black, 1980). Such indicators are influenced by the quality and availability of data which may however not be readily accessible in many African countries. Comparisons can also be made of life expectancy and potential years of life lost due to premature deaths. Per capita rates of expenditure can be examined by region and the availability of other resources such as doctors, nurses and health facilities. This information is more likely to be readily available than health status data.

The Lorenz curve and the Gini co-efficient were developed as methods meant to compare income distribution within populations. The diagonal line of the Lorenz curve implies perfect equality in income distribution and the further the real line is from the diagonal the more unequal the income is distributed. The Gini co-efficient expresses this numerically with a range between 0 and 1. Zero representing perfect equality of income distribution and 1 perfect inequality, meaning that one individual receives all the income. The same technique has been applied to analyze the distribution of health service resources.

The illness concentration curve is a refinement of the Lorenz approach. In this curve the horizontal axis measures socio-economic status (social class) rather than income. The illness concentration curve first ranks individuals according to their ability to pay beginning with the poorest. Usually the curve shows that illness is concentrated amongst the lower income groups.

Despite the tremendous efforts made by the government to improve equity in access to health and health care, achieving equity still remains an elusive goal. It is important to appreciate that the health sector on its own cannot resolve the problem of equity in health. The unequal distribution of wealth at the macro-economic level influences the fundamentals in the distribution of wealth and thus the whole equation on equity. Policies at this level influence social and economic opportunities as well as determining the extent and distribution of poverty in society.

Weak participatory democracy at the local level is a constraint to access to opportunities for the creation of wealth. This affects women, the aged, children and other marginalized members of society much more than the other groups. It is therefore crucial that local health committees or similar structures become involved in determining and managing user fee and other exemption mechanisms.

In order to tackle the problem of equity the government and its partners must first of all be able to identify the problem of inequity, quantify it, monitor and evaluate any interventions aimed at resolving it. It is thus important to develop an information system which will make it easy to detect any such inequities. It should be possible for the data that is collected to be disaggregated according to social groups, gender and age at the national and sub-national levels. It must also be possible to monitor and analyze resource allocations according to social needs and their geographical distribution.

Information flow must be regular and able to establish the experiences of different social groups in their attempts to gain access to health services. The reasons for the low utilization of essential services must be fully explored and measures to redress such imbalances put in place. Any assessment of this nature must include how well each group is doing with respect to selected indicators and the extent of the gaps between the groups. Such information must be presented as clearly and as simply as possible for both lay and professional audiences to be able to understand and appreciate.

In strengthening its health information system the MOHCW put in place a system of health profiles that are produced at the national, provincial and district levels on an annual basis. Unfortunately data from poverty assessment studies has not been regularly fed into this information system. The Demographic Health Surveys are a rich source of information which includes several indictors aggregated by gender, socio-economic status and other characteristics.

Box 11.1. A selection of indicators to monitor equity

- Children's growth and nutritional status.
- Child mortality rates.
- Life expectancy at birth.
- Maternal Mortality rates.
- Access to food supply.
- Adequacy homes.
- Poverty (income, expenditures and economic assets).
- Educational attainment.
- Income inequality in society.
- The burden of payment for health care, the proportion of household total expenditures that goes to pay for health care services.
- Indicators of health care resource allocation.
- Public expenditures on health care, including the private sector.
- Distribution of qualified health care personnel.
- Distribution of health care facilities at the primary, secondary, tertiary and quaternary levels and their budgetary allocation.
- Availability of essential drugs at facilities.
- Indicators of utilization and quality of health care.
- Immunization coverage.
- Reproductive health coverage:-
  - Antenatal care.
  - Safe delivery coverage.
  - Contraceptive prevalence.

Conclusions and the way forward

The socio-economic difficulties faced by the government of Zimbabwe and indeed many African governments are a serious challenge to the achievement of equity in health and health care. Within the sector there is still inequity in the allocation of resources between curative and preventive services and between the different levels of the health delivery system. At the macro level the per capita expenditure on high-income individuals in the private sector is at least ten times more than that on middle and low-income users of public sector services.

Central to the sector's ten year National Health Strategy (1997-2007) is the development of a needs based resource allocation formula and the decentralization of budget management to the district level. Experience with the initial attempts at formulating a resource allocation formula within the MOHCW indicates that whilst it was a sound approach to needs based resource allocation it was biased towards hospital care, insensitive to equity and only applicable to the public sector. The MOHCW and its stakeholders have reached a consensus and endorsed the need to develop a new budget allocation formula that will ensure equity and reduce allocative inefficiencies and move resources towards areas of greatest need.

From a democratic perspective, in pursuing its objective of achieving equity, the MOHCW has demonstrated its concern for justice for all individuals as far as the opportunities to achieve individual well being are concerned. The concept of equity is however paradoxical in its nature. For each decision that is made to divide something equally (resources and services) there is another decision that will distribute something unequally somewhere in the system. The distribution of resources equally between regions or districts does not necessarily translate into equitably distributed health or health care, (in Saltman et al, (Eds) 1999).

Review questions

1. Most countries in Africa have cited equity as one of the goals of their public health systems. Critically analyze the strategies that some of these countries have put in place in order to achieve equity in access to health care and health services.
2. It is generally agreed that some elements of health reforms have adverse effects on equity. Discuss concrete examples of such reform elements.
3. Design a strategy for the ministry of health to monitor the effects of health reforms on equity.
4. In what ways do government subsidies to the private sector adversely affect equity, if at all?
5. Discuss the challenges that developing countries face in trying to achieve equity in health. How can these be best resolved?

12

MONITORING AND EVALUATING HEALTH REFORMS

Introduction

The decision to implement health sector reforms is a fundamental policy decision with a potential for both positive and negative outcomes. Unfortunately, in most cases decisions to embark on health reforms are often not based on objective evidence or any assessment of the situation prior to the reforms. There is no evidence in the case in Zimbabwe that any baseline information was collected to assess the situation prior the implementation of the country's health reforms.

The adoption of reforms must be backed by objective evidence which must be analyzed in order to inform any decision making processes related to the reform process. Such information must be easily digestible, user friendly, easily understood and usable by all stakeholders, including those without any training in the area of reforms. It should not be necessary for one to have prior experience in the policy development processes in order to objectively appreciate the impact of health sector reforms. Monitoring and evaluation of the reform process must include both qualitative and quantitative indicators. Any indicators that are adopted for this purpose must be adapted and made relevant to the local situation. In evaluating reforms it must be accepted that reforms constitute a process of social change which is value laden and conflict ridden.

Some objectives to consider in establishing an evaluation framework for health reforms include:

- The promotion and application of policy analysis within ministries of health.
- Improvement in the understanding of the effects of specific health reforms on sector objectives such as improving quality, efficiency, equity, sustainability and acceptability to both clients and providers.
- Identification of specific policy, institutional, managerial and extra-sectoral conditions necessary for reforms to achieve their intended effects. (WHO/SHS/NHP95.10).

Some issues to consider when evaluating reforms:

- Recognition of the fact that values, stakeholders and their perspectives hold significant importance over the content and process of reform.
- That judgment as to whether the reforms are effective or not depends on understanding societal goals and values as well as the explicit objectives of the reforms themselves.
- That the successful implementation of reforms requires good and practical managerial skills and effective data collection and dissemination strategies.
- That the institutional capacity necessary for successful reform is not only a set of skills but also a set of principles that govern relationships among the different partners within the process.

The evaluation of health reforms should use routinely available information as well as data collected specifically to determine if the effects can indeed be attributed to specific policy changes. The analysis must demonstrate causality on the basis of detailed analyses of other possible explanatory factors. The monitoring and evaluation process must follow the footsteps and pace of implementation of the reforms, which are usually in one of several forms:

- Passage of legal or regulatory instruments.
- Alteration of bureaucratic structures e.g. restructuring of the organization and its establishment.
- Changing resource allocation strategies in order to support the policy process.
- Dealing with human resources development issues.

♦ The dissemination of information to the public and stakeholders with an interest in the reforms.

♦ Development of guidelines for staff that will be responsible for implementing the reform policy.

Critical areas to consider in evaluating health sector reforms:

♦ Efficiency: the extent to which the costs of a given package of services or reforms are minimized.

♦ Responsiveness: the extent to which services treat people in a decent manner in order to meet their individual wishes and preferences as part of the quality of services.

♦ Choice: allowing people to decide what services or providers they want to use.

♦ Equity: the extent to which services should be open to everyone according to need irrespective of factors such as income, socioeconomic status, gender or ethnic origin.

♦ Health impact: the attribution of the impact of health reforms on health status is rather remote. It is therefore imperative to undertake a thorough analysis of all other possible contributing factors than to take the impact of health reforms for granted.

Box 12.1   Indicator framework for monitoring health reforms

Baseline and Process Indicators:
- Accessibility - geographical and economic.
- Seasonal variability in utilization of services.
- Availability of manpower, health facilities, standard equipment and essential drugs.
- Expenditures on health - public and private sector.
- Appropriateness of referrals.
- Contributions from community.
- Functionality of community participatory health committees.

Indicators of Input:
- Number of facilities by level of the health system that are rehabilitated or built by year.
- Proportion of facilities fully staffed with appropriately trained health workers.
- Implementation of a performance based pay and reward system.
- Proportion of facilities by level which are fully stocked with essential drugs.

Indicators of Output:
- Coverage – antenatal, institutional delivery, growth monitoring, immunization.
- Contraceptive prevalence rate among women 15-49 years old.
- Women at risk of unwanted pregnancy.
- Maternal mortality – institutional.
- Outpatient consultations per year.
- Bed occupancy rates - by level.
- Number of health workers trained – per year and per training institution.
- Training dropout rate - by level and by training institution.
- Regularity of supervision.
- Functionality of the transport system.

Indicators of Outcome:
- Maternal mortality rate.
- Infant mortality rate.
- Under five mortality rate.
- Low birth weight rate.
- Prevalence rates for selected marker diseases.
- Incidence rates of specific diseases.
- Client satisfaction with health services.

Table 12.1 Issues to consider in developing health reform policies.

Implementation strategy	Policy clarification
• A plan to guide those people responsible for implementing the strategy. • Definition of lines of authority for the implementation process. • Outline of implementation timelines. • Decisions on how implementation will proceed, e.g. pilot versus program development.	• Clarification of policy language. • Target groups identified. • Identification of persons responsible for implementation. • Operational rules or regulations prepared. • Laws adopted.
Program development • Guidelines for action or procedures developed. • Training provided to responsible groups. • New responsibilities and lines of authority defined.	**Resource allocation** • Budget requirements prepared. • Potential sources of funding identified. • Internal procedures for handling funds identified. • Changes in staffing patterns, equipment allocation or infrastructure defined and acted upon.
Social awareness and mobilization • All stakeholders, including the general public, informed about policy. • Media briefed. • Community oriented groups briefed. • Public information prepared.	**Response of consumers to changes in health services.** • Economic access. • Geographical access. • Willingness to pay. • Affordability of services.
Epidemiological consequences of health reforms. • Incidence and prevalence. • Utilization rates: admission rates, discharge rates, *bed occupancy rates, **bed turnover rates, ***average length of stay (ALOS). • Burden of disease and disease profiles.	**Changes in service delivery as a result of health reforms:** • Additional resources for the health sector. • Effective use of resources. • Changes in quality of services.
Financial management issues • Mobilization of additional resources. • Collection and management of revenue. • Transparency. • Pool funding.	

*Bed occupancy rates = ALOS x Turnover/365 x beds
**Bed turnover rates = admissions (or discharges + deaths)/beds
***Average length of stay (ALOS) = inpatient days/admissions (or discharges plus deaths)

Proposed framework for assessing health reforms

There are several qualitative and quantitative indicators that can be adapted for use in monitoring progress, outcome, output and the long term impact of the reform process. These can be a combination of existing indicators and other situational indicators relevant to the reform process. Outcome indicators help in strategically thinking about key results that are meant to be achieved. They also verify intended positive change, e.g. an outcome indicator for an advocacy activity aimed at policy change in governance may include observing the passage of a law and monitoring if the law is backed by an allocation of resources. An output indicator verifies the production of outputs or tangible results which are usually delivered in a short time frame.

Describing the health system

1. Is there a document that describes the strategic direction of the sector?
2. Details of actors within the health sector.
   - Types of clients or patients.
   - Presence of third party payers - health insurance schemes.
   - Effectiveness of the government as a regulator.
   - Availability of not-for-profit providers - missions and NGOs.
   - Range of public sector providers - MOH, other government ministries and local authorities.
   - Levels of the health delivery system.
   - Others.
3. Interactions within the sector.
   - Efficiency of the referral system.
   - Payment for services - types of insurance schemes, user fees.
   - Contributions towards insurance schemes.
   - Modalities of payment for insurance claims.
   - Regulation of insurers.
   - Free health services.
4. Exemption mechanisms operating for cost recovery through user fees.
5. Population coverage.
   - National Health Accounts - public and private expenditures per capita.
   - General health indicators.

- Resource ratios for each segment of the population - by geographical region, socio-economic groups.
  - Physicians, nurses, etc. per population.
  - Hospital beds per population.
  - Service coverage.
  - Equity.

Describing the socio-economic context

1. Social indicators - economic, education, housing and cultural.
2. Health status indicators - morbidity, mortality, QALYS and DALYS.
3. Governance issues:
   - Structure of government.
   - Role of the state in health provision.
   - Economic policies.
   - Social policies.

Eliciting reasons for undertaking the reforms

1 Objectives of the health reforms.
   - Describe the situation to be achieved after the reforms have been implemented.
2 What are the reasons for the reforms?
   - Describe the critical situations that are the driving force for the reform.
   - Economic - cost containment, value for money, economic crises and chronic scarcity of resources.
   - Political - political reforms, etc.
   - Ideological - market, reduction of the role of the state and public private mix.
   - Epidemiological transition.
   - Other problems requiring solutions - efficiency, equity and quality.

Describing interactions within the sector

1. Roles and interplay between stakeholders.
   - Diverse interest groups and motivation.
   - How they affect agenda setting.
   - Policy formulation process.
   - Formulation and implementation of public policy.
   - Democratic versus authoritarian implementation.

2. What scale of reform is to be implemented?
- Timing - short-term versus long term.
- Procedure - technocratic control versus consensus building.
- Proposed scale - pilot model versus full-scale countrywide.

Identifying critical elements of reforms

What are the proposed institutional arrangements for regulation, financing and delivery of services?

Health Financing:
- What are the sources of health finance currently in place - user fees, private insurance and social insurance?
- Is there a choice of financiers available?

Decentralization:
- Are there policy documents on decentralization?
- What are the administrative levels or structures currently in place?
- Do local government structures coincide with those of the health sector?
- Is there a regulatory framework - administrative, legal instrument or any contractual arrangements to support decentralization?

Organizational Restructuring:
- Are there any plans or proposals for restructuring?
- What are the existing levels and institutions?
- What are the proposed new levels and institutions?
- Are there plans to abolish existing levels and institutions?
- What administrative levels are currently in place: regional, provincial, district and village?
- What development structures are in place?
    - District development committees.
    - Provincial development committees.
    - Ward development committees?
    - Village development committees.
    - District health boards.
    - Hospital boards.
    - Others.

Identifying responsibilities of the various administrative levels or institutions:

- Allocation of resources.
- Performance linked contract.
- Decisions on capital budget.
- Authority to hire and fire staff.
- Setting of salary levels.
- Do they retain the revenue they collect?
  - At what level is the responsibility to prepare plans?
  - How much freedom do local managers have to transfer funds between line items and programs?
  - Is there any formula for the allocation of resources equitably and rationally?
  - What are the current responsibilities of the following administrative levels within the health sector – national, provincial, district and other institutions (hospitals)?

Do the large national referral hospitals have any autonomy?

- Provision of global budgets.
- Raising additional funds.
- Authority to manage their institutions and staff.

Assessing quality of care issues:

- Does the health sector have a client or patients' charter?
- Is there a quality assurance framework or program within the health sector?
- Is evidence based medicine being practiced?
- Are there standards of care and practice that have been developed?
  - Who is responsible for the development of standards?
  - In which particular areas have standards been developed?
  - How are the standards being monitored?
- Are there any protocols or guidelines that have been developed for the management of specific conditions?
- Are there any specific initiatives on clinical or medical audit at the hospital level?
- Is there an established system for handling patients and clients complaints within the health sector?

Private and public sector collaboration:

- Is there a private medical sector in the country?
  - None.
  - Private for profit: - general practitioners, private clinics, private hospitals, nursing and maternity homes and private pharmacies.
  - Private not for profit: - NGOs, missions.
  - Others.
- Is there any legislation that regulates the operations of the private medical sector?
- What regulatory mechanisms are in place in relation to?
  - Quality of care (minimum standards).
  - Quantity of care (regulation of the establishment of private facilities).
  - Price of care (fee schedules).
- Are health workers in the public sector allowed to do private practice? Describe arrangements in place.
- Are private practitioners allowed to practice and offer services in public health facilities or to admit patients into government facilities?
- Do government hospitals have private wards or beds?
- Is there provision for the licensing and inspection of (accreditation) health facilities in general?
- What is the licensing authority?
- What incentives or disincentives are there in relation to the operations of the private sector?
- Are there any services that the ministry has outsourced?
- What funding arrangements are there between the government and mission institutions, local authorities and the private for profit sector?

The objective of the above framework is to provide a tool that will guide and ensure that the process of monitoring and evaluation is comprehensive, objective, regular, institutionalized and sustainable, at the same time being able to feed back into the decision making process. All stakeholders must be involved in monitoring and evaluation and ensure that their interests are recognized and accommodated. Each country is expected to adapt the indicators to suite its own circumstances. Once the selection of "common" indicators is agreed it should be possible to undertake comparative analyses of different countries that are implementing health sector reforms.

A comparison of the impact of health reforms in different countries has the possibility of providing answers as to whether reform policies have improved or impeded the performance of the health sector in the different country settings. At a meeting on "Achieving Evidence Based Health Sector Reforms in Sub-Saharan Africa", in Arusha, Tanzania in 1995, countries in the African Region agreed to rely on objective information to guide their decision making processes in their reform process. Objective information is invariably necessary in planning and implementing health sector reforms as well as in monitoring their impact in the achievement of health objectives.

Health systems research is a unique tool for obtaining the necessary evidence on health sector reforms. The list of indicators that has been outlined above provides an enriched pool of indicators which if adopted could facilitate the implementation of evidence-based reforms.

The public sector policy analysis process

Reforms are a fundamental policy change which requires a thorough understanding and the identification of alternative options to achieve policy objectives in an efficient and effective manner. In analyzing health reform policies the policy analyst can organize his/her work into four major steps:

Description

This stage consists of observing, describing and recording facts through the application of research techniques and listening attentively. As in any epidemiological inquiry, to find out *who, what, where, when and why?*

♦ Who – are the key parties, interest groups involved or affected by the reforms; who is making what proposal or asking for the analysis?

♦ What – is the proposal, key issues, and what is the expected outcome? What is the origin of the problem? Is it related to other issues? What is the political context and what are the financial implications?

♦ Where – do the reforms have regional, national or international dimensions?

♦ When – are the reforms related to an election period or end of term of government? When is the decision required? Implementation period for the reform?

- Why – is the reform issue before government? What is actually wrong and why are people concerned?

Analysis

Sifting through the facts identified in order to diagnose the problem, understand the constraints on any proposed solutions. Analysis involves examining the current situation, the objectives, available options and barriers.

- Identifying key issues and their root causes.
- Analyzing policy issues in relation to other policies or positions –policy issues may be linked to other positions with strong public support or strong backers.
- Determining the parties involved or affected by the policy decision – their interests, history or organization (political parties)
- Examining relationship between parties – good, bad, distant and how the policy affects these
- Exploring the origins of the policy- who are the proponents?
- Interests of groups or organizations that give rise to the positions they take on the policy – are there common patterns?
- Analyzing timeframes that may be relevant to the policy – when the new policy is to be implemented, deadlines and related milestones. Is it a crisis or anticipated crisis?
- What are the theoretical assumptions behind the policy analysis, especially causative relations – how valid are they?
- Documentation of public views on reforms issues - consensus or marked differences of opinion, are these changing or likely to change in the future?
- What are the quantifiable costs and benefits to the policy? Who will pay for the policy implementation? Are there opportunities for recovery of costs?
- Which administrative levels drive the policy reform – provincial or national/ does issue require cabinet, Treasury or other collective approvals?
- What are the legal considerations – constitutional or otherwise?

Assessing options

The analysis at this stage should facilitate the adoption of potential options and possible constraints to the achievement of reform objectives.

♦ Setting realistic options on the way forward
  ♦ Paradigm shifts – based on theoretical considerations - competing theories
  ♦ Conventional options – brainstorming and creativity
  ♦ Process options – the white paper approach, the preferred option.
♦ Evaluating the list of possible scenarios to achieve the primary objective, based on ;
  ♦ Legitimacy – will the outcome of the reform process be acceptable to government supporters, ideology, morality, legality and conventional knowledge; consistent with government policy, practice, standards, fair and reasonable?
  ♦ Feasibility – affected by technology (computers, telephones), organizational and administrative considerations (e.g. decentralization), financial and human resources, available time frame, and cooperation of the public?
  ♦ Affordability – how much it will cost, who pays, do benefits outweigh the costs. What are the costs of not implementing the reforms?
  ♦ Communicability – can the policy be communicated to stakeholders; can it be defended before the public, parliament and the public? What is the view of the media?
♦ Support – to what extent does the policy reform have support from parties, groups and individuals? What is the reaction of the general public? Key decision makers should be identified – ministers, political advisors and outside advisors.
♦ Summation – based on above criteria of legitimacy, affordability, communicability and support assess likely options.

Providing the advice

Provide clear, succinct and thoughtful advice and recommend the mostly likely option that meets the needs of the client:
  ♦ What commitments the proposal requires?
  ♦ Whose responsibility is it to make decisions? Who has to act?
  ♦ What are the next steps?
  ♦ The time frame for decisions, negotiations and implementation?
  ♦ What resources are required and where will they come from?

Review questions

1. Why is it considered essential to monitor and evaluate the implementation of health sector reforms? Justify your response.

2. Describe the limitations of using health status indicators to assess the impact of health sector reforms? Suggest a more appropriate selection of indicators and justify your choice.

3. Review the chapter on "Decentralization of Health Services" and conduct a policy analysis of this reform policy.

13

GENERAL CONCLUSIONS AND THE WAY FORWARD

Introduction

The period between the dawn of the 1990s and the mid 2000s saw the reversal and decline of Zimbabwe's achievements in health service provision. This is also the period during which the country's economy experienced a rapid decline, characterized by negative GDP growth rates estimated at -0.2% in 1997, -5.1% in 2000 and -8.9% in 2001 and a hyperinflation rate of over 600% in the first quarter of 2004, reaching 11 000 000% by the third quarter of 2008 and 231 million percent by September of the same year. The situation was exacerbated by the HIV/AIDS epidemic, the effects of the chaotic land reform program and the withdrawal of overseas development assistance to the country. The early 1990s experienced the warning signs of a health sector under pressure from declining expenditures, deteriorating social conditions and an economic meltdown, evident even to the man in the street who openly complained about the deteriorating quality of health services at public health institutions.

A summary of articles on the state of the health delivery system in Zimbabwe paints a very gloomy picture; *".....three years of economic free fall and inflation, now averaging 620% per annum, have left Zimbabwe desperately short of even basic drugs and medical equipment..... Government clinics now have no working radios, refrigerators and trained medical workers.... Zimbabwe's immunization program once exemplary, now provides coverage of less than 70% .... Zimbabwe was the only country in Sub-Saharan Africa which could buy all its own vaccines.... but by 2001 it could not afford it ....*

The Chairman of Zimbabwe's Parliamentary Portfolio Committee on Health and Child Welfare reiterated that in the 2003-04 financial year the health sector needed a budget allocation of US$ 10.3 million to resuscitate critical areas of service delivery to deal with problems related to drug procurement, a crumbling infrastructure and retention of skilled personnel.... *"Drug levels are currently at 40% of national requirements and the sector is operating with 45% of the required staffing levels.... The National Pharmaceutical Company which requires US$ 4 million per month for drug purchases has received only US$ 3 million in 9 months...... Harare Central hospital which has an annual intake of 180 nursing students failed to open its school of nursing on the 4th January 2004 because of an acute shortage of nurse tutors....."*

In an attempt to respond to popular concerns and to prevent further and rapid deterioration in the health sector the MOHCW started implementing health sector reforms in the early 1990s. The reforms involved a complex transition which required synchronized action in health financing, public and private collaboration, human resources development and the development of effective regulatory instruments and mechanisms within the health sector. The reform package developed by the health sector in Zimbabwe consisted of the following elements:

- ◆ Organizational restructuring; decentralization and the establishment of semi-autonomous institutions.
- ◆ Health financing (cost recovery and Social Health Insurance).
- ◆ Contracting out of noncore services.
- ◆ Management strengthening.
- ◆ Regulation of the health sector.
- ◆ Private and public collaboration.

Health reforms in Zimbabwe were multi-faceted, largely considered to be home grown, though also driven by a set of universal factors which included:

- ◆ Macroeconomic conditions of economic recession, the Economic Structural Adjustment Program and conditionality attached to these such as; reduction of expenditures on social services, introduction of market reforms, reduction of the role of the state in service provision and public-private collaboration.
- ◆ Increasing levels of poverty, inadequate social safety nets and poor access to social services by vulnerable groups.
- ◆ Excessive dependency on external aid which forced the government to accept conditional cooperation agreements, loans and grants requiring the country to undertake structural reforms.
- ◆ Increased work load on an underfunded public health sector due to the HIV/AIDS epidemic; an adult HIV sero-prevalence rate of between 25% and 30%.

♦ A massive flight of skills from the public health sector resulting in vacancy rates of up to 55% for doctors and 31.4% for nurses in 2002.

The major objectives and outcome areas for the reform agenda in Zimbabwe were:
   ♦ Increased technical and allocative efficiency.
   ♦ Improved health status of the population.
   ♦ Improved equity.
   ♦ Improved quality of care.

In analyzing the context and content of health reforms in Zimbabwe, it is pertinent to consider the fact that, like in most situations, reforms are driven by a mixture of internal and external forces and/or agencies. A major driving force behind most reforms is the requirement by multilateral and/or bilateral aid agencies for changes in government systems for financial management, accountability and monitoring and evaluation before any resources can be committed or transferred to a particular government.

To date it is not objectively possible to state if the health sector reforms in Zimbabwe achieved the intended objectives. This is mainly because no specific evaluation or assessment has been undertaken to determine their outcome and long term impact.

Achievements and constraints in reforming the health sector in Zimbabwe

The impact of health reforms on the public health system

Zimbabwe's reform agenda consisted of a mix of financial, social, technical, political and organizational restructuring goals and objectives. Because no baseline information was collected on the areas targeted for reform, it is difficult to objectively conclude if the reforms were successful or not. Furthermore, factors that have an influence on the health sector go beyond those directly related to the sector itself or the reform process. This means therefore that there is a potential problem of attribution, especially as to which factors influence the performance of the health sector and when they actually do so.

A major reason for undertaking health reforms was to respond to and arrest the deteriorating indicators of morbidity and mortality in the country. The proposal revolved around strengthening the health system by instituting health reform initiatives that would reinforce and strengthen the implementation of core public health functions and capabilities. A review of the reform elements implemented reveals that most of them focused on structural and process issues; which in themselves do not have a direct and tangible impact on health status.

The assessment of health sector reforms has used, as proxy, results from studies conducted to assess the outcome and impact of service and program delivery during the reform period, though these were not specifically intended to link the performance of the health delivery system to the reform process. These studies indicate that during the decade the reforms were being implemented, outcome and impact health indicators continued to deteriorate.

With regards patient related services, proxy indicators for quality of health care services continued to deteriorate. During the same period evidence indicates that the quality of care at public hospitals deteriorated significantly. The poor performance of the economy led to increased levels of poverty, drug shortages, brain drain, non-functional medical equipment and a deteriorating health infrastructure. The poor economic situation militated against effective implementation of some of the health financing reforms aimed at increasing the allocation of resources to the health sector.

One is inclined to conclude that the state of the economy made it impossible for the reforms to achieve their intended objectives. A more objective but controversial assessment of the health system in Zimbabwe is contained in the WHO Performance Report of 2000 which ranked the performance of the country's health system at 155 out of 191 WHO member states. The report stated that the health delivery system was not responsive enough to patient needs and that physical access to health care was not equitable.

From these analyses it is reasonable to infer that the quality of services at public health institutions deteriorated, that the health status of the population declined, that patients continued to shun public health facilities and that the work force was not motivated and continued to leave the public health sector. From a process point of view, there was notable progress in decentralization, contracting-out and regulation of the health sector, though the impact of these particular reforms on the health system is not clear.

It is important to note that during the period the reforms were implemented the political and socioeconomic landscape of the country deteriorated significantly. There is enough evidence in literature that socioeconomic status is a significant determinant of health and health status, in particular the levels of income, employment opportunities and poverty. The prevailing unstable and unpredictable environment made it very difficult to guarantee a positive impact of health reforms on health status. Since policies in other sectors such as education, food security and safe water can influence the health status of the population, it is essential to undertake simultaneous evaluations of policies in these sectors.

Mobilization of resources for the health sector

Another objective of the government's health reforms was to increase health sector financing and financing options for the sector through health financing reform initiatives. It was expected that more resources would be made available and in a more predictable manner to, and within, the health sector. This was expected to be achieved through increased public health spending by the government and development partners and the introduction of a flexible source of funds at the operational level of the health system. Facts on the ground indicated that health demands and the cost of health services continued to escalate, mainly as a result of several factors which include; the natural population increase, escalation in the costs of inputs for health service delivery and an increased burden of disease from HIV/AIDS and opportunistic infections. The introduction of the ART program was another major cost driver for the health sector.

The government did not significantly increase the proportion of total government expenditures on health. The 15% level agreed in the Abuja Declaration has not been achieved to date. The financial resources made available to the sector did not increase adequately enough to match the increasing demand for health services. On the contrary, resources allocated to the health sector declined by more than 30% during the period of the reforms. Poor management at the macroeconomic level which resulted in negative economic growth rates contributed significantly to this state of affairs. Competing demands on the meager government budget, some of which were not entirely justified, hyperinflation, the devaluation of the country's currency and the shortage of foreign currency are other contributing factors. With the imposition of economic sanctions on the country, previous sources of overseas development assistance to the country literally dried up as of the year 2000, declining to less than 5% of public health expenditures.

Whilst the minimum package of interventions necessary to support the basic health needs of a developing country, including the maintenance of the infrastructure necessary to support its delivery, is estimated to cost between US$ 30 and US$ 40 per capita, Zimbabwe was spending less US$ 10 per capita per annum. Overall, one can conclude that the health reforms implemented at the time did not achieve the intended objective to increase the levels of health financing in Zimbabwe, considering, of course, intervening circumstances.

Cost recovery and other financing policies

As part of the reform process fees charged at government institutions were revised upwards to levels charged by the private sector, to reflect the economic costs of providing health in Zimbabwe. This policy move, combined with the establishment of the Health Service Fund (HSF) and the decision to allow institutions to retain revenue from user fees, led to a significant increase in the revenue collected at institutional level. There is evidence that as institutions began to use revenue from user fees the availability of essential drugs and supplies improved.

The increase in user fee levels impacted negatively on patient initiated utilization of health services by vulnerable groups. Poor people either did not have the money to pay or they were simply deterred and intimidated by the user fee policy itself. Apart from the exemption mechanisms not being publicized, their implementation was largely ineffective in protecting the poor. The plight of the poor in accessing health services is likely to suffer further as a result of the establishment of semi-autonomous hospitals which have the potential to implement regressive admission policies at their institutions. The successful implementation of the user fee policy at Health Center level in particular was affected by the high administrative costs of the process. The administrative costs at this level were actually higher than the revenue collected. A comprehensive user fee policy has been developed which also includes exemptions for maternal and child health services and the treatment of pensioners and the elderly at public health institutions. The treatment of tuberculosis at public and private institutions is free.

Up until towards the end of the year 2008 the Social Health Insurance (SHI) scheme which has been in the pipeline since the 1980s had not been established. By way of progress, an Act of parliament was enacted in 2007 to provide for the establishment of the SHI scheme. The lack of progress has partly been attributed to concerns by stakeholders on the economic down turn and its impact on the incomes of employees as well as the lengthy bureaucracy within relevant government departments.

In terms of earmarked taxes, the AIDS levy was successfully introduced in 2000 and has since provided invaluable support for the country's multi sectoral HIV/AIDS intervention efforts.

Decentralization of health services

Despite the fact that there is a lot of skepticism on the added value of decentralization this has been one of the most popular reforms being implemented across the divide. Experience with health sector reforms in Senegal reveal that decentralization reforms in that country led to widespread breakdown of the health system (Grundman, 2000). In Zambia when decentralization was implemented, the district level experienced less funding than they had received before the reforms (Chita, 2000). In the majority of cases in which decentralization reforms resulted in negative outcomes, poor implementation has been blamed for the failures. It is important to note that conclusions from literature on the decentralization of health services in African countries indicate that this policy reform has not achieved all its intended benefits.

In Zimbabwe poor coordination within government made it difficult to transform the policy on decentralization into reality. For example, there was no agreement as to how financial resources for the delivery of social services would flow from treasury to the RDCs. The Public Service Commission did not develop the modalities for transferring staff to RDCs and new recruitment procedures to be used in a decentralized form of government. Health workers were opposed to being employed by RDCs mainly because RDCs had a poor reputation with regards the management of council finances, staff salaries and health infrastructure.

Notable achievements in the implementation of the decentralization policy in Zimbabwe include:

- ♦ The development of an institutional framework for the devolution process within government which was largely agreed to.
- ♦ The health sector strategy to devolve health services to RDCs was approved by government and the association of RDCs of Zimbabwe.
- ♦ The Health Services Fund to manage a flexible pool of funds at national, provincial and district levels was established.
- ♦ A capacity building program for RDCs and District Health Management Teams was approved and implemented.
- ♦ Hospital Management Boards were established.
- ♦ Semi-autonomous hospitals were established.

Progress in the decentralization of health services to RDCs stalled as a result of the withdrawal of donor support to the overall decentralization program in government as well as specific support to the health reform program. The capacity building program for RDCs stopped also as a result of the termination of donor support. It is uncertain when the process is likely to resume in earnest, considering anticipated changes in government. The longer it takes to resuscitate the reform process, the more certain is the loss of institutional memory on the process. With a loss of institutional memory it becomes necessary to revisit the consensus building process, capacity building and baseline assessment of the reform situation. A more conducive social and political environment for change, sound leadership and stability in government over an extended period of time will be necessary if any meaningful change can be achieved, this time around.

New Public Management issues

Public management issues are driven more by the need to improve efficiencies in public sector management than by the need to improve the health status of the population.

Contracting out and commercialization

The government of Zimbabwe successfully commercialized the Drugs Control Council into a semi-autonomous and self financing Medicines Control Authority of Zimbabwe (MCAZ). The commercialization of the Government Medical Stores (GMS) was also finalized when a new company, Natpharm, was established. Each organization is managed by a CEO who is accountable to a management board. The viability of Natpharm has been affected by the country's critical shortage of foreign currency, making the company to rely on government grants and commodity support from donors, rather than being self-sustaining.

Hospital cleaning, hospital security, laundry and grounds maintenance at the five central hospitals, one provincial hospital and one general hospital were successfully subcontracted to private companies. The anticipated cost savings did not immediately materialize as contract costs exceeded initial estimates. The process has however reduced the opportunity costs resulting from the employment and supervision of unskilled staff in the public sector. The quality of services provided by contracted parties, though generally considered satisfactory, has varied by institution. It also became evident that the public sector did not have the capacity to design water tight contracts and to monitor them. The contracting-out of non-core services is now a permanent feature of the Ministry of Health that requires perfecting and, where possible, extension to district level.

Hospital autonomy

In 2000, in line with the Medical Services Act, the Minister of Health and Child Welfare appointed Hospital Management Boards to oversee the work of CEOs at the country's central hospitals. Management Boards at provincial hospitals are earmarked for appointment in the not too distant future. All central hospitals have appointed Chief Executive Officers to replace Medical Superintendents. The rest of the central hospital management team consists of the Director of Finance, the Director of Clinical Services and the Director of Operations. The conditions of service for the CEO and his/her directors are determined by the board and are based on 3-year performance contracts. The employment conditions of the rest of the hospital staff are determined by the Health Service Board. The next natural step is for the hospital Management Boards to be empowered to determine the conditions of services of the rest of the staff, under the guidance the Health Service Board. Management Boards should normally be able to determine the conditions of service for staff, hire, discipline and fire staff, as necessary. The legal framework that establishes this board should ideally have provided for the transfer and management of staff, movable and immovable assets of central and provincial hospitals from the government to the management boards.

There is anecdotal evidence that some aspects of the quality of hospital management at some of the central hospitals has improved. The combination of semi-autonomous status and contracting out seems to have resulted in improved cleanliness in some of these hospitals. The retention of revenue from user fee had an enormous impact initially until the hyperinflationary environment spoiled the party. The quality of care at these institutions continued to deteriorate for other reasons than the granting of semi-autonomous status. The contracts of the CEOs are not monitored, nor is the performance of CEOs appraised. Unfortunately, the civil service perception of permanence in positions of employment has slowly developed amongst the CEOs and led to complacence, with no institutional or personal incentives for improved performance and accountability.

The regulatory environment

The Medical Services Act and the Health Professions Act empower the Ministry of Health and Child Welfare to assume its rightful role as the regulator, to ensure the provision of quality health care, encourage fair play, correct market failures and maintain acceptable professional standards of practice. Independent professional councils proposed under the new Health Professions Act have been successfully established. In order to operate, public and private health facilities are accredited and inspected on a regular basis by the Health Professions Authority. Under the new Act, health insurance schemes operate only if they are registered by the Ministry of Health. According to the Act all insurance schemes are required to provide the core health service package as the minimum benefit package to their members. The Medicines Control Authority of Zimbabwe (MCAZ) is the designated regulating arm for the pharmaceutical industry.

Practical problems in this area include a lack of capacity in some of the professional councils to finance their operations on a sustainable basis. This often leads to inadequate capacity to carry out inspections on a regular basis and to follow up on decisions made during inspections.

Organizational restructuring

The Ministry of Health has undertaken several attempts to restructure and align its organizational structure to its roles and responsibilities, especially within a devolved health delivery system. Unfortunately such attempts have not been preceded by any functional reviews of the organization. The restructuring process has meant that semi-autonomous central and provincial hospitals do not fall under the direct management control of the central Ministry of Health. Within the hospitals, the post of CEO (a general manager) has replaced that of the Medical Superintendent as the head of the central hospital. The posts of Clinical Director, Director of Operations and Director of Finance have been created to underpin the CEO. The CEOs do not report to the Secretary for Health but are accountable to their respective Hospital Management Boards. Technically speaking, these institutions constitute the provider arm of the health sector, the Ministry of Health (headquarters) being the purchaser of services. Similar accountability relationships apply to the MCAZ, ZNFPC and Natpharm. Similar arrangements are expected to govern the management of the National Institute of Research (formerly the Blair Research Institute) and the Government Analyst Laboratory. The Health Service Board was established as part of the reform process to give effect to de-linking the health sector from the Public Service Commission.

A major reorganization of the Ministry of Health took place in 2000 whereby three new functional divisions were established at the ministry's headquarters: Technical Support, Finance, and Policy and Planning. The post of Chief Nursing Officer replaced that of Director of Nursing. A Quality Assurance unit was also established. The other major restructuring process took place in 2007 whereby some of the positions that prevailed prior to the 2000 reorganization where re-established; Curative Services, Preventive Services and the Director of Nursing. Of significance at policy level was the establishment of a unit responsible for Traditional Medicine.

The health work force

Yet another objective of the health reforms was to improve the availability, motivation and performance of the health work force in the public health sector and to put in place measures to retain staff. The achievement of this objective was however frustrated by the continued deterioration in the country's economy. The HIV/AIDS epidemic on the other hand increased the natural attrition of health workers through AIDS related deaths. The continued flight of skills meant that those health workers remaining in the service had an even greater workload, which increased their frustration and lowered their morale. The following are some of the reform initiatives undertaken in the area of human resources for health:

- De-linkage of health workers from the Public Service Commission through the establishment of a Health Service Board.
- Proposals to empower Hospital Management Boards to set conditions of service, hire, discipline and fire staff.
- The introduction of new cadres of health workers, e.g. the Primary Care Nurse, to alleviate the shortage of staff at rural health facilities.
- The establishment of a second medical school.
- Proposals to re-profile the role of the Clinical Nursing Officer to take a greater role in the management of patients.
- Employment of health workers on performance contracts:
  - Nurse trainees recruited on contract.
  - The CEO and directors at central hospitals employed on 3- year performance contracts.
  - Junior Resident Medical Officers (JRMOs) employed on contract.
  - Consultants yet to be employed on contract. (2008)

- The Health Professions Act reviewed to facilitate effective regulation of professional practice.
- Decentralization of Registered General Nurses training to Provincial, General and other hospitals.

In the final analysis the health sector was not able to achieve all the reform objectives in this area. Whilst the number of nurses trained was almost doubled and a new nurse cadre introduced, the rate of attrition also increased significantly and the shortage of nurses, especially in rural areas persists. There was no significant improvement in the numbers of medical doctors employed in the public health sector, especially in the rural areas. This was largely the result of continued deterioration in the conditions of service in the public sector coupled with a poor work environment. The Health Service Board did not receive the necessary financial support from the government to improve the conditions of service for health workers. The establishment of semi-autonomous hospitals is also likely to attract health workers from rural areas to these institutions if they are allowed to develop more favorable conditions of service for their staff. Some attractive retention schemes for health workers have been implemented in the public sector, unfortunately in a rather disjointed manner.

Conclusions on the impact of health reforms

It is evident from these analyses that not enough objective information is available to establish if health reforms in Zimbabwe achieved their intended objectives. What is clear however is that literally all aspects of the health delivery system in Zimbabwe continued to deteriorate over the decade that the health sector was implementing the reforms. The dilemma, though, is that whilst the reforms were also aimed at addressing health sector problems resulting from economic recession, the root cause of the problem persisted as the economy of the country continued its down ward spiral.

Triangulation of information collected from different sources suggests that the quality of care at public health institutions and the health status of the population have been on the decline, at least since the late 1990s until 2008. This is despite the fact that some specific health indicators have remained better than regional averages. Policies to diversify sources of health financing have had mixed results. At institutional level cost recovery and the retention of revenue from user fees significantly improved local revenue generation. Earmarked taxation in the form of the AIDS Trust

Fund was successfully introduced in 1999 and has mobilized resources that have over the years supported HIV/AIDS prevention and mitigation efforts. The HIV/AIDS Trust Fund was instrumental in supporting the introduction of the ART program in Zimbabwe. The user fee policy is unpopular and has proven to be a threat to the achievement of equity.

The process to introduce the sub-contracting of non-core services was completed though its benefits are not yet very apparent in the health sector. It terms of civil service reforms the implementation of subcontracting reduced the government salary bill by transferring these costs to another budget sub item.

The reforms did not improve equity in resource allocation within the sector. Disparities in per capita resource (budgetary, human resources, drugs, number of beds) allocations continue between and within provinces. The poor continue to be exposed to substandard health care and health facilities. The reforms have also not adequately addressed capacity in human resources planning and management within the health sector.

Reforms have however brought about a fundamental shift in management relationships within the public health sector through the establishment of semi-autonomous hospitals. These institutions are no longer under the direct management control of the Ministry of Health bureaucracy. The establishment of the Health Service Board introduced a paradigm shift in the management of government employees as the determination of conditions of service for health workers is no longer the responsibility of the PSC.

The reforms in Zimbabwe were incremental in their nature and mainly led by "reform architects" within the Ministry of Health. However with the advent of an unstable political environment leading to the 2002 presidential elections and beyond some senior civil servants toned down some of the reform elements considered to be a threat to the political and election process. The withdrawal of donor support to the reform process, more pressing economic problems and severe budgetary constraints have relegated health sector reforms to the bottom of the priority list of government. In the author's view, this should have been the most opportune time for a more concerted effort to implementing the health reform process.

Some weaknesses in the reform process

Situation analysis

The Ministry of Health did not undertake any situation analysis prior to undertaking its health reform process. As a result the design of the reform strategy was based on intuition and any relevant information available from studies not specifically tailored for this purpose. Apart from the design and implementation process of the reform program relying heavily on external technical assistance, most of the information used was based on regional and international experience considered to be relevant to the country situation.

Reform plan for the sector

Even though a concept paper for the health reforms had been developed at the inception of the reform process there was initially no schedule of events or milestones to be achieved or monitored during the process of reform. However, as the reform process unfolded and development partners began to fully participate in the process, a plan of action emerged. A benchmark system was developed and put in place to monitor progress in the implementation of the reforms.

Stakeholder participation

Consultations are considered an essential ingredient for successful reforms. It is important that there is local ownership and an all inclusive process. An analysis of the process in Zimbabwe leads one to conclude that the health reform agenda was largely top-down and driven by Ministry of Health technocrats. The central Ministry of Health led the process with minimum participation by staff at the operational level. Donors seem to have been involved much more than Ministry of Health staff. However some of the internal processes of the reform process seem to have been undertaken with the necessary levels of consultation. For example, there were consultations on the Social Health Insurance scheme with the National Association of Medical Aid Societies (NAMAS) and the Zimbabwe Congress of Trade Unions (ZCTU) being actively involved. ZIMA, ZINA, Association of Health Funders (formerly NAMAS) and the Association of Private Hospitals of Zimbabwe were involved in the formulation of the Medical Services Act. The Association of Urban Councils and the Association of Rural District Councils actively participated in the development of the decentralization strategy of the Ministry of Health. The review of the Medical, Dental and Allied Professions Act was undertaken with the full participation of all the health professional groups, NGOs as well as interested civil society groups.

Consideration of financial implications of the reform agenda

The costs of implementing the reform program were not fully assessed at the inception of the health reform process. As a result not all available options of financing the reforms were exploited. When the reforms were in full swing they were at the mercy of two major donors, DANIDA and the EU. Because the government did not explicitly contribute financial resources to the reform process, this gave the impression that the reforms were more a result of pressure from donors than a government initiative. As a result when DANIDA unilaterally terminated its support to the government of Zimbabwe the implementation of the major aspects of the reform program also came to an end.

Communications strategy

Despite the production of a Ministry of Health quarterly newsletter, *Lifelines*, the communication strategy on health reforms proved to be an uphill struggle. The advocacy strategy on reforms was thus ineffective in disseminating the message of reform across to all the stakeholders. Little or no information on the reforms reached the majority of staffs within the health sector at district and sub district levels. Civil society groups and the private sector were completely left out of the information loop on health reforms. The result was that there was a lot of ignorance about the reform process. The little that stakeholders knew seemed to alienate them from the Ministry of Health. The general public was also of the opinion that not much was being done to arrest the rapid decline in the quality of health services in the public sector. This was because both the general public and the private sector were not really aware of the reform initiatives that the Ministry of Health had put in place to try and reverse the deteriorating conditions in the public health sector. The health sector did not undertake any media briefings to counter these adverse reports.

The introduction of new procedures and rules

New reform or policy initiatives usually require new legislation, new rules and procedures to back them. In the case of the health reforms in Zimbabwe, when this was done, obsolete regulations were not immediately reviewed, causing confusion in some cases. A good example is the introduction of the Health Service Fund (HSF) which required the introduction of commercial accounting procedures. After the HSF started operating existing government accounting procedures remained in force for some time, making it very difficult for the districts to operate the HSF.

Furthermore, HSF manuals and guidelines were introduced late, long after the HSF had become operational.

The need for an enabling environment

Political stability, political will and trust between development partners and the government are often highlighted as being essential ingredients for successful implementation and outcome of reforms. The fact that reforms in Zimbabwe were implemented during a politically and economically turbulent period in the country's history makes it very difficult to clearly define the impact which can be attributed directly to them as opposed to those effects of other intervening factors. It is also difficult to ascertain if the developments in the health sector would have been much worse than they are had the reforms not been implemented.

There is however no doubt that the meltdown in the country's economy contributed directly and indirectly to the deterioration of the health system in Zimbabwe. The adverse socio-economic environment diverted the attention of the health sector from pursuing and building on some of the achievements of the reform agenda. The rift between development partners and the government of Zimbabwe dealt a significant blow to the support the reform process was receiving from donors. The withdrawal of financial and technical support by DANIDA and the EU, in particular, affected the operations of the Health Services Fund which had become an efficient conduit for the flow of finances to support district operations.

In 1999 the health sector in Zimbabwe resisted pressure from the World Bank and other development partners to embark on a SWAp. This was the period the health sector was developing its National Health Strategy (1997-2007). The Ministry of Health was of the opinion that the consultative processes in planning, budgeting, monitoring and evaluation were already based on sector wide thinking. Furthermore, like-minded donors and multilateral organizations were withdrawing overseas development assistance and calling for the isolation of the country. Under these circumstances it was in the best interest of the country for the government to deal with donors on an individual rather than a collective basis. After all, the spirit behind the SWAp is a coordinated approach based on trust - and there was no trust between the government and donors!

The way forward for the health sector in Zimbabwe

Improving the economic and political environment

Unless the social, political and economic environment in Zimbabwe improves, the future of the health sector in Zimbabwe remains bleak. Any attempt to improve the health system must do so from several fronts. First and foremost there must be a conviction and the political will to increase public health expenditures to at least US$34 per capita. Due cognizance must be taken that this amount of expenditures only covers basic care, including ARV therapy, and the infrastructure necessary to deliver it. As these estimates do not cover specialist and referral services, it will be necessary to estimate the additional financial requirements to provide referral and specialist services.

There must be additional commitment to a new and sound economic order for the country and a deliberate strategy to eliminate poverty, reduce unemployment rates and strengthen social safety nets and coping mechanisms for the poor. The prevalence rate of extreme poverty estimated to be 38.9% in 2004 is an obvious constraint to health development. When heads of households for poor people become ill their entire household becomes in jeopardy as they lose their income and incur very high health costs. Good health contributes to the development of a country through; higher productivity, improved human capital, higher rates of national savings and improved demographics. More effort must be invested in empowering the poor and civil society groups and to increase their participation in health planning and implementation processes.

Strengthening partnerships in the health sector

Any proposals to further market orientation of the public health sector in Zimbabwe must be considered with caution. There is little evidence that market oriented health care systems are more efficient than public health care systems. The truth of the matter is that in a market oriented health care system it is probably considered profitable to produce unnecessary care. Furthermore, where there are profit oriented voluntary insurance schemes, transaction costs (inefficiencies) may be as high as 40% in some cases. There is compelling evidence that public health care systems can guarantee equity and thus be considered more efficient compared to market oriented systems. Where there are inefficiencies in public health systems these can and should be resolved through the adoption of appropriate public health policies.

The above arguments do not mean that the government should exclude the development of a viable and complementary private for profit sector. The private-for-profit medical sector is necessary to ensure the health market has choices and for those who can afford and are willing to pay for their own health care, to exercise that right unhindered. There must however be a well regulated environment and no subsidies of the private medical sector by the public sector. In addition to regulating the private sector the government must pursue a collaborative approach in engaging this sector. Several options for such collaboration are available:

+ Integrating private practitioners into the public sector.
+ Provision of incentives for private practitioners to provide preventive services.
+ Contracting private-for-profit institutions and private-not-for-profit institutions e.g. NGOs and missions to offer health services to populations located in areas where the government does not have its own facilities.
+ Efficient management of the privileges granted to public sector health workers to do private practice.

Visionary health sector leadership

The public health sector is expected to lead the national health development process by providing the strategic vision and direction for the sector based on the expectations of the people. The government must also ensure that every individual is guaranteed access to quality health care and that every citizen is protected against poverty precipitated by illness. It is therefore the responsibility of the government to work towards achieving universal access to health and health care by its people, to increase national resources allocated to the health sector, to implement risk pooling and removal of economic barriers to access to health care. The building of partnerships between the state and other providers of health is one means to ensure sustained health service delivery coverage.

A turnaround strategy for the sector will require visionary leadership, an understanding of current global, regional and national health policies and issues, the capacity to set a credible strategic direction for the sector and a capacity for creativity. The health sector leadership must clearly articulate the central objectives of the organization and those responsibilities to be devolved to the operational level. Such a transformation will require a complete paradigm shift, from an administrative culture to a management culture, which must permeate throughout the organization. The concept of general management must be clearly understood to avoid mis-understandings between general managers and professional staff within the sector. It must be clear that professional management deals with the internal management of the responsibilities and workload of profession-als within specific departments. It deals with the management concerns of clinicians within their respective specialties.

The policy process, which is led by the government, must address some of the core public health functions as well as strengthening support systems for the health sector. The main priority is to strengthen the health system by developing strategies and initiatives on: health technologies, essential medicines, workforce planning and development, investment in develop-ing the health delivery platform, addressing governance issues (regulation, accreditation and health legislation) and health financing.

In the technical area of curative and public health programming, sev-eral areas must be addressed; the development and enforcement of norms, standards and quality assurance in the delivery of disease interventions across the spectrum of health promotion, prevention, treatment and care and rehabilitation. In particular, it is crucial to address behaviors and life-styles of individuals and communities, to provide water and sanitation, nutrition, and to deal with epidemics and disasters by ensuring adequate measures for preparedness and control.

Development of Human Resources for Health

Development partners have demonstrated their willingness to assist with the resolution of the Human Resources for Health crisis in devel-oping countries. In order to benefit from this goodwill the Ministry of Health has to develop a comprehensive human resources development plan with all the costs of implementation clearly articulated, including a financial gap analysis.

The role, objectives and responsibilities of the Health Service Board must be clearly and understood. The board must be supported with ade-quate financial resources to support its operations and the implementation of its recommendations on improved conditions of services for health workers. Without adequate resources, the Health Service Board is no dif-ferent from the Public Service Commission. It must be perfectly clear that the mere existence of a Health Service Board will not in itself improve the conditions and well being of health workers.

According to Cassels (1995) when the employment of health workers is taken out of the civil service, government may lose the normal control of the civil service in terms of reducing overall public sector spending. Furthermore, to make any meaningful change, compensation for loss of government conditions of service must be substantial if it is to ensure that health workers are not disadvantaged by the new conditions of service under a Health Service Board.

Pursuing the reform agenda

Judging from the lack of both strategic and operational capacity at all levels of the health delivery system, an informed and cautious approach to the reform agenda is advised. In further pursuing the decentralization of health services to local authorities, government must guarantee the availability of adequate financial support to RDCs and ensure the availability of acceptable capacity within the RDCs to effectively provide social services.

Considering the current state of the health sector in Zimbabwe and the inability of the government to finance the sector, another intense phase of health reforms cannot be avoided. This next phase of the reform agenda is likely to be more rapid and radical. Donors are likely to pressure the government to:

- Improve accountability in the use of resources
- Commit to the decentralization process
  - The Health Service Fund will come in handy for channeling and managing development assistance
- Implement the Sector Wide Approach (SWAp).
- Strengthen private and public collaboration
- Enter into contractual relationships with mission institutions
- Involve civil society, NGOs, etc. in the health development process
- Develop a comprehensive human resources for health development plan.

Improving aid effectiveness at country level

The government has to strengthen its capacity to coordinate development partners who are willing to support efforts to reform the health delivery system. The Sector Wide Approach (SWAp) to health development is one popular approach among the development community. The Ministry of Health is encouraged to acquaint itself with the SWAp, the Paris Declaration and Accra Agenda for Action for improving aid effectiveness, if it is to benefit from significant overseas development assistance. The sector already has a national health strategic framework, which needs updating and a Health Services Fund which forms a credible basis for pooling donor and government funds at national and district levels. The SWAp approach has the potential to strengthen district support systems in planning, budgeting, procurement, and monitoring and evaluation.

Donors will probably try at all costs not to place any explicit conditionality for the assistance but will, to the extent possible, abide by the Paris Declaration and the Accra Agenda for Action in achieving aid effectiveness. Whilst development assistance will be forthcoming, it is unlikely to be a walk in the park.

The ultimate goal is to achieve demonstrable improvements in the health status of each and every member of society. Peculiar circumstances and capacities in each country determine the best local approach to health reforms. Whereas reforms in developed countries seek ways to contain costs those in African countries seek means to raise additional resources. Both reform environments however aim to achieve increased efficiencies in the utilization of resources. Because reforms require major changes and have objectives that often conflict with political and societal values they will, in most cases than not, be opposed. Experience shows that the identification of leaders who are committed to reforms positively influences the course of the reform process. After all, the reform agenda is always in a state of flux with situations likely to change any minute depending on the prevailing political temperature.

The question to answer is: "Will the health sector in Zimbabwe be able, once more, to join the rest of the world and achieve targets set for health related Millennium Development Goals, as stated in Table 13.1? This is the challenge faced by most if not all health systems in Africa.

Table 13.1 Progress on health related millennium development goals (2008)

Goals and Targets of the Millennium Declaration	Indicators for monitoring Progress	1995 – 1999 Baseline level	ZDHS 2005-06 level	2015 Target
Goal 4: Reduce child mortality				
	Under-five mortality rate.	102 deaths per 1 000	82 deaths per 1 000	34 per 1000
	Infant mortality rate.	53 deaths per 1000 live births	60 deaths per 1 000 live births	
Reduce by 2/3 between 1990 and 2015.	Proportion of one-year old children immunized against measles.	71%	65.6%	90%
	Proportion of children under the age of five years malnourished	13%		7%
Goal 5: Improve maternal health				
Reduce by ¾, between 1990 and 2015, the MMR	Maternal mortality ratio.	570-695 deaths per 100 000 live births	555 deaths per 100 000 live births	174 deaths per 100 000 live births
	Proportion of births attended by skilled health personnel.	30 - 72%	68%	100%
Goal 6: Combat HIV/AIDS, malaria and other diseases				
Have halted by 2015 and begun to reverse the spread of HIV/AIDS.	HIV prevalence among 15-24 pregnant women.	32%	18%	<16%
	Condom use rate			
	Contraceptive prevalence rate		58%	
	Number of children orphaned by HIV/AIDS.			
	Incidence rate of malaria.	122/1000 persons		64/1 000 persons
Have halted by 2015 and begun to reverse the incidence of malaria and other major diseases.	Prevalence and death rates associated with tuberculosis.			
	Proportion of population in malaria risk areas using effective measures for malaria prevention and treatment			
	Proportion of tuberculosis cases detected and cured under directly observed treatment, short-course (DOTS)			
	Tuberculosis incidence rate	399/100 000 population		121/100 000 population
Goal 8: Develop a Global Partnership for development				
In cooperation with pharmaceutical companies, provide access to affordable essential drugs in developing countries.	Proportion of population with access to affordable, essential drugs on a sustainable basis.			

The following tables summarize some of the critical activities that need to be considered at the policy, strategic and operational levels of the health system in order to revamp the health delivery system in Zimbabwe. The revival of the health sector will depend to a large extent on the stabilization of the political environment which is expected to create a conducive atmosphere for sustained economic growth. Economic growth is in turn expected to facilitate increased government expenditures on health and education and thus provide resources to invest in strengthening the health delivery system. Addressing governance and accountability issues provides the necessary confidence for development partners to invest their resources in the country's health and other sectors.

At service delivery level health sector priorities should focus on areas that contribute most to poor health and the burden of disease in Zimbabwe such as child health conditions, women's health, HIV/AIDS, infectious diseases and nutrition. The major causes of disease in each of these areas are well known and simple, cost effective and affordable interventions are available. Major causes of ill health in children include pneumonia, diarrhea, malaria and measles. Major interventions in this area include the provision of immunizations, oral rehydration therapy, newborn resuscitation, Nevirapine, water, sanitation and hygiene. In the area of women's health an affordable and comprehensive package of reproductive health interventions is available to be complemented by improved access to emergency obstetric care, contraceptives, the prevention, diagnosis and treatment of Sexually Transmitted Infections (STI). An effective package of interventions for HIV/AIDS prevention and improved access to treatment and care is available. Resources have recently been made available for interventions in the area of neglected infectious diseases such as intestinal helminthes, trachoma, schistosomiasis, leprosy, African trypanosomiasis, in addition to tuberculosis and malaria. Nutrition, which recognizes food as a health intervention, is yet another priority area for the health sector in terms of providing food supplementation for school children, children under the age of 5 years, orphans, feeding of pregnant women, and nutrition support to the treatment of tuberculosis, HIV/AIDS and palliative care.

For effective implementation, these programs must be delivered in an integrated manner and as part of the overall health delivery system, which must be appropriately strengthened. This will involve increasing population access to identified cost effective health interventions, the development of health infrastructure, strengthening of health support systems such as the efficient deployment and supervision of human resources, improved management, logistics, health information systems, disease surveillance, monitoring and evaluation and equipment.

Table 13.2 Establishment of a stable economic environment

Priority Area	Actions Areas	Specific Areas of action	Time Frame
Socio-Economic Development	Macro-Economic Policies.	Implement a sound Economic Recovery Program – sustained economic growth	Medium to long Term
	Poverty Reduction.	Focus on Poverty Reduction in terms of policies, strategies and activities to reduce poverty – social safety nets, social assistance programs, and improved capacity to identify the poor and respond to their needs (social targeting).	Immediate to Medium Term
	Overseas Development Assistance (ODA)	Put in place an effective coordination mechanism for the management of overall development assistance to the country.	Immediate

Table 13.3 Addressing governance and accountability issues

Priority Area	Actions Areas	Specific Areas of action	Time Frame
Governance and Accountability	Elimination of corruption.	Establish a stable political environment, accountability to citizens, accountability within public institutions, responsible utilization of resources	Immediate.
	Effective management of Overseas Development Assistance	Design and implement a harmonized framework for coordinated management of development assistance to the health sector – through the Sector Wide Approach (SWAp); General Budget Support	Immediate to long Term
		All parties to ODA to implement and monitor recommendations of the Paris Declaration to ensure improved aid effectiveness. Adherence to the Accra Agenda for Action on aid Effectiveness	Immediate to Medium
	Visionary leadership	Develop and adopt a common vision and mission for the sector – development of a Health Sector Strategic Plan.	Immediate to long term
		Build capacity for health sector leadership, capacity to steer a strategic direction for the health sector, build partnerships for health, effectively regulate the sector and coordinate development partners to ensure support and convergence on country priorities and attainment of tangible results.	Immediate to long term

Table 13.4 Strengthening systems within the health sector

Priority Area	Actions Areas	Specific Areas of action	Time Frame
Health Systems Strengthening	Strategic and operational planning	Conduct a health sector analysis/ assessment and identify key system constraints.	Immediate
		Plan for the health sector (public & private) in context of national socio-development plan, PRSP, MTEF and MDG approach.	Immediate
		Develop a single national health policy and strategy to guide both the public and private health sectors.	Immediate
		Develop and fully cost an all-inclusive health program of work that covers the whole sector and ensure all stake-holders buy into this single framework.	Immediate to Medium Term.
	Service delivery	Develop an affordable comprehensive, essential package of health services targeted at the most vulnerable groups (the poor), delivered by the public sector and complemented by the private sector.	Immediate to Medium Term.
		Strengthen the referral system to support the PHC package. Rehabilitate and equip all central and provincial hospitals	Medium to Long Term
		Strengthen capacity and improve the quality of diagnostic and public laboratory network	Immediate to Medium Term
	Restructuring the health sector	Undertake a Functional review and restructure the health ministry to respond effectively to current needs of the health sector.	Immediate to Medium Term
		Strength existing health management structures and insti-tutions and build appropriate capacity at local level within the MOH in line with the decentralization process.	Medium to Long Term.
		Assess and strengthen the capacity of RDCS and Urban Councils to take up new health service delivery respon-sibilities.	Medium Term
		Define, legislate for and consolidate the roles and responsi-bilities of the various levels of the health delivery system. Define policies that will ensure the sustainability and effec-tive functioning of semi-autonomous hospitals.	Immediate
		Advocate for the harmonization of legislation related to the roles and responsibilities of local government institutions in a decentralized environment.	Immediate to Medium Term
	Health Financing and Financial Management.	Develop a health financing policy for the sector and focus on increasing government investment in the health sector.	Immediate to Long Term
		Develop and implement a strategy and plan to strengthen financial management and ensure transparency and accountability within the sector. Strengthen the manage-ment of the Health Service Fund at all levels	Immediate to Medium Term.
		Undertake regular National Health Accounts and health sector expenditure reviews.	Ongoing.
		Advocate for the finalization of the process to establish a Social Health Insurance Scheme.	Medium term.
		Design and implement sustainable strategies for private and public collaboration.	Immediate to Medium Term.

Priority Area	Actions Areas	Specific Areas of action	Time Frame
	Regulation of the health sector.	Strengthen and consolidate the regulatory role of the MO-HCW, function and capacity of Health Professions Authority and other regulatory bodies.	Immediate to medium term
		Provide a once off financial bail out for the Health Professions Authority	
		Improve health sector capacity to formulate, analyze and enforce policies.	Medium term
	District Health System	Consolidate the composition, role and function of District Health Management Teams (DHMTs).	Immediate.
		Strengthen district level capacity for coordination, operational planning and budgeting, financial management, program implementation, service delivery and monitoring and evaluation.	Immediate to long Term.
		Consolidate the utilization of the Health Service Fund (HSF), especially at the district level and the implementation of community based health activities	Immediate to medium term
	Community Participation	Increase the space for communities and civil society groups to engage and hold providers of health services accountable – strengthen the various health committees, local governance structures, etc.	Immediate to Long Term.
	Human Resources for Health	Transform and strengthen the "personnel unit" of MOHCW into a fully fledged Human Resources Department.	Immediate to Medium Term
		Develop and cost human resources for health policy, strategy and plan, and information system. Solicit for international support for the development of HRH	Immediate to long term
		Together with relevant stakeholders, develop, implement and monitor a training policy and strategy for the sector.	Immediate to Medium Term
		Strengthen and consolidate the role, operations and independence of the Health Service Board.	Immediate
		Develop a short-term strategy to address shortages of HRH – a comprehensive package of incentives to retain health professionals. Solicit for support from development partners to finance the scheme sector wide	Immediate.
	Procurement, distribution and management of supplies.	Conduct an emergency assessment of essential drugs and supplies requirement and initiate an emergency procurement and distribution plan and strategy for the sector.	Immediate
		Quantify and cost total sectoral needs for drugs and other essential supplies and develop annualized procurement plans.	Immediate
		Provide once off capitalization to enable Natpharm to procure drugs and other supplies and sell them at a reasonable return to the public and private sectors.	Immediate
		Assessment of health sector requirements for technical assistance (TA) and development of a TA procurement plan and budget for demand driven Technical Assistance (TA).	Immediate to medium term

Priority Area	Actions Areas	Specific Areas of action	Time Frame
	Procurement, distribution and management of supplies	Develop and implement a fully fledged Zimbabwe Essential Drugs Action Plan (ZEDAP) for rational use of essential drugs.	Immediate to long term
		Provide financial bailout for the recapitalization of the Medicines Control Authority of Zimbabwe.	
	Physical Assets Management and Essential Health Technology	Develop and cost an investment policy, strategy and plan for health sector-rehabilitation, facility upgrading and construction.	Immediate to Medium Term
		Update the 1999 health facilities database and GIS map. Map out gaps in the distribution of health facilities resulting from new settlement patterns	Medium Term.
		Develop policies to guide the management of physical assets in the health sector.	Medium to Long Term
		Consider options to outsource physical assets management.	Medium term
		Update the standard equipment lists for each level of the health delivery system in line with developments in the service package to be delivered.	Immediate
		Update the national equipment database.	Immediate
		Quantify, cost and undertake emergency procurement of basic medical equipment.	Immediate to Medium Term
		Develop and enforce a transport management policy and procure the necessary transport requirements for the health sector.	Immediate to Medium Term
		Update IT hard ware and soft ware for routine Health Information and surveillance information systems.	
		Develop a common monitoring, assessment and evaluation strategy and framework based on joint evaluation procedures, common indicators and a Sector Wide Approach.	Immediate
		Maintain a sustainable epidemiological database and epidemic response system.	Immediate
		Update and implement the policy on essential health research.	Immediate to medium term
	Quality Assurance	Develop and implement a Quality Assurance program for health services.	Immediate to Medium Term.

Review questions

1. From the analysis of the Zimbabwe Health System outlined in the previous chapters, is the reform strategy adopted the best way to improve the performance of the sector?

2. One of the weaknesses cited in the design and implementation of the reforms in Zimbabwe is the lack of adequate consultations and involvement of the public and professional bodies. Discuss.

3. Health reforms in African countries have been considered to be the result of the conditionality of Economic Structural Adjustment Programs. Justify and/or discredit this statement.

4. The reform agenda in Zimbabwe has not achieved its objectives. Discuss.

APPENDIX 1

THE CORE HEALTH SERVICE PACKAGE FOR ZIMBABWE

Background

The Ministry of Health and Child Welfare and its stakeholders developed the following core health service package in 1994.

Objectives

+ To define a cost effective package of services targeted at the poor which would be made available at all times at the various levels of the health delivery system.
+ To define the minimum standards for physical infrastructure, staffing, equipment and supplies required to deliver the package at each level of the health system.
+ To define a package that is both essential and yet affordable to both the government and the consumer.
+ To develop simple indicators to monitor progress in the implementation of the package, its quality, access and impact on the health status of the population.

Organization of the health delivery system

The Zimbabwe health delivery system has since the country's independence been organized into four hierarchical levels forming the referral system.

+ The Primary level consisting of community health services which link with the formal health delivery system at the health center (RHC) level.

- The Secondary level which consists of the District Hospital, in some cases mission hospitals, as the first referral level which is supported by the operations of the District Health Management Team (DHMT). The DHMT coordinates a network of primary health facilities; NGO clinics, RHCs, Council clinics and private clinics within the district.
- The Tertiary level consisting of the Provincial Hospital which provides selected specialist referral services to district and mission hospitals. The Provincial Medical Directors' offices support public health programs and oversee the operations of all health providers within the province.
- The Quaternary level which consists of 5 (national) specialist referral hospitals which are also teaching hospitals.

Community based health services

These are incremental activities undertaken by the following categories of health workers:

Village Health Workers (VHW) and Farm Health Workers (FHW) responsible for:
- Health promotion for selected program areas.
- Community based growth monitoring.
- Community mobilization - health campaigns etc.
- Collection of community based health information.
- Supervision of community based supplementary feeding schemes.
- First aid treatment.
- Support to home based care activities.
- Participation in local health committee structures.

Community Based Distributors (CBD)
- Initiating certain contraceptive methods and supplying contraceptives including condoms.
- Promotion, prevention and control activities on STIs, HIV/AIDS, FP, MCH etc.

Traditional Midwives
- Perform normal deliveries.
- Attend upgrading courses undertaken by the MOHCW.
- Encouraged to refer pregnant women for ANC and delivery at health facilities.

- Promote breast feeding, FP, EPI, baby hygiene, HIV/AIDS messages etc.
- Receive and use delivery kits from the MOHCW.

Traditional health practitioners
- Practice of traditional medicine under the Traditional Health Practitioners Act.
- Health promotion - HIV/AIDS, FP etc.
- Referral of patients to health centers.
- Collaborate in research

Health center based activities

Health Promotion and Preventive services
Promotion activities
- Organization of IEC activities in partnership with NGOs, communities, civil society groups, etc.
- Outreach activities including educational campaigns on various program areas.
- Supervision of VHW, FHW, and CBDs, etc.

Preventive services
- Child Health Services:
  - Growth monitoring and nutrition surveillance.
  - EPI, prevention of malaria and diarrheal diseases, promotion of the use ORT/SSS, etc.
- Reproductive health
  - ANC and PNC.
  - Safe motherhood initiatives.
  - FP: oral contraceptives, condoms and spermicides.
  - Promotion of breast feeding practices, STIs, HIV/AIDS prevention and control.
  - Counseling services for STIs, HIV AIDS etc.
  - Supervision of Traditional Midwives.
  - Micronutrient supplementation for pregnant women.
  - Disease surveillance
  - Investigation, control and notification of disease outbreaks.
  - Collection of appropriate information - integrated disease surveillance.
- Environmental health services
  - Citing and support to communities to construct toilets, waste disposal dumps, protected wells, etc.

♦ Inspection of food handling premises.
♦ Construction, protection and upkeep of small rural water supplies.

♦ Outreach services
  ♦ Domiciliary visits on EPI, growth monitoring, IEC, FP etc.
  ♦ Support to community based health workers.
  ♦ School health programs.

Curative services

♦ Child Health
  ♦ Integrated Management of Childhood Illnesses.
  ♦ Treatment of Acute Respiratory Infections.
  ♦ Prevention and treatment of diarrheal diseases (CDD).
  ♦ Use of ORT or Sugar Salt Solution (SSS).
  ♦ Nutrition rehabilitation.
  ♦ Treatment of minor injuries and locally endemic conditions.

♦ Reproductive health
  ♦ Antenatal and Postnatal care.
  ♦ Provision of Essential Obstetric Care.
  ♦ Early referral of abnormal pregnancies.
  ♦ Syndromic management of STIs and opportunistic infections.
  ♦ Support to home-based care activities.

♦ Chronic diseases
  ♦ Maintenance of chronic disease registers.
  ♦ Re supply of drugs to patients with chronic diseases.
  ♦ Contact tracing of TB (DOTS) and other chronic disease patients.

♦ Minor clinical procedures
  ♦ Suturing minor lacerations, episiotomy.
  ♦ Assessment, incision and drainage of minor abscesses.
  ♦ Insertion of Intra Uterine contraceptive Devices (where a nurse has been trained).
  ♦ Urinalysis for protein.
  ♦ Hemoglobin estimation.

♦ Rehabilitation services
  ♦ Identification of at risk babies post delivery
  ♦ Education of mothers on at risk babies
  ♦ Keeping a register of disabled persons within the catchment area.

♦ Staffing requirements
  ♦ Standard staffing levels:
  ♦ 2 Nurses/Midwives
  ♦ 1 Environmental Health Technician (EHT) per ward.
  ♦ 1 Nurse Aide.
  ♦ 1 General hand.

- ◆ Flexible staffing levels
  - ◆ 1 Nurse for 28 new patients per day.
  - ◆ A work load of at least 52 new patients daily requires 2 nurses (midwives)
  - ◆ A work load of 120 new patients daily requires 4 nurses (2 of which are midwives).
- ◆ Support services
  - ◆ Health center committee - meets once a month.
  - ◆ Health Center Team meeting - monthly or as necessary.
  - ◆ Attend District Health Team meetings - quarterly.
  - ◆ Receive regular supervision - monthly.
- ◆ Basic infrastructure
  - ◆ A standard Rural Health Center as per Family Health Project 1
  - ◆ Land size 10 000 square meters.
  - ◆ Running water, electricity from main grid or solar power.
  - ◆ Radio communications/telephone -24 hour link to district hospital as well as with Ambulance.
  - ◆ 3 staff houses (F14 rural).
  - ◆ Refrigerator.
  - ◆ 1 placenta disposal pit.
  - ◆ 1 refuse pit.
  - ◆ 3 Blair toilets
  - ◆ Perimeter fence.
  - ◆ Equipment according to the standard equipment list.
  - ◆ A postal bag where possible.

District Core Health Services

Promotive and Preventive Services

Maternal and Child Health Services

- ◆ Reproductive health services, IEC on - STIs, FP, HIV/AIDS, ANC, PNC etc.
- ◆ Providing counseling services - STI, HIV/AIDS etc.
- ◆ Adolescent and youth health services.
- ◆ Comprehensive Essential Obstetric Care.
- ◆ Growth Monitoring.
- ◆ Immunization.
- ◆ Other outreach services.

Nutrition

- ◆ Community based nutrition programs - growth monitoring, therapeutic and supplementary feeding schemes.

- Promotion of safe breast-feeding practices.
- Promoting baby friendly hospital initiatives.
- Prevention of micronutrient deficiencies - Vitamin A, Iodine and Iron.

Environmental health services
- Support to communities in the construction of Blair toilets.
- Food safety control: ensure food handlers undergo medical examinations.
- Vermin control.
- Investigation of food outbreaks.
- Food sampling.
- Inspection of premises.
- Waste disposal.
- Meat inspection.
- Water quality - sampling of drinking water supplies.

Prevention and control of Communicable Diseases
- Epidemic preparedness and control activities.
- Epidemic disease surveillance.
- Notification of diseases in terms of the Public Health Act.
- Reporting of reportable or sentinel conditions - measles, neonatal tetanus, malaria, polio, dysentery etc.
- Notification of notifiable diseases.

Health Information
- Collection, analysis and use of health information.

Oral health services
- Oral health campaigns

Outreach services
- Immunizations.
- Psychiatric services.
- School health program.
- Home based care.
- Information, education and communication activities.
- Educational/information campaigns - HIV/AIDS, STIs, Malaria, EPI, cholera, etc.

Curative care services

These services include those listed under the Health Center level but require more experienced staff and more sophisticated equipment. The services are provided to patients referred from RHCs, clinics, mission hospitals, rural hospitals and private clinics. This level also deals with patients who are referred back from provincial and central hospitals. Occasionally there are those patients who bypass the health center and come straight to the district hospital. Emergencies are attended to irrespective of referral status.

Clinical services

- Outpatient and inpatient services, accident and emergencies.
- Diagnosis and treatment of acute and chronic medical and pediatric conditions which include:-
  - IMCI and CDD.
  - Hypertension.
  - Diabètes mellitus.
  - ARI.
  - Malaria.
  - TB.
  - Measles.
  - Malnutrition.
  - Treatment of opportunistic infections.
  - Treatment of eye conditions.
  - Etc.
- Medical procedures:-
  - Lumbar puncture.
  - Blood transfusion.
  - Electro cardiogram.
- Common surgical procedures:-
  - Emergency laparotomy for acute abdomen.
  - Treatment of simple fractures.
  - Circumcision.
  - Repair of hernias.
  - Relief of acute urinary retention.
  - Appendicectomy.
  - Chest drainage.
  - Venous cut down.
- Comprehensive essential obstetric care.
  - Normal and complicated deliveries.
  - Caesarian sections.
  - Vacuum extraction.
  - Induction of labor.
- Special care of babies
  - Phototherapy.
  - Care of preterm babies.

- Management of common gynecological conditions including:
    - Laparotomy (emergency).
    - Repair of ruptured uterus.
    - Tubal-ligation.
    - Dilatation and curettage.
    - Evacuation of uterus.
    - Post abortion care.
    - PAP smear.
    - Cervical biopsy.
- Oral health services
    - Scaling, filling and extraction of teeth.
- Rehabilitation services
    - Assessment and physiotherapy for clients.
    - Provision of aids and appliances.
    - Counseling.
- Eye services
    - Treatment of eye conditions.
    - Eye surgery by visiting eye specialists.

Diagnostic services

Radiology services

- Basic radiological examinations - chest, abdomen, spine (thoracic, lumbar and cervical), skull, pelvis and hip.
- Ultrasound scans.

Laboratory services

- Blood investigations:
    - Hemoglobin.
    - White cell count.
    - Differential cell count.
    - ESR.
- Biochemistry:
    - Urine chemistry - glucose, protein levels.
    - Blood chemistry - glucose, potassium, urea.
    - Cerebrospinal fluid - glucose, protein.
- Bacteriology and parasitological examinations.
    - Sputum for AAFB.
    - Stool microscopy.
    - Malaria parasites.
    - Urine for parasites e.g. Schistosoma hematobium.
- Blood transfusion services:
    - A.B.O and Rhesus grouping.
    - Cross matching of blood.
    - Blood bank.

- Serological testing.
  - RPR test for syphilis.
  - HIV testing.
  - Pregnancy testing.

Pharmacy services
- Dispensing of drugs and other supplies.
- Support to the health centers and mission institutions.

Forensic services
- Mortuary services.
- Post mortems.

Support systems and management structures

District Health Management Team consisting of:
- District Medical Officer (DMO).
- District Nursing Officer (DNO).
- District Environmental Health Officer (DEHO).
- District Health Service Administrator (DHSA).
- District Pharmacist (DP).
- Hospital Matron.
- Co-opted members.

Functions
- Main executive body for district health services.
- Coordinates district planning and implementation activities.
- Monitoring and supervision of service delivery.
- Ensures efficient and effective use of resources.

District Health Team

Composition:
- District Health Management Team members.
- Representatives from each of the district's health facilities - RDC, mission, NGOs and private sector.
- The Hospital Matron.
- Health Information Clerk.
- Executive Officer (health) from the RDC.

Functions
- Undertake planning, budgeting and implementation.
- Maintain links with community, government departments and other health related agencies within the district.

- ◆ Joint decision making on running health services in the district.
- ◆ Development of management norms.
- ◆ Ensuring adequate support is given to health service units within the district.

Hospital Executive

Composition:
- ◆ DMO.
- ◆ Government Medical Officer.
- ◆ Hospital Matron.
- ◆ DHSA.
- ◆ Pharmacist.
- ◆ Co-opted members from within the hospital.

Community Health Council - composition and functions as per the Medical Services Act, (S.I. 208 of 2001).

District Development Committee - all district heads of government departments and chaired by the Council Chief Executive.

Transport requirements at the district level

Standard transport requirements include:
- ◆ Two (2) 4 x4 wheel drive ambulances.
- ◆ One (1) 2 wheel drive vehicle utility.
- ◆ One minibus in selected districts with training schools.
- ◆ Three (3) light four wheel drive utility vehicles for outreach/ supervision/disease control.
- ◆ One (1) trailer.
- ◆ One (1) motor cycle.

Basic Infrastructure for a district hospital

The structure is as per specifications in the Family Health Project 2. The size would normally vary depending on the catchment population, expected work load and contiguity of other facilities. The bed capacity ranges from 52 - 140 beds, depending on the catchment population.

The following departments constitute minimum requirements for a standard district hospital:

- Administration block.
- Outpatient department, consultation rooms and MCH department.
- Emergency department.
- Pharmacy and dispensary department.
- Maternal and child health department.
- Standard acute wards: male, female, pediatric.
- Maternity ward.
- Labor ward.
- Operating theater.
- X-ray department.
- Kitchen (and dining hall where there is a training school).
- Laundry.
- Central supplies stores/department.
- Incinerator.
- Mortuary.
- Waiting mothers' shelter.
- Laboratory.
- MCH/FP training unit.
- Dental unit.

APPENDIX 2

GLOSSARY OF TERMS

Allocative Efficiency - refers to the allocation of resources in order to produce goods that have the highest value to consumers.

Beveridge Model - in this model the health system is predominantly tax financed and consists of a publicly operated comprehensive health service.

Bismarck Model - in this model the health service is predominantly financed by social insurance. Financing and delivery are institutionally separated and contractual arrangements govern the relationships.

Block Contract - can be likened to a budget for a defined service where the purchaser agrees to pay a fee in exchange for access to a broadly defined range of services.

Capacity (Operational) - the institutional abilities that make it possible to carry out those activities that result in the delivery of services in a system.

Capacity (Strategic) - this is the institutional ability to carry out all those responsibilities in the health sector that are accorded to government. These do not include operational activities of the actual delivery of services.

Capitation - fixed payment which is made to a provider per person (enrolled in an insurance scheme).

Civil Service Reforms - reforms concerned with changing the role of the state and introducing "new public management" which is associated with "down-sizing", identification of targets for personnel numbers, training and setting of performance criteria and improving remuneration, often by payment of "top ups" by donors.

Community Financing - contributions by individuals, family beneficiaries or community groups to support a part of the costs of health services.

Conditionality - a situation where donors or other parties induce partner governments to adopt policies or programs that they would otherwise not adopt on their own. This is usually achieved through requiring the recipient countries to agree to undertake certain specified actions before any financial aid can be released.

Contracting out - shifting partial or complete responsibility for the provision of clinical or non-clinical services to the private sector whilst the responsibility for financing remains with the public sector.

Cost and Value Contract - payment for specific services is more explicitly related to the services offered e.g. specified number of patients per specialty.

Core Health Service Package - see Minimum Health Care Package.

Cost-effective interventions - those health interventions that have a comparative advantage with respect to costs per unit of consequence or outcome.

Co-payment - the amount of money that the beneficiary of an insurance scheme must pay for each service used.

Cost per case Contract - a single cost is set for each item of service. Requires a lot of cost information which is usually not readily available in most developing countries.

Coverage Exclusions - services that are not covered in the benefit package of public or private insurance plans. Individuals are left liable for their full costs or the costs over and above what is covered.

Decentralization - in general terms it is the transfer of authority or dispersal of power in public planning, management and decision making from the national level to sub national levels, or more generally from higher to lower levels of government. (Rondinelli, 1981).

Deconcentration - decision-making is transferred to a lower administrative level.

Devolution - decision-making is transferred to a lower political level.

Delegation - tasks are allocated to actors at a lower organizational level.

Deductible - the amount that must be paid out of pocket before benefits of the insurance scheme become effective.

De-linkage - from the public service implies removing staff management issues of a government department (ministry of health) from the Public Service Commission to some other authoritative body like a Health Service Board. This means that people who are not in the public service e.g. private sector, NGOs or newly created autonomous service providers such as statutory authorities will provide services meant for the public.

Demand - represents the subset of wants that individuals are willing to act upon. Demand thus requires a willingness to sacrifice time, money or goods in exchange for the product or service.

Earmarked (health) tax - a section of national or local taxation is identified specifically for the purposes of spending on health services or health care generally, e.g. the AIDS levy in Zimbabwe.

Equity - generally reflects the concern to distribute health care fairly in recognition of differences in health need.

Equity (vertical) - refers to a situation where the distribution of the burden to pay for health care should reflect differences in ability to pay.

Externalities - these are negative or positive utilities accruing to an individual from another person's consumption, e.g. if the majority in a community are vaccinated against an infectious disease, the resulting head immunity benefits those who have not been vaccinated.

Equal expenditure per capita - implies that providing the same services will cost more in some areas than others.

Equal access per capita - may mean different things including equal number of doctors per capita and equal average distance to a health facility per capita.

Equal expenditure for equal needs or demand - planners need to take into account factors which influence need or demand for services.

Equal access for equal needs - takes into account problems discussed in the above notions of equity excerpt the possibility that people may tend to use services differently.

Equal utilization for equal needs - since utilization is determined by both supply and demand achieving this measure of equity implies positive discrimination to overcome factors which determine demand.

Equal health status - this implies even more positive discrimination to overcome factors which negatively affect health status but operate outside the health sector (Barbara McPake, 1991).

Equity (horizontal) - refers to a situation in which only those who benefit from/use health care should pay for it.

Essential Health Care Package - see Minimum Health Care Package.

General Management - follows the logic that at the operational or strategic levels all top professional officers are responsible to a general manager, e.g. general managers who are the heads of clinical specialties are normally doctors. Other professions thus have to accept responsibility to the chiefs of each of these units.

Gini-Coefficient - describes the income distribution in a population in numerical terms. One (1) representing perfect inequality and zero (0) perfect equality of income distribution.

Gross National Product - this is the sum of consumption expenditures, gross investment and government spending.

Health Insurance - a means by which risks or uncertain events are shared between many people. Premiums are paid to an insurance institution which compensates any insured victim of the event for any financial loss resulting from the event. It helps in lessening and spreading the risks.

Health Sector - a coherent set of activities which can be relatively distinguished in terms of policies, institutions and finances and which need to be looked at together to make a meaningful assessment i.e. the entire network of public, private and voluntary institutions financed and managed or regulated by the ministry of health.

Health Sector Reform - a sustained process of fundamental change in policy and institutional arrangements guided by the government and designed to improve the functioning and performance of the health sector and ultimately the health status of the population.

Health Service Commission or Board - this refers to a legislated entity with the responsibility for providing guidelines on the recruitment, discipline, promotion, discharge and the determination and review of the conditions of service for health staff. Its role is mainly to facilitate de-linkage of the health sector from the Public Service Commission.

Hospital Efficiency - refers either to:
The efficient allocation of resources to hospitals in relation to other levels of care e.g. persons tending to self refer to hospitals where unit costs are much higher cause inefficiencies in these hospitals.
OR
The efficient internal management of available resources by individual hospitals i.e. technical efficiency - the purchase for example of very costly high technology equipment would be hard to justify in a context of budget constraints.

Information asymmetry - the differential in uncertainty between the physician (provider of health services) and the patient with respect to the efficiency of treatment.

Integration of service delivery - this implies the bringing together of otherwise independent administrative structures and functions in health delivery in such a way as to combine them into one whole, e.g. inter-sectoral planning, allocating resources to multipurpose programs as opposed to special projects, training staff in multiple areas, conducting multipurpose supervision visits etc.

Job Evaluation - an approach to measuring the content, intensity and qualitative nature of a job, usually undertaken for the purposes of remuneration and more appropriate job design and redesign within an organization.

Lock-in-effect - in policy development the term refers to a situation whereby preexisting policy frameworks affect the extent to which new policies can be adopted e.g. in an environment where there has not been any viable private health sector it may not be possible to immediately adopt policies that relate to the private health sector.

Market failure - a situation whereby individuals consulting a medical practitioner put their faith in the health provider with little information as to what the quality of treatment to expect. In a perfect world doctors would do what patients would wish them to do if they were fully informed. Providers may however have other motives of their own such as maintaining certain levels of income by prescribing excessive medication and ordering unnecessary tests to boost their income. In such cases the choice of patients is limited by a lack of adequate information.

Memorandum of Understanding (MoU) - in the context of a SWAp this is a document that encapsulates the agreements reached between the government and several development partners in the joint funding of a sectoral program. The document which is usually not legally binding provides for, amongst other things, the following:
+ How funds will be used.
+ How donor funds will be channeled.
+ Arrangements for the procurement of goods and services.
+ Mechanisms for conflict resolution.
+ Monitoring and evaluation processes.

Minimum Health Care Package - a package of health services that is composed of cost effective interventions which are supposed to prevent and control the main causes of disease burden, usually in low income countries.

Moral hazard - the tendency for individuals, once insured, to behave in such a way as to increase the likelihood or size of the risk against which they are insured.

National Health Accounts - a tool for describing and analyzing the financing of national health systems which presents opportunities for policy recommendations aimed at the performance of the health system in both aggregate and subsystem terms.

Need - this term is applied in reference to professionally determined indications of ill health.

Non-excludability - a situation whereby if a service is provided it is not possible to exclude those who have not contributed towards the cost of the good from benefiting from it, e.g. vector control activities.

Non-rivalry - refers to public goods in which the benefit gained by one person does not reduce the benefit others can get.

Outcome (health) - refers to the results of a medical intervention in terms of changes in the patient's current and future health status which can be attributed to a particular health care intervention.

Ownership - combinations of commitment, technical and administrative capacity to conceive, negotiate and implement, e.g. ownership of the reform process.

Pareto-optimality - a state where there are no possible changes which could be made without making at least one individual worse off.

Patient's Charter - an approach that sets out national and local standards to improve the quality of care provided to patients by empowering citizens to participate actively in monitoring those standards of care. The objective is to achieve a better service that is much more consumer friendly (to patients), that guarantees rights to access to services without any discrimination, the right to be treated with dignity and to have any complaints about the health services investigated and a timely response provided by local management. Such entitlements are generally not legally binding.

Policy (health) - this refers to the process by which laws and regulations concerning health care (and its provision) emerge or the effect of such output upon society in terms of health status and well being.

Pooled funding (Basket Funding) - this is a concept in which a fund account is operated for the purposes of health development and consists of revenue from several development partners, the government and revenue from user fees all managed from one basket or as a pool of funds. Ideally this pool of funds is supposed to be flexible in its utilization and not necessarily earmarked. The participating parties usually agree on the modalities for the management of the funds as well as the accounting procedures.

Poverty Reduction Strategy - what has become an integral part of World Bank and IMF concessionary lending and promotes the development of strategies that focus on poverty reduction and are characterized by country ownership, the broad representation of civil society and the participation of the poor in their design.

Pre-payment schemes - these are voluntary lump sum payments by households for services provided by local health facilities when a user fee system is in place - they usually operate on a cash basis but may be in kind. Coverage may apply to the entire household.

Private Health Insurance - as opposed to Social Health Insurance is based on voluntary contributions which may vary for individuals or groups.

Private-not-for-profit sector - consists of private health institutions genuinely motivated by altruism (missions and NGOs). In some cases such institutions charge token user fees at the same time receiving subsidies and subventions from the state.

Privatization - tasks are transferred from public ownership into private ownership.

Process (health) - this refers to the interaction between practitioner and patient which includes clinical interventions and the use of treatments and investigations.

Professional management - in an institution such as a hospital the medical or nursing professions have their own hierarchy, the top of which cannot be countermanded by somebody from another profession or from outside the realm of professions altogether. Such management deals with issues of a professional nature within a clinical department.

Provider influence - the tendency for decisions made by providers to reflect not only the patient's preferences but also the provider's own ulterior motives for a reasonable income by for example over prescribing or ordering unnecessary tests.

Public - what the government or the state owns.

Public goods - health services whose benefits accrue to all members of society including those who have not contributed towards the cost of the goods.

Public Service Commission (PSC) - usually established in terms of a country's constitution and is responsible for the appointment, dismissal and discipline of persons working in the civil service. The Public Service Commission is the employer of civil servants but not necessarily all public servants. The day-to-day management of staff issues is the responsibility of individual government departments.

Public and private collaboration - this refers to formal or informal cooperation between the public (governmental) and private (voluntary and for profit) sectors in the provision and financing of health services.

Purchaser-Provider split - the separation of the roles and responsibilities of the purchaser of health services from that of the provider of services, e.g. the functions of the central ministry of health (purchaser) and those of local authorities or autonomous hospitals (providers).

Quality Adjusted Life Years (QALYS) - the number of years of life gained from an intervention as adjusted by a measure of their quality e.g. chronic illness where treatment enables survival for a certain period of time at a less than optimal state of health.

Quality Assurance Program - a set of activities that are carried out to set standards and to monitor and improve performance so that the care provided is as effective and as safe as possible.

Rationing of health services - a process of distributing health services (scarce goods) by political or administrative rather than economic means in a population. In practical terms this translates to all receiving a little bit of everything or some getting something and others getting something else based on some predetermined criteria.

Referral system - the structure and design of a health delivery system that allows for the movement or flow of patients based on the severity of the illness, the necessary treatment and the sophistication of services within the system itself. For example the flow of patients from the primary level or the General Practitioner to the District hospital, tertiary and central hospitals levels for better and more appropriate levels of care.

Re-profiling the health work force - involves changes in skills mix, for example replacing doctors at the high level of expertise with less specialized workers at lower remuneration, e.g. clinical officers. The objective is usually to save costs by ensuring that cheaper employees do as much as possible.

Resources - classically, land, labor and capital including reference to inputs into health services production such as time, goods, equipment, buildings, specialized knowledge, etc.

Retention of revenue - this refers to a policy in which revenue accruing from user fees is retained at the point collection, usually a health facility, and is used for health improvement at the point of collection. This is in contrast to the policy whereby all revenue collected at government institutions reverted to the central treasury or central government.

Sector Wide Approach (SWAp) - a method of working between the government and development partners in which significant funding for the sector supports a single sector policy and expenditure program. The government which is in the driving seat adopts common approaches across the sector in collaboration with its partners.

Semi-autonomous (health) institutions - these are previously public owned and managed (government) institutions which have been granted independent management status on the basis of a legal instrument. New management structures are established consisting of a Chief Executive who is responsible to a Management Board which is in turn responsible to the minister responsible for health. Such institutions have a legal right to sue and be sued, to hire and fire staff and to determine staff conditions of service without reference to the Public Service Commission. These institutions however remain part of the public sector.

Service Agreement - a contractual arrangement (between for example, the central ministry of health and private providers) which states the service standards to be provided by specifying the quality and levels of services to be expected as well as the avenues for redress and compensation where services fail to meet the standards.

Social Health Insurance - an insurance scheme organized by the state and usually financed by the imposition of mandatory insurance payments on employed workers as a proportion of their wages and imposing similar or higher payroll tax on their employers. Other groups in non-formal employment can be included on the basis of some measures of income or wealth.

Structural Adjustment Programs - programs or policies aimed at changing the structure of the economy so as to improve the balance of trade and the efficiency of the economy over the medium term.

Supplier induced demand - arises from patients' reliance on providers for information about their need for demand specific services - this is one of the reasons why fee for service reimbursement causes cost escalation in the health sector.

SWAp - see Sector Wide Approach.

Taxation (progressive) - this refers to taxation that falls more heavily on the rich than the poor and is thus considered to be equitable.

Taxation (regressive) - this refers to taxation that falls heavily on the poor than the rich and is thus considered inequitable.

Technical efficiency - this term refers to the concept of achieving greater productivity for a given amount of resources.

Transaction costs - these are costs of running markets as opposed to the direct management of providers or services.

User fees - payments consumers make directly to health care providers.

APPENDIX 3

ABBREVIATIONS

AAFB	Alcohol Acid Fast Bacilli.
AFRO/WHO	World Health Organization Regional Office for Africa.
AIDS	Acquired Immune-Deficiency Syndrome
ANC	Antenatal Care
ARI	Acute Respiratory Infection
ART	Antiretroviral Therapy
ARVT	Antiretroviral Therapy.
BSc	Bachelor of Science Degree
CBCC	Capacity Building Coordination Committee
CDR	Crude Death Rate
CEO	Chief Executive Officer.
CHBC	Community Home-Based Care
CWGH	Community Working Group on Health.
CSO	Central Statistics Office
DALY	Disability Adjusted Life Years.
DANIDA	Danish International Development Agency.
DCC	Drugs Control Council.
DD	Deputy Director
DDC	District Development Committee
DEHO	District Environmental Officer
DHE	District Health Executive
DHMB	District Health Management Board
DFID	Department for International Development (UK)
DHMT	District Health Management Team
DHS	District Health System
DHSA	District Health Services Administrator
DMO	District Medical Officer
DNO	District Nursing Officer

ECG	Electrocardiogram
ECSA	East Central and Southern Africa
EDF	European Development Fund
EDLIZ	Essential Drug List for Zimbabwe
EHP	Essential Health Package
EHT	Environmental Health Technician
EPI	Expanded Program on Immunization
ESAP	Economic Structural Adjustment Program
EU	European Union
FP	Family Planning
GAVI	Global Alliance for Vaccines and Immunizations
GDP	Gross Domestic Product
GFATM	Global Fund to fight AIDS, Tuberculosis and Malaria
GM	Growth Monitoring
GMS	Government Medical Stores
GOZ	Government of Zimbabwe
HB	Hepatitis B virus
HIPC	Highly Indebted Poor Country
HIV	Human Immunodeficiency Virus
HMB	Hospital Management Board
HNP	Health, Nutrition and Population
HPA	Health Professions Authority
HPC	Health Professions Council
HQ	Headquarters
HRH	Human Resources for Health
HSF	Health Services Fund
HSPS	Health Sector Program Support
HSR	Health Sector Reform
ICHE	Institute of Continuing Health Education
IEC	Information, Education and Communication
IHP	International Development Partnership
IMF	International Monetary Fund
IMR	Infant Mortality Rate
JRMO	Junior Resident Medical Officer
KAP	Knowledge, Attitudes and Practices
LIC	Low Income Country
Mash	Mashonaland
Mat	Matebeleland
MCH	Maternal and Child Health

MCAZ	Medicines Control Authority of Zimbabwe
MDG	Millennium Development Goal
MFED	Ministry of Finance and Economic Development
MILGRUD	Ministry of Local Government and Rural Development
MLGNH	Ministry of Local Government and National Housing
MLS	Medical Laboratory Scientist
MMR	Maternal Mortality Rate
MOFED	Ministry of Finance and Economic Development
MOH	Ministry of Health
MOHCW	Ministry of Health and Child Welfare
MoU	Memorandum of Understanding
MPH	Masters Degree in Public Health
MTEF	Medium Term Expenditure Framework
MTP	Medium Term Plan
NAC	National AIDS Council
NACP	National AIDS Coordination Program
NAMAS	National Association of Medical Aid Societies
NGO	Non-Governmental Organization
NHA	National Health Accounts
NPA	National Program of Action (Child Survival Program)
NSSA	National Social Security Agency
NUST	National University of Science and Technology
ODA	Overseas Development Agency (UK) (now DFID)
ODA	Overseas Development Assistance
OED	Organization for Economic Development
OPD	Out Patient Department
PCN	Primary Care Nurse
PDC	Provincial Development Committee
PEHO	Provincial Environmental Officer
PEPFAR	U.S. President's Emergency Plan for AIDS Relief
PER	Public Expenditure Review
PHC	Primary Health Care
PHSA	Provincial Health Services Administrator
PMD	Provincial Medical Director
PMCTC	Prevention of Mother to Child Transmission (of HIV)
PNC	Post Natal Care
PNO	Provincial Nursing Officer
PSC	Public Service Commission
PSIP	Public Sector Investment Program

RDCCBP	Rural District Council Capacity Building Program
RGN	Registered General Nurse
RHC	Rural Health Center
RVS	Relative Value Schedule
SAP	Structural Adjustment Program
SCN	State Certified Nurse
SDF	Social Dimensions Fund
SDU	Strategic Development Unit
SHI	Social Health Insurance
SI	Statutory Instrument
SSB	Salary Service Bureau
STD	Sexually Transmitted Diseases
STEP	Short Term Emergency Program (HIV/AIDS).
STI	Sexually Transmitted Infections.
SWAp	Sector Wide Approach
TB	Tuberculosis
TBA	Traditional Birth Attendant
TFR	Total Fertility Rate
TMT	Top Management Team (MOHCW)
TOR	Terms of Reference
TOT	Trainer of Trainers
UNDP	United Nations Development Program
UNGASS	United Nations General Assembly Special Session
UNICEF	United Nations Children's Fund
USAID	(US Official Development Assistance Agency)
US$	United States Dollar
UZ	University of Zimbabwe
VIDCO	Village Development Committee
VHW	Village Health Worker
WHO	World Health Organization
ZACH	Zimbabwe Association of Church Related Hospitals
ZEDAP	Zimbabwe Essential Drugs Action Program
ZD	Zimbabwe Dollar.
ZNFPC	Zimbabwe National Family Planning Council
ZIMA	Zimbabwe Medical Association
ZIMPREST	Zimbabwe Program for Economic and Social Transformation
ZINA	Zimbabwe Nurses Association.
ZNASP	Zimbabwe National AIDS Strategic Plan

BIBLIOGRAPHY

Aday, L. A., et al (1980). Health Care in the US: Equitable for whom? Beverly Hills. Sage.

African Development Bank (2005); Economic Research Working Paper Series Number 81: Reorienting Public Management in Africa: Selected Issues and Some Country Experiences (November 2005)

Akin, J,. Hutchinson, P., and Strumpt, K, 2001; Decentralized and government provision of public goods: the public health sector in Uganda. Draft Paper, MEASURE EVALUATION. Carolina Population Center, University of North Carolina. March 2001.

Backstrom, C.H., & Hirsch-Cesar (1989). Survey Research. McMillan Publishing.

Birch, S., & Abelson, J. (1993a). Is reasonable access what we want? Implications of, and challenges to, current Canadian Policy on equity in Health Care. International Journal of Health Services. 23(4), 629-652.

Black, D., (1980). Inequalities in Health: A Report of a Research Working Group. London. DHSS.

Bobadilla, J. C., et al (1995). The Minimum Package of Health Services: Criteria, Methods and Data. World Bank Group.

Bossert, T., (1998). Analyzing the decentralization of health systems in Developing Countries: Decision Space, Innovative and Performance. Social Science Medicine 47(10), 1513-1527.

Brown, A., et al (2001). The Status of Sector Wide Approaches. Working Paper 142. Overseas Development Institute.

Cassels, A., (1997). A guide to Sector Wide Approaches for health development: concepts, issues and working arrangements. WHO/DANIDA/DFID and EU. WHO/ARA/97.12

CBCC (1999). First Joint Government of Zimbabwe/Donor Review Report, 1st October 1996-30th June 1998. Incorporating the Second 6 monthly Review Report.

Chai, Y. M., (1995). The interaction effect of information asymmetry and decentralization on manager's job satisfaction: A research note. Human Relations 48 (6).

Chatora R *et al*, (2006). Policies and Plans for Human Resources for Health: Guidelines for Countries in the WHO African Region. WHO/AFRO.

Chatora R, (2003). Migration of Health Professionals. Presentation at 38th Regional Health Ministers' Conference. Livingstone, Zambia, (17-21 November).

Cheema, G.S., & Rondinelli, D.A. (1983). Decentralization and Development: Policy Implementation in developing countries. Sage. Beverley Hills. California.

Chikanda,A, (2005). Medical Leave: The exodus of Health Professionals from Zimbabwe. Southern African Migration Project.

Chita, B., et al (2000). Decentralization of Health Systems in Zambia. Partnerships for Health Reform Technical Report. Bethesda: PHR, (forthcoming).

Conyers, D., (1965). Decentralization, the latest fashion in development administration. Public Administration Development. 3, 97-109.

Collins, C. et. al. (2008). Exploring SWAp's contribution to the efficient allocation and use of resources in the health sector in Zambia. Health Policy and Planning 2008 23(4):244-251.

Collins, C., and Green, A. (1993). Decentralization and Primary Health Care in Developing Countries: Ten Key Questions. Journal of Management in Medicine 7(2), 58-68.

Collins, C., and Green, A. (1994). Decentralization and Primary Health Care: Some Negative Implications in Developing Countries. International Journal of Health Services 24(3), 459-475.

Collins, T., and Higgins, L. (June 2000). Sector Wide Approaches with a focus on Partnership. Seminar Report. Ireland Aid.

Community Working Group on Health (CWGH). (May 1998). Report of a Meeting of Community Based Organizations on Communication and Information on Health. Zimbabwe.

Cyler, A., (1991). Equity in Health Care Policy. Unpublished working Paper. Department of Health Administration, University of Toronto.

DANIDA, Ministry of Foreign Affairs. (8th October, 1997). Internal Technical Review Working Paper: Zimbabwe Health Sector, 1997-98.

Daniels, N. (1982). Equity of Access to Health Care: Some Conceptual and Ethical Issues. Millbank Memorial Fund. Quarterly. 60, 51-81.

Deville, L. (1998). Review of the Health Sector for Zimbabwe. Study to Assist Programming for the 8th EDF Assistance to the Health Sector: by Health Research for Action, (HERA).

Dhliwayo, R. (2001). The Impact of Public Expenditure Management under ESAP on Basic Social Services: Health and Education. Department of Economics, University of Zimbabwe.

DFID (2003). Promoting Institutional and Organizational Development: A Source Book of Tools and Techniques.

DFID/Health Systems Resource Center. (2001). Measuring health sector performance at country level. Report of a DFID Workshop.

Dranove D., & White, W.D. (1987). Agency and the Organization of Health Care Delivery. Inquiry. 24, 405-415.

Dusault,G, & Dubois, C (2003). Human Resources for Health Policies: A Critical Component in Health Policies. Human Resources for Health 2003, 1:1 (14 April 2003): http://www.human-resources-health.com/content/1/1/1.

England, R. (1998). Health Sector Reform: Human Resources Issues: a Briefing Note on Public Service Commissions in the Commonwealth. Institute for Health Sector Development.

European Commission (EC) and Government of Zimbabwe (GOZ). (1995). Framework of Cooperation, National Indicative Program 1996-2000.

Fesler, J.W. (1965). Approaches to the understanding of decentralization. Journal of Politics 27(2), 536-566.

Forster, M. (2000). New Approaches to Development Co-operation: What can we learn from experience with implementing Sector Wide Approaches? Working Paper 140. Overseas Development Institute: Center for Aid and Public Expenditure.

Forster, Mick and Adrian Fozzard (2000). Aid and Public Expenditure (DFID Economists' Manual). London: Overseas Development Institute.

Gaidzano, R (1999). Voting with their feet: Migrant Zimbabwe Nurses and Doctors in the era of Structural Adjustment. Research Report No. 111. Nordiska Afrikainstitutet.

Gilson, et al (1994). Local government decentralization and the health sector in Tanzania. Public Administration and Development 14, 451-477.

Gould, Jeremy, et al. (1998). How Sectoral Programs Work. (Policy Papers 1/1998). Helsinki: University, Institute of Developing Studies.

Government of Zimbabwe (GOZ)/Ministry of Health (MOH). (1984). Planning for Equity in Health: A Sectoral Review and Policy Statement. Government Printers.

Government of Zimbabwe (GOZ)/Public Service Commission (PSC). (1998). Framework for the Second Phase of the Public Service Commission Reform Program.

Government of Zimbabwe (GOZ)/ZIMPREST. (1998). Zimbabwe Program for Economic and Social Transformation 1996-2000. Government Printers.

GOZ/CBCC. (1998). An outline of the decentralization implementation Strategy. (Unpublished).

Government of Zimbabwe. Budget estimates for years ending December, 1998, 1999, 2000 and 2001.

Government of Zimbabwe. (1991). Drugs and Allied Substances Control Regulations.

Government of Zimbabwe. (1996). The Public Service of Zimbabwe, Confidential Appraisal Report Form.

Government of Zimbabwe. (1992). Zimbabwe National Program of Action for Children.

Griffin, C. C, and R. Paul Shaw. (1995). Health Insurance in Sub-Saharan Africa: Aims, Findings, Policy Implications: In R. Shaw and Martha Ainsworth, eds., Financing Health Services through User Fees and Insurance: Case Studies from Sub Saharan Africa. Discussion Paper no. 294. Washington Technical Department.

Grundman, C. (2000). Decentralization of Health Services in Senegal. Bethesda, MD: Partnerships for Health Reform Technical Report, (forthcoming).

Grythen, et al. (1995). Can a Public Health Care System achieve Equity? The Norwegian Experience. Medical Care. 33(9), 938-951.

Gwatkin, D., et al. (2000). Socio-economic differences in Health, Nutrition and Population in Zimbabwe. HNP/Poverty Thematic Group/World Bank.

Hansard. Parliament of Zimbabwe. 8th December 1994.

Harris, R.L. (1983). Centralization and Decentralization in Latin America. In Cheema, GS, Decentralization and Development (pp. 183-203), Sage: Beverly Hills. California.

Health Research for Action (HERA), January 2004: Mid-Term Review of the Health Sector Support Programs I and II, Zimbabwe

Hongoro, C., Chirove, J. and Musonza, T.G. (1997). A Study on regulating the Private Medical Sector in Zimbabwe. Ministry of Health and Child Welfare. (MOHCW).

Hutton, G. (2000). Indicators for Monitoring Health Sector Reform and the Sector Wide Approach. Presentation at Sector Wide Approach in Health Conference "Moving from Policy to Practice", Royal Tropical Institute, Amsterdam, 27-28 November 2000.

Institute for Health Sector Reform (IHSD): Issues Note (2000). Improving Health Systems by Measuring Health Status. Is WHO serious? IHSD.

Katele, K. (1997). Towards an Equity-Oriented Policy of Decentralization in Health Systems under conditions of turbulence: The case of Zambia. WHO/ARA/97.2

KPMG Management Consultants. (October 1996). Social Health Insurance Study. MOHCW/USAID.

Lambo, E., et al. (2001). A Tool for Country Level Monitoring and Evaluation of Health Sector Reform. International Management Consultants/WHO/AFRO.

Lauglo, M., & Molutsi, P. (1994). Decentralization and Health Systems Performance. The Botswana Case Study. Centre for Partnership in Decentralization. DIS and The University of Botswana.

Lenneiye, N. (2000). Quest for a Corporate African Leadership: Public Sector Case Studies from Southern Africa. Nehanda Publishers (Private) Ltd. Harare. Zimbabwe.

Lowenson, R., Chikumbirike, T., et al. (1999). Report from Participatory Research in four Districts of Zimbabwe. TARSC/CWGH. Monograph 18.99.

Lowenson, R. (1991). Challenges to Equity in Zimbabwe health and health care: A Zimbabwean case study. Social Science Medicine. 32 (10), 1079-1088.

Luiz, J., & Araujo, C. (1997). Attempts to Decentralize in Recent Brazilian Health Policy: Issues and Problems, 1988-1994. International Journal of Health Services 27(1), 109-124.

Martinez, J. (2007). HLSP Policy Brief: "The Global Fund operating in a SWAp through a common fund: Issues and lessons from Mozambique". Available online at http://www.hlspinstitute.org , accessed on 26 August 2008.

Mastillica, M. (1999). Health Care Reform in Croatia. In Health Care Reforms in Central and Eastern European Countries. European Public Health Association, Department of Social Medicine, University Medical Soros Foundation. Debrecen.

McPake, et al. (1990). Evaluation of the Bamako Initiative: Background Paper. London School of Hygiene and Tropical Medicine. LHHT/ODA.

Mills, A. et al. (1990). Health System Decentralization: concepts, issues and country experiences. WHO, Geneva.

Mills A., Hongoro, C. & Bromberg, J. (1997). Improving the Efficiency of District Hospitals: Is Contracting an Option? Trop. Med. Int. Hlth. 2(2), 116-126.

Ministry of Health and Child Welfare (MOHCW). Zimbabwe. (1989). Corporate Plan and Action Plan.

Ministry of Health and Child Welfare, (MOHCW). Zimbabwe. (1995). Job Descriptions for Medical Doctors in Government Institutions. MOHCW.

Ministry of Health and Child Welfare, (MOHCW). Zimbabwe. (March 1995). District Core Health Services for Zimbabwe. MOHCW.

Ministry of Health and Child Welfare, (MOHCW). Zimbabwe. (1995). ZEDAP, Private Sector Essential Drugs Survey.

Ministry of Health and Child Welfare, (MOHCW). Zimbabwe. (1995). Health Sector Reform in Zimbabwe: Concept Paper on Decentralization.

Ministry of Health and Child Welfare, (MOHCW). Zimbabwe. (1996). Position Paper for the Commencement of General Nurse Training in Provincial Schools and Increasing the establishment at Central Hospital Training Schools. MOHCW.

Ministry of Health and Child Welfare, (MOHCW). Zimbabwe. (1996). Zimbabwe Health Service Indicators Handbook.

Ministry of Health and Child Welfare (MOHCW)/DANIDA. (1997). Annual Sector Review Agreement: Health.

Ministry of Health and Child Welfare. (MOHCW). (June 1997). HIV/AIDS in Zimbabwe: Background, Projections, Impact and Interventions. MOHCW.

Ministry of Health and Child Welfare,(MOHCW). (1998). Index of established posts, 1996-97.

Ministry of Health and Child Welfare, (MOHCW). Zimbabwe. (1999). National Health Strategy for Zimbabwe, 1997-2007.

Ministry of Health and Child Welfare, (MOHCW). Zimbabwe. National Health Profiles for 1995, 1996, 1997 and 1999.

Ministry of Health and Child Welfare (MOHCW). Zimbabwe. Directorate of Pharmacy. (2000). Public Sector Survey 2000: Report on the Public Sector Survey carried out in February 2000.

Ministry of Health and Child Welfare,(MOHCW). Zimbabwe. (2001). Report of the Secretary for Health and Child Welfare: Year ended 2000.

Ministry of Health and Child Welfare, (MOHCW). Zimbabwe. (2001). Organization and Functions: Working for Equity and Quality. MOHCW.

Mooney, G. (1987). What does equity in health mean? World Health Statistics. 40.

Morris, S. (1980). Health Economics for Nurses. An Introductory Guide. Prentice Hall. Nursing Series. 86-108.

Mudyarabikwa, O. (2000). Examination of Public Sector subsidies to the Private Health Sector: A Zimbabwe Case Study. Equinet Policy Series No. 8.

Musgrave, R.A., & Musgrave, P.B. (1989). Public Finance in Theory and Practice. McGraw-Hill. New York.

Mwaluko, G.M.P., et al. (1996). Health Sector Reforms in Eastern and Southern Africa: A Training Manual for District and Other Health Workers. Biomedical Research and Training Institute (BRTI).

Nagarajan, P. (2001). Sub-Saharan Africa: Towards health-led economic development. In the "Financial Daily" (July 14, 2001). Available at: http://www.thehindubusinessline.com/businessline/2001/07/14/stories/041420ju.htm.

National Association of Medical Aid Societies (NAMAS). (November 1996). Private Clinic Project. NAMAS.

Norton, A., Conway, T. & Forster, M. (2001). Social Protection Concepts and Approaches: Implications for Policy and Practice in International Development. Working Paper 143. Overseas Development Institute.

Okuonzi, L. (1995). Decentralization and Health Systems Change: Uganda. ARA/WHO.

Ortendahl, C. (2007). The Uganda health SWAp: new approaches for a more balanced aid architecture? The challenges of the Uganda health Sector Wide Approach. Available online at: www.eldis.org/go/display&type=Document&id =35563 - Cached .

Paul, S. (1995). Capacity Building for Health Sector Reform. WHO/ SHS/95.8.

Paton, C., (2000). Impact of Market forces on Health Systems: Scientific Evaluation of the Effects of the Introduction of Market forces into the Health Systems (Final Report). European Health Management Association.

Paton, C. (1996). Health Policy and Management: The Health Care Agenda in a British Political Context. Chapman and Hill.

Paton, C. (1992). Competition and Planning in the NHS: The Consequences of the NHS Reforms. Stangley Thornes (Publishers) Ltd.

Putman, R.D. (1993). Making Democracy Work: Civic Traditions in Modern Italy. Princeton University Press. Princeton.

Pratt, J.W. & Zeckhauser, R.J. (1991.) Principals and Agents: The Structure of Business. Harvard Business School Press. Boston.

Prud'homme, R. (1995). On the Dangers of Decentralization. World Bank Transportation, Water and Urban Development Department.

Reed and Associates/Ministry of Health and Child Welfare, Zimbabwe. (1996). Prevailing Attitudes towards the Zimbabwe Health System: A study among clients and providers. MOHCW.

Reed, G. and Frank, M. The Cuban Approach to health care, Origins, Results and Current Challenges. American Association for World Health, 1997. Online and available at: www.medicc.org/embargo.php.

Rondinelli, D.A. (1983). Decentralization of development administration in East Africa. In Cheema, GS, and Rondinelli, DA (eds.) Decentralization and Development. Sage: Beverley Hills. California. 77-126.

Sachs, J, Why Prioritize when there isn't enough money. Bulletin of Medicus Mundi Switzerland. No. 91, December 2003. Available online at:

http://www.medicusmundi.ch/mms/services/bulletin/bulletin200304/kap02/09_wikler.html

Sachs, J.D. (2001). Macroeconomics and Health: Investing in Health for Economic Development. A Report of the Commission on Macroeconomics and Health. WHO.

Saltman, R. (1995). Applying Planned Market Logic to Developing Countries' Health Systems: an Initial Exploration. WHO/SHS/95.7

Saltman, R.B., Figueras, J. & Sakellaries, C. (1999). In Critical Challenges for Health Care Reform in Europe (Eds). Open University Press.

Sanders, D. (1990). Equity in Health: Zimbabwe Nine Years on: Journal of Social Development in Africa. 5(1), 5-22.

Schieber, G., (2007). Presentation at a Senior Policy Seminar in Thailand on: "Overview of Health Financing". Online and available at:

http://siteresources.worldbank.org/INTTHAILAND/Resources/333200-1089943634036/475256-1151398858396/Overview_of_Health_Financing_WB.ppt.

Schwartz, J.B., Zwizwai, B.M. (May 1995). Economics of the Health Sector in Zimbabwe. USAID.

Segall, M. (1983). Planning and politics of resource allocation for Primary Health Care: Promotion of meaningful national policy. Social Science and Medicine 17, 1947-1960.

Sen, K., & Koivusalo, M. (1998). Health Reforms in Developing Countries. International Journal of Health Planning and Management 13, 199-215.

Sikosana, P.L., et al. (1997). Health Sector Reforms in Sub-Saharan Africa: An analysis of Experiences, Information Gaps and Research Needs. WHO/ARA/CC/97.2.

Stilwell, *et.al.* (2003). Human Resources for Health 1:**8**: Available at: http://www.human-resources-health.com/content/1/1/8/table/T4.

TARSCO/MOHCW/EQUITY GAUGE. (2001). Proposal for Including Equity into Resource Allocation in Health. Report of a study on inclusion of equity indicators in the resource allocation formula for Ministry of Health funds in Zimbabwe.

United Nations Economic Commission, (2007): Economic Report for Africa (2007). Available at: http://www.iss.co.za/dynamic/administration/file_manager/file_links/ERA2007Full.pdf.

United Nations Development Program: Poverty Report 2000: Overcoming Human Poverty.

USAID, (2007), Zimbabwe: Economic Performance Assessment. A Bench mark Study. Available online at: http://www.nathaninc.com/nathan2/files/ccLibrary-Files/Filename/000000000210/Zimbabwe_Country_Analytic_Report.pdf

UNFPA (2003) statistics available at: www.unfpa.org/profile/zimbawe.cfm.

Whitehead, M. (1992). The concepts and principles of equity in health. International Journal of Health Services. 22(3), 429-445.

WHO/SHS/NHP. 95.10. (1995). Evaluation of Health Financing Reforms. Report on Consultations.

WHO/ARA/96.1. Equity in Health and Health Care. WHO/SIDA Initiative.

WHO/SHS/NHP/95.2 (1995). Decentralization and Health Systems change: A framework for analysis. [Revised working document].

World Bank (2006). Global Monitoring Report 2006: Strengthening Mutual Accountability-Aid, Trade, and Governance. Washington DC: World Bank.

World Bank. (1996). Understanding Poverty and Human Resources in Zimbabwe. Changes in the 1990s and Directions for the Future. A Dimensions Paper: Human Development Group, Eastern and Southern Africa. World Bank.

World Bank. (1994). Better Health in Africa. A World Bank Publication.

World Bank. (1993). World Development Report. 122-3. A World Bank Publication.

World Bank, OED. (1999). Meeting Health Care Challenges in Zimbabwe.

Ziken International. (1994). Role of Rural District Councils in the Provision, Management and Maintenance of Health Care in Zimbabwe.

Zimbabwe Association of Church Related Hospitals. (April 1991). The State of Zimbabwe's Mission Hospitals and Clinics. ZACH.

INDEX

E

F

G

H

I

R

S

Z